PRINCIPLES OF CLINICAL LABORATORY MANAGEMENT

A Study Guide and Workbook

Jane Hudson, PhD, MT(ASCP)SM, CLS(NCA)

Senior Editor

The University of Southern Mississippi

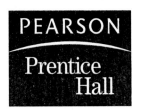

Upper Saddle River, New Jersey 07458

Library of Congress Cataloging-in-Publication Data

Principles of clinical laboratory management: a study guide and workbook / [edited by] Jane Hudson.
   p. cm.
   Includes index.
   ISBN 0-13-049538-7 (pbk.)
   1. Medical laboratories—Management.   I. Hudson, Jane, 1947–
   R860 P75 2004

610'.28'4—dc22   2003016835

Publisher: Julie Levin Alexander   **Production Managing Editor:** Patrick Walsh
Assistant to Publisher: Regina Bruno   **Production Liaison:** Alex Ivchenko
CLS Series Editor: Elizabeth A. Zeibig   **Production Editor:** Marty Sopher/Lithokraft
Senior Acquisitions Editor: Mark Cohen   **Manufacturing Manager:** Ilene Sanford
Associate Editor: Melissa Kerian   **Manufacturing Buyer:** Pat Brown
Editorial Assistant: Mary Ellen Ruitenberg   **Design Director:** Cheryl Asherman
Senior Marketing Manager: Nicole Benson   **Senior Design Coordinator:** Christopher Weigand
Marketing Assistant: Janet Ryerson   **Composition:** Lithokraft
Channel Marketing Manager: Rachele Strober   **Printing and Binding:** Banta Corporation
Director of Production and Manufacturing: Bruce Johnson   **Cover Printer:** Phoenix Color Corp.

Notice: The authors and the publisher of this textbook have taken care that the information and technical recommendations contained herein are based on research and expert consultation, and are accurate and compatible with the standards generally accepted at the time of publication. Nevertheless, as new information becomes available, changes in clinical and technical practices become necessary. The reader is advised to carefully consult manufacturers' instructions and information material for all supplies and equipment before use, and to consult with a health care professional as necessary. This advice is especially important when using new supplies or equipment for clinical purposes. The authors and publisher disclaim all responsibility for any liability, loss, injury, or damage incurred as a consequence, directly or indirectly, of the use and applications of any of the contents of this volume.

Copyright © 2004 by Pearson Education, Inc., Upper Saddle River, New Jersey, 07458.
Pearson Prentice Hall. All rights reserved. Printed in the United States of America. This publication is protected by Copyright and permission should be obtained from the publisher prior to any prohibited reproduction, storage in a retrieval system, or transmission in any form or by any means, electronic, mechanical, photocopying, recording, or likewise. For information regarding permission(s), write to: Rights and Permissions Department.

Pearson Prentice Hall™ is a trademark of Pearson Education, Inc.
Pearson® is a registered trademark of Pearson plc
Prentice Hall® is a registered trademark of Pearson Education, Inc.

Pearson Education LTD., London   Pearson Education Australia PTY, Limited
Pearson Education Singapore, Pte. Ltd   Pearson Education North Asia Ltd
Pearson Education, Canada, Ltd   Pearson Educación de Mexico, S.A. de C.V.
Pearson Education–Japan   Pearson Education Malaysia, Pte. Ltd
Pearson Education, Upper Saddle River, New Jersey

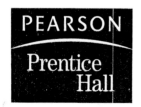

21 22 23 24 25   V036   16 15 14
ISBN 0-13-049538-7

PRINCIPLES OF CLINICAL LABORATORY MANAGEMENT

A Study Guide and Workbook

Dedication

To the many unseen laboratory professionals that strive daily to provide quality patient care and to our profession, which is enjoyable, provides professional friendships, provides our livelihood, and allows us an opportunity to contribute to the welfare of our patients.

Contents

Foreword	xi
Preface	xiii
Editors and Authors	xv
Acknowledgments	xix

SECTION I MANAGEMENT ISSUES REGARDING THE WORKFORCE

Chapter 1	**Professionalism** Jane Hudson, PhD, MT(ASCP)SM, CLS(NCA)		1
Chapter 2	**Professional Ethics** Jane Hudson, PhD, MT(ASCP)SM, CLS(NCA)		4
Chapter 3	**The Resumé** Paula Holland, MEd, MT(ASCP)		9
Chapter 4	**Job Description and Job Advertisement** Paula Holland, MEd, MT(ASCP)		18
Chapter 5	**Employment Interview and Selection Process** Paula Holland, MEd, MT(ASCP)		26
Chapter 6	**Employee Evaluation** Jane Hudson, PhD, MT(ASCP)SM, CLS(NCA)		33
Chapter 7	**Employee Correction and Discipline** Jane Hudson, PhD, MT(ASCP)SM, CLS(NCA)		41
Chapter 8	**Celebrating Diversity** David Thrash, BS, MT(ASCP), CLS(NCA)		44
Chapter 9	**Change** Jane Hudson, PhD, MT(ASCP)SM, CLS(NCA)		51
Chapter 10	**Stress Management** Eric Hogue, MS, MT(ASCP), CLS(NCA)		55

SECTION II MANAGEMENT ISSUES REGARDING COMMUNICATION

Chapter 11	**Professional Writing** Mary Lux, PhD, MT(ASCP), CLS(NCA)	**61**
Chapter 12	**Communications and Interpersonal Relationships** John Curry, MEd, MT(ASCP)DLM	**68**
Chapter 13	**Motivation** Jane Hudson, PhD, MT(ASCP)SM, CLS(NCA)	**73**
Chapter 14	**Leadership** Jane Hudson, PhD, MT(ASCP)SM, CLS(NCA)	**78**
Chapter 15	**Team Building** Paula Holland, MEd, MT(ASCP)	**85**
Chapter 16	**Conflict Management** Jane Hudson, PhD, MT(ASCP)SM, CLS(NCA)	**91**
Chapter 17	**Telephone Etiquette** Beth Parham White, BS, MT(ASCP), CLS(NCA)	**95**
Chapter 18	**Customer Satisfaction/Public Relations Program** John Curry, MEd, MT(ASCP)DLM	**99**

SECTION III MANAGEMENT ISSUES REGARDING THE WORK

Chapter 19	**Clinical Laboratory Safety** Hermolee Thomas Barnes, MEd, MT(ASCP)	**103**
Chapter 20	**Marketing and Development of an Outreach Program** Greg Hatten, BS, MT(ASCP)BB	**112**
Chapter 21	**Writing Procedures in the NCCLS Format** Beth Parham White, BS, MT(ASCP), CLS(NCA)	**116**
Chapter 22	**Laboratory Budgeting and Finance** Sandi Thames, BS, MT(ASCP), CLS(NCA)	**121**
Chapter 23	**Fraud and Abuse** Hassan Aziz, PhD, CLS(NCA)	**129**
Chapter 24	**Workload Recording** Dixie Daniels, BS, MT(ASCP)	**134**
Chapter 25	**Purchasing** Eric Reed, BS, MT(ASCP)	**140**
Chapter 26	**Employee Scheduling** Kathy Shields, MHS, MT(ASCP)	**148**
Chapter 27	**Evaluation of New Test Methods – The Comparison Study** David Thrash, BS, MT(ASCP), CLS(NCA) Margot Hall, PhD, FAIC, CChem MRSC	**155**

Chapter 28	**Quality Control** Margot Hall, PhD, FAIC, CChem MRSC	**165**
Chapter 29	**Quality Management** Gayle Curtis, MS, MT(ASCP), CPHQ	**177**
Chapter 30	**Problem Solving** Sabrina Bryant, MS, MT(ASCP), CLS(NCA)	**184**
Chapter 31	**Preanalytical, Analytical, and Postanalytical Phases** Jane Hudson, PhD, MT(ASCP)SM, CLS(NCA)	**189**
Chapter 32	**Instrument Selection** Carolyn Beck, EdD, MT(ASCP)SBB	**194**
Chapter 33	**Establishing Preventive and Corrective Maintenance Programs** Carolyn Beck, EdD, MT(ASCP)SBB	**201**
Chapter 34	**Organization and Time Management** Hermolee Thomas Barnes, MEd, MT(ASCP)	**208**
Chapter 35	**The Laboratory Information System: Choosing the Right One** Beth Parham White, BS, MT(ASCP), CLS(NCA)	**212**
Chapter 36	**Epidemiology in the Clinical Laboratory** Margaret McDonald, PhD, MT(ASCP)	**217**
Chapter 37	**Accreditation** John Curry, MEd, MT(ASCP)DLM	**227**
Chapter 38	**Legal Considerations** Jane Hudson, PhD, MT(ASCP)SM, CLS(NCA)	**232**
Chapter 39	**Consulting** Jane Hudson, PhD, MT(ASCP)SM, CLS(NCA)	**237**
Chapter 40	**Establishment of a Continuing Education Program** David Thrash, BS, MT(ASCP), CLS(NCA)	**241**
Chapter 41	**Construction and Delivery of an Instructional Unit** Claudia Miller, PhD, MT(ASCP), CLS(NCA)	**247**
Chapter 42	**Measurement and Evaluation Strategies for an Instructional Unit** Claudia Miller, PhD, MT(ASCP), CLS(NCA)	**255**

Answers for Questions and Case Commentaries   **265**

Index   **335**

Foreword

The editors and authors of *Principles of Laboratory Management: A Study Guide and Workbook* present detailed information on a variety of management topics in a clear and concise format. The topic summaries followed by review questions, exercises, and case studies provide stimulating and challenging experiences for learners. The mixture of theoretical information and practical application allow learners to analyze management situations and determine appropriate actions.

Principles of Laboratory Management: A Study Guide and Workbook is part of Prentice Hall's Clinical Laboratory Science series of textbooks, which is designed to balance theory and practical applications in a method that is engaging and useful to students. Furthermore, the books in this series are designed to foster various kinds of learning and some of the titles will be accompanied by computer applications.

We hope that this book, as well as the entire series, proves to be a valuable educational resource.

Elizabeth A. Zeibig
CLS Series Editor
Prentice Hall Health

Preface

In the current rapidly changing health care environment, the role of medical technology/clinical laboratory science personnel is expanding. An increased awareness of the business aspects of health care is expected. Therefore, the entry level laboratory practitioner must be cognizant of the financial, personnel, operational, and marketing issues affecting the laboratory in order to successfully perform and compete in this continuously changing environment.

Principles of Clinical Laboratory Management: A Study Guide and Workbook was designed to allow the learner to develop basic management competencies through a variety of learning experiences. The book can be used in a classroom situation or as a self-tutorial instructional manual. Each chapter is divided as follows:

- **Objectives**: competencies that should be attained upon completion of each chapter. The objectives are leveled (I, II, and III) as a guide to the learner regarding the depth of comprehension that should be attained. Level I indicates an ability to recall the material, Level II indicates the ability to apply the material, and Level III indicates the ability to solve problems in new situations.

- **Topic Summary**: a brief introductory narrative regarding the topic. Selected terms and phrases are in bold-faced type to emphasize a concept. Subheadings are used as appropriate based on the chapter topic. The learner may gain more information regarding the topic by reviewing the bibliography and internet sources as well as other management materials.

- **Bibliography**: suggested readings to enhance knowledge regarding the topic.

- **Internet Resources**: resources available on the Web. Although the authors have found these sites to be helpful, the authors do not endorse any site.

- **Questions**: a method for the learner to engage in reviewing the narrative information. The questions specifically address the cognitive skills. Each question is coded to the corresponding objective and level for easy reference.

- **Exercises**: activities in which the learner might engage to enhance knowledge of the topic. These exercises address the psychomotor and cognitive skills of the learner and correspond to pertinent chapter objectives. Exercise objectives primarily address the higher taxonomic levels.

- **Cases**: available to stimulate the learner's problem-solving abilities regarding the topic. The cases are a level III learning activity, correspond to a pertinent chapter objective, and address primarily the cognitive domain; however, some may address the psychomotor domain.

At the end of the book, the learner will find

- **Answers**: for the chapter questions.
- **Commentaries**: a discussion by the author of the cases. The learner should understand that, primarily, the commentaries present only one possible viewpoint of the case solutions and that other solutions may be valid. In fact, the authors encourage the learner to explore alternative solutions as a means of developing better problem-solving skills.

Editors and Authors

Senior Editor

Jane Hudson, PhD, MT(ASCP)SM, CLS(NCA)
Chairperson and Professor
Department of Medical Technology
The University of Southern Mississippi
Hattiesburg, Mississippi

Editors

Paula G. Holland, MEd, MT(ASCP)
Education Coordinator
Singing River Hospital
Pascagoula, Mississippi

David S. Thrash, BS, MT(ASCP), CLS(NCA)
Education Program Leader, CLS/CLT
Forrest General Hospital
Hattiesburg, Mississippi

Beth Parham White, BS, MT(ASCP), CLS(NCA)
Clinical Educator, Laboratory
Memorial Hospital at Gulfport
Gulfport, Mississippi

Authors

Hassan Aziz, PhD, CLS(NCA)
Assistant Professor
Armstrong Atlantic State University
Savannah, Georgia

Hermolee Thomas Barnes, MEd, MT(ASCP)
Clinical Educator for Diagnostic Services (Ret.)
Memorial Hospital at Gulfport
Gulfport, Mississippi

Carolyn Beck, EdD, MT(ASCP)SBB
Associate Professor
Department of Medical Technology
The University of Southern Mississippi
Hattiesburg, Mississippi

Sabrina Bryant, MS, MT(ASCP), CLS(NCA)
Instructor
Department of Medical Technology
The University of Southern Mississippi
Hattiesburg, Mississippi

John R. Curry, MEd, MT(ASCP)DLM
Laboratory Director
Memorial Hospital at Gulfport
Gulfport, Mississippi

Gayle Curtis, MS, MT(ASCP), CPHQ
Director, Quality Management Services (Ret.)
Forrest General Hospital
Hattiesburg, Mississippi

Dixie P. Daniels, BS, MT(ASCP)
Director of Laboratory
Gulf Coast Medical Center
Biloxi, Mississippi

Margot Hall, PhD, FAIC, CChem MRSC
Professor
Department of Medical Technology
The University of Southern Mississippi
Hattiesburg, Mississippi

Greg M. Hatten, BS, MT(ASCP)BB
Lab Outreach Coordinator
Singing River Hospital
Pascagoula, Mississippi

Eric Hogue, MS, MT(ASCP), CLS(NCA)
Medical Technologist
Hattiesburg Clinic
Hattiesburg, Mississippi

Paula Holland, MEd, MT(ASCP)
Education Coordinator
Singing River Hospital
Pascagoula, Mississippi

Jane Hudson, PhD, MT(ASCP)SM, CLS(NCA)
Chairperson and Professor
Department of Medical Technology
The University of Southern Mississippi
Hattiesburg, Mississippi

Mary Lux, PhD, MT(ASCP), CLS(NCA)
Professor
Department of Medical Technology
The University of Southern Mississippi
Hattiesburg, Mississippi

Margaret McDonald, PhD, MT(ASCP)
Director
U.S. Outcomes Research
Pfizer Global Pharmaceuticals
New York, New York

Claudia E. Miller, PhD, MT(ASCP), CLS(NCA)
Professor
National-Louis University
Health Studies Department
Evanston, Illinois

Eric Reed, BS, MT(ASCP)
Director of Laboratory
Singing River Hospital
Pascagoula, Mississippi

Kathy Shields, MHS, MT(ASCP)
Laboratory Director
River Oaks Health System
Rankin Medical Center
Jackson, Mississippi

Sandi Thames, BS, MT(ASCP), CLS(NCA)
Chief Technologist
Laboratory Services
Forrest General Hospital
Hattiesburg, Mississippi

David S. Thrash, BS, MT(ASCP), CLS(NCA)
Education Program Leader, CLS/CLT
Forrest General Hospital
Hattiesburg, Mississippi

Beth Parham White, BS, MT(ASCP), CLS(NCA)
Clinical Educator, Laboratory
Memorial Hospital at Gulfport
Gulfport, Mississippi

Acknowledgments

The staff at Pearson Prentice Hall have been very helpful. Beth Zeibig, CLS Series Editor, critiqued the book and offered many excellent suggestions. Melissa Kerian was always available to advise regarding format. Mark Cohen was instrumental in initiation of the project. Marty Sopher, production editor at Lithokraft, efficiently coordinated the book design and proof approval with the twenty authors. The authors would also like to thank the family members and friends who have provided encouragement during this project.

Reviewers

Joan Aldrich, PhD
Associate Professor
University of Texas Southwestern Medical Center
Department of Medical Laboratory Sciences
Dallas, Texas

James Aumer, MS, MT(ASCP)
Program Director
Rochester Institute of Technology
Medical Technology Program
Rochester, New York

Mary Banman, MT(ASCP), NCA(CLS)
Clinical Education Coordinator and Instructor
University of North Dakota
School of Medicine and Health Science
Department of Pathology
Grand Forks, North Dakota

Cheryl G. Davis, MS, CLS(NCA)
Assistant Professor
Tuskegee University
Department of Medical Technology
Tuskegee, Alabama

David Falleur, MEd
Chair and Associate Professor
Southwest Texas State University
Department of Clinical Laboratory Science
San Marcos, Texas

Lynn M. Glazener, MS, MT(ASCP)
Instructor
Texas A&M University—Corpus Christi
Department of Clinical Laboratory Science
Corpus Christi, Texas

Susan S. Graham, MS, MT(ASCP)SH
Assistant Professor and Chair
SUNY Upstate Medical University
Department of Clinical Laboratory Science
Syracuse, New York

Kenneth E. Griswold, PhD
Professor and Coordinator
Louisiana Technical University
Program in Medical Technology
Ruston, Louisiana

Jean Holter, EdD
Professor and Program Director
West Virginia University
Medical Technology Program
Morgantown, West Virginia

Jeanne Isabel, MSEd
Associate Professor
Northern Illinois University
Clinical Laboratory Science Program
DeKalb, Illinois

Leta Stewart, MS, DLM(ASCP), MT(ASCP), CLS(NCA)
Director of Laboratory Services
OSF Saint Anthony Medical Center
School of Clinical Laboratory Science
Rockford, IL

SECTION I MANAGEMENT ISSUES REGARDING THE WORKFORCE

Chapter 1

Professionalism

Jane Hudson, Ph.D., MT(ASCP)SM, CLS(NCA)

OBJECTIVES

Upon completion of this chapter the learner will be able to

1. Define the terms *profession, professional*, and *professionalism*. *(Level I)*
2. Identify one function of each of the following organizations: American Society for Clinical Laboratory Science (ASCLS), National Credentialing Agency for Laboratory Personnel, Inc. (NCA), and National Accrediting Agency for Clinical Laboratory Sciences (NAACLS). *(Level I)*
3. Defend the importance of the profession, characteristics of a professional, and the need for professionalism. *(Level III)*
4. Recommend appropriate professional behavior, given case situations. *(Level III)*

TOPIC SUMMARY

Medical technology/clinical laboratory science qualifies as a profession according to the characteristics of a profession described by Lindberg and associates and later by Clerc. The American Society for Clinical Laboratory Science (ASCLS), **a professional organization**, has provided the professional **Body of Knowledge** that defines the scope of practice and the **Code of Ethics** that **advocate standards of excellence**. Also, through the professional organization, medical technologists/clinical laboratory scientists strive to **promote the profession's recognition and dignity**. The National Credentialing Agency for Laboratory Personnel, Inc. (NCA) has developed and employed a national certification examination for **entry into the profession**. The National Accrediting Agency for Clinical Laboratory Sciences (NAACLS) has established **criteria for educational programs**. The bold-faced items listed previously are essential characteristics that must be present for a vocation to be classified as a profession.

Therefore, medical technology/clinical laboratory science is a profession, and those of us who practice it are professionals. Our professionalism is judged by the professional quality with which we practice the profession. It is imperative that we develop the skills necessary for professionals to exhibit. What are those skills? We immediately identify competency regarding technical skills. Indeed, without outstanding technical skills, we would never be identified as professionals. But we must understand and develop competency in our total scope of practice, which includes roles such as technical expert, communicator, manager, consultant, team member, motivator, leader, salesperson, evaluator, problem solver, advisor, educator, and so on in order to provide maximum benefits to our patients, our colleagues, and our profession. The manner in which the scope of practice is performed is a responsibility of each practitioner. When we choose to provide quality in our total scope of practice, we are acting as professionals and exhibiting professionalism.

Important in the development of the professional is membership in a professional organization. Professional organizations for medical technology/clinical laboratory science are typically divided into generalist and specialist professional organizations. Examples of generalist professional organizations include the ASCLS, American Society of Clinical Pathology (ASCP), American Medical Technologists (AMT), and International Society for Clinical Laboratory Technology (ISCLT). Examples of specialist professional organizations for medical technology/clinical laboratory science include the American Society for Microbiology (ASM) and the American Association of Clinical Chemistry (AACC). Professional organizations enhance professionalism by providing members with current literature, continuing education, networking opportunities, and representation regarding health-care issues that impact both the professional and our clients.

The professional demonstrates professionalism by obtaining certification at entry level and enhancing entry-level knowledge through continuing education activities. Certification agencies include the NCA the ASCP Board of Registry, and others. Generalist and/or specialist examinations are offered.

Professional membership, certification, and continuing education activities are three ways in which professionals indicate commitment to providing quality in the total scope of practice.

Bibliography

Clerc, Jeanne M. 1992. *An introduction to clinical laboratory science.* St. Louis, Mo.: Mosby Year Book.

Lindberg, D. S., M. B. Stevenson, and F. Fisher 1984. *Williams's introduction to the profession of medical technology.* 4th ed. Philadelphia: Lea & Febiger.

Internet Resources

National Accrediting Agency for Clinical Laboratory Sciences. <www.naacls.org>
American Society for Clinical Laboratory Science. <www.ascls.org>
American Society of Clinical Pathology. <www.ascp.org>
American Association of Blood Banks. <www.aabb.org>
American Society of Hematology. <www.hematology.org>
American Society for Microbiology. <www.asmusa.org/>

QUESTIONS

1. Define: *(Objective 1, Level I)*

    Profession:

    Professional:

    Professionalism:

2. Identify one function of each of the following organizations: *(Objective 2, Level I)*

    ASCLS:

    NCA:

    NAACLS:

EXERCISES

Completion of the exercises will enhance your knowledge of professionalism. *(Objective 3, Level III)*

1. Attend the Student Forum meeting in your state and/or attend the ASCLS affiliate meeting in your state. Summarize in writing your thoughts regarding the profession, the professionals you met, and how the meeting enhanced your understanding of the profession.

2. Interview a medical technologist/clinical laboratory scientist who exemplifies professionalism. Ask the individual to define *professional* and *professionalism* and to identify specific behaviors of professionals. Ask how unprofessional behavior is harmful to coworkers, patients, and the profession. Write a report identifying the characteristics that this person exhibits and that you wish to adopt.

3. Interview professionals in other fields (e.g., pharmacist, physical therapist, nurse, physician, occupational therapist, etc.) and ask them to describe *professionalism*. Write a summary of their comments.

CASES

Following are two cases addressing the actions of the laboratory professional. Using the information given, individually or as a group recommend appropriate professional behavior for the case. *(Objective 4, Level III)*

1. A physician comes to the hematology laboratory yelling about not receiving his test results in a timely manner. You are the medical technologist/clinical laboratory scientist in charge of the hematology laboratory and have the responsibility of responding to him. Describe how you would exhibit professional behavior in this situation.

2. You have the responsibility of implementing a new test procedure in your laboratory. There are two procedures that could be used. One procedure is of high quality, very accurate, and cost effective, but your laboratory will not make as much money as the second procedure, which has reasonable quality and accuracy. What decision do you believe would exhibit professionalism? Justify your answer.

Chapter 2

Professional Ethics

Jane Hudson, Ph.D., MT(ASCP)SM, CLS(NCA)

OBJECTIVES

Upon completion of this chapter the learner will be able to

1. Define *medical ethics*. *(Level I)*
2. Discuss the three duties of the medical technologist/clinical laboratory scientist as stated in the American Society for Clinical Laboratory Science Code of Ethics. *(Level II)*
3. Identify the five ethical principles. *(Level I)*
4. Discuss the difference between the deontological and the teleological ethical theories. *(Level II)*
5. Analyze an ethical situation as stated in the exercises. *(Level III)*
6. Choose the most appropriate ethical approach in given case studies. *(Level III)*

TOPIC SUMMARY

Ethics is a study of standards of conduct and moral judgment. Medical ethics applies this study to the practice of medicine. Standards are used as a basis of judging value, and morals relate to right and wrong conduct. Thus, medical ethics is a study of standards used as a basis of judgment regarding right and wrong conduct in the practice of medicine. Professional ethics refers to a specific profession, in this case, medical technology/clinical laboratory science. One of the characteristics of a profession is formulation of a code of ethics. The American Society for Clinical Laboratory Science (ASCLS) has developed and published the following professional Code of Ethics:

Code of Ethics of the American Society for Clinical Laboratory Science

PREAMBLE

The Code of Ethics of the American Society for Clinical Laboratory Science (ASCLS) sets forth the principles and standards by which clinical laboratory professionals practice their profession.

I. DUTY TO THE PATIENT

Clinical laboratory professionals are accountable for the quality and integrity of the laboratory services they provide. This obligation includes maintaining individual competence in judgement and performance and striving to safeguard the patient from incompetent or illegal practice by others.

Clinical laboratory professionals maintain high standards of practice. They exercise sound judgement in establishing, performing, and evaluating laboratory testing.

Clinical laboratory professionals maintain strict confidentiality of patient information and test results. They safeguard the dignity and privacy of patients and provide accurate information to other health care professionals about the services they provide.

II. DUTY TO COLLEAGUES AND THE PROFESSION

Clinical laboratory professionals uphold and maintain the dignity and respect of our profession and strive to maintain a reputation of honesty, integrity, and reliability. They contribute to the advancement of the profession by improving the body of knowledge, adopting scientific advances that benefit the patient, maintaining high standards of practice and education, and seeking fair socioeconomic working conditions for members of the profession.

Clinical laboratory professionals actively strive to establish cooperative and respectful working relationships with other health professionals with the primary purpose of ensuring a high standard of care for the patients they serve.

III. DUTY TO SOCIETY

As practitioners of an autonomous profession, clinical laboratory professionals have the responsibility to contribute from their sphere of professional competence to the general well being of the community.

Clinical laboratory professionals comply with relevant laws and regulations pertaining to the practice of clinical laboratory science and actively seek, within the dictates of their consciences, to change those which do not meet the high standards of care and practice to which the profession is committed.

PLEDGE TO THE PROFESSION

As a clinical laboratory professional, I strive to:

- Maintain and promote standards of excellence in performing and advancing the art and science of my profession;
- Preserve the dignity and privacy of patients;
- Uphold and maintain the dignity and respect of our profession;
- Seek to establish cooperative and respectful working relationships with other health professionals; and
- Contribute to the general well being of the community.

I will actively demonstrate my commitment to these responsibilities throughout my professional life.

(American Society for Clinical Laboratory Science. 1995. *Code of Ethics*)

Two major ethical theories for consideration when discussing professional ethics are deontological and teleological. Five ethical principles (associated with both the deontological and teleological ethical theories) to consider are

1. Justice—impartiality; fairness.
2. Autonomy—self-governing.
3. Veracity—truthfulness; honesty.
4. Fidelity—a faithful devotion to one's vows.
5. Beneficence—doing good/Nonmaleficence—doing no harm.

Immanuel Kant is usually associated with the deontological approach, which advocates that right and wrong are inherent, action is independent of consequences, and the means are more valuable than the end results. When considering the different ethical principles, the deontological approach would advocate positions as follows:

Ethical Principle	Position
Justice	It is wrong to deny anyone.
Autonomy	A person's beliefs should always be respected.
Veracity	Truth-telling is always right.
Fidelity	Breaking promises or confidentiality is always wrong.
Beneficence/Nonmaleficence.	Consequences not considered.

The teleological approach is associated most commonly with Jeremy Bentham and John Stuart Mill. This approach advocates that the end results are more valuable than the means, and actions should be those that produce the most benefit (i.e., if good consequences, the action is right; if bad consequences, the action is wrong). The teleological approach would advocate the following positions in relation to the five aforementioned ethical principles:

Ethical Principle	Position
Justice	Deny someone if more good than harm is done.
Autonomy	Respect a person's beliefs only when more good than harm will be done.
Veracity	Truth-telling is right only when more good than harm occurs.
Fidelity	Consequences determine whether one should break a promise or confidentiality.
Beneficence/Nonmaleficence	Consider consequences—if they are primarily good, then action should be taken.

Following is an example of the application of these two ethical approaches to a patient situation:

A patient has a terminal illness, and the decision has to be made whether to tell the patient of the illness. The pure deontological approach would advocate telling the patient regardless of the consequences, whereas the pure teleological approach would advocate telling the patient only if the consequences would be beneficial. These two major ethical theories, deontological and teleological, are a basis to begin the decision-making process; however, an individual may employ both or a mixture of the two theories when actually making an ethical decision. One may take the deontological position regarding one situation and the teleological position regarding another situation.

Ruth Purtilo (1999) has described three types of ethical problems that can occur. These are defined as follows:

1. Ethical distress—one recognizes what the course of action should be, but a barrier to the action exists, thus inhibiting obtaining the desired results.
2. Ethical dilemma—one must make a decision between two courses of action with two different outcomes.
3. Locus of authority—one must decide who has the authority to make the decision.

Purtilo also presents six practical steps in the ethical decision-making process. First, gather all the facts regarding the situation, so that the decision is made using all available information. Second, decide whether the situation is ethical distress, ethical dilemma, or locus of authority. Third, determine whether the deontological or teleological approach is to be used. Fourth, seek all practical solutions. Fifth, implement the solutions selected. And sixth, evaluate the results.

BIBLIOGRAPHY

American Society for Clinical Laboratory Science. 1995. *Code of ethics.* (Available from American Society for Clinical Laboratory Science, 7910 Woodmont Ave., Suite 530, Bethesda, MD, 20814.)

Clerc, Jeanne M. 1992. *An introduction to clinical laboratory science.* St. Louis, Mo.: Mosby Year Book.

Gauthier, Candace C. *Professional issues—Medical ethics for the clinical laboratorian.* (Available from the American Society for Clinical Laboratory Science, 7910 Woodmont Ave., Suite 530, Bethesda, MD, 20814.)

Heath, P., and Schneewind, J.B., (eds.). 1997. *Immanuel Kant lectures on ethics.* Trans. Peter Health. Cambridge, UK: Cambridge University Press.

Immanuel Kant lectures on ethics. Trans. Louis Infield. 1963. New York: Harper & Row.

Kant's critique of practical reason and other works on the theory of ethics. Trans. Thomas Kingsmill Abbott. 1923. London: Langmans, Green and Co.

Mill, John Stuart. 1969. *Essays on ethics, religion and society.* Ed. J. M. Robson. Toronto, Canada: University of Toronto Press.

Purtilo, Ruth. 1999. *Ethical dimensions in the health professions.* 3d ed. Philadelphia: W. B. Saunders Company.

Veatch, Robert M., and Harley E. Flack. 1997. *Case studies in allied health ethics.* Upper Saddle River, N.J.: Prentice Hall.

The works of Jeremy Bentham. 1962. Reproduced from the Bowring Ed. of 1838–1843, vol. 8, pp.128, 209–210, 289. New York: Russell and Russell, Inc.

INTERNET RESOURCES

The American Society for Clinical Laboratory Science. <www.ascls.org>

Genethics.ca. <www.genethics.ca>

Issues in Health Care. <www.geocities.com/hotsprings/3872/>

QUESTIONS

1. Medical ethics is defined as _____. *(Objective 1, Level I)*
2. Name and discuss the three duties of the medical technologist/clinical laboratory scientist as stated in the ASCLS Code of Ethics. *(Objective 2, Level II)*
3. Which of the following is NOT an ethical principle? *(Objective 3, Level I)*
    a. Justice
    b. Honesty
    c. Autonomy
    d. Veracity
    e. Fidelity
4. Discuss differences between the deontological and the teleological ethical theories. *(Objective 4, Level II)*

EXERCISES

Completion of the exercises will enhance your knowledge of professional ethics. *(Objective 5, Level III)*

1. Identify and record specific ethical situations in the laboratory. As the situations are presented, the group evaluates each situation by identifying the ethical problem, the ethical approach, practical alternatives, and how the situations relate to the professional code of ethics.

2. Develop a case study regarding an ethical situation and evaluate the study identifying the ethical problem, the ethical approach, practical alternatives, and how the situation relates to the professional code of ethics.

CASES

Following are five cases involving professional ethics. Using the information given, answer the five questions given with each case. *(Objective 6, Level III)* A group may decide to work together and select the best answers as determined by group consensus.

1. Presently, a screening test for the antibody of a deadly agent is being performed on all blood units, because the agent is transmitted via transfusions. If the antigen test for this agent is added to the workup, approximately 5 additional donors with the agent will be identified each year and eliminated as donors (5 donors out of 25 million total blood donors per year). The cost to add the antigen test is expected to be approximately $60 million per year. Should the antigen test be added?
   a. What is the ethical problem?
   b. Which ethical approach should be used?
   c. What are the practical alternatives?
   d. Does the professional Code of Ethics address this situation? If so, how?
   e. What would you do?

2. You enter a patient's room, introduce yourself, and state that you are from the laboratory and have come to draw some blood. The patient refuses to have blood drawn due to religious reasons. You know that the test for which the blood is requested is critical to the health, even life, of the patient. Should you insist upon drawing the blood?
   a. What is the ethical problem?
   b. Which ethical approach should be used?
   c. What are the practical alternatives?
   d. Does the Professional Code of Ethics address this situation? If so, how?
   e. What would you do?

3. One of the tests performed on a forty-seven-year-old male on admission was carcinoembryonic antigen (CEA). You performed the test and know that the CEA level is elevated. You then go to his room to draw blood for additional studies. The patient tells you his history of cancer and that he has decided it is better to die while feeling good than to live and suffer. He finishes by asking you if the preceding day's tests were normal. Do you believe that the patient should be told the truth?
   a. What is the ethical problem?
   b. Which ethical approach should be used?
   c. What are the practical alternatives?
   d. Does the Professional Code of Ethics address this situation? If so, how?
   e. What would you do?

4. Your best friend is dating an individual on which you performed an HIV test. The test was positive. Should you tell your best friend?
   a. What is the ethical problem?
   b. Which ethical approach should be used?
   c. What are the practical alternatives?
   d. Does the Professional Code of Ethics address this situation? If so, how?
   e. What would you do?

5. You work the night shift with one other tech in a 300-bed community hospital. You know your coworker and some of the evening shift techs are faking the quality control (QC). You talk to the supervisor about the matter and are told "You just do your work and mind your own business." It does not appear anyone wants to take the QC issue seriously, yet you know that errors could be avoided and better patient results provided if QC was performed appropriately. What should be done?
   a. What is the ethical problem?
   b. What ethical approach should be used?
   c. What are the practical alternatives?
   d. Does the Professional Code of Ethics address this situation? If so, how?
   e. What would you do?

Chapter 3

The Resumé

Paula Holland, M.Ed., MT(ASCP)

OBJECTIVES

Upon completion of this chapter the learner will be able to

1. Define the purpose of the resumé. *(Level I)*
2. Name two resumé format types. *(Level I)*
3. Discuss the appropriate use of each resumé format identified in Objective 2. *(Level II)*
4. Discuss the contents of a cover letter. *(Level II)*
5. Construct your resumé. *(Level III)*
6. Construct your cover letter for a position you wish to pursue. *(Level III)*
7. Given a resumé, examine it in terms of items included, format, spelling, and sentence structure, and propose suggestions for improvement. *(Level III)*

TOPIC SUMMARY

The Resumé

What does it take to prepare the best resumé? Realizing the intent of preparing a resumé is the first step in its development. In the context of today's business language, a resumé is the key tool or vehicle one uses to advertise his or her services when seeking employment. To be successful in marketing these skills, it is important to accent strengths in order to attract the attention of the person(s) who will read the resumé. The parts of a resumé are (in specific cases, some items may not apply):

- The candidate's name, residential address, and phone number (including e-mail address)
- Career objective
- Educational qualifications
- Work experience
- Graduate course work
- Military experience
- Certification(s)
- Professional memberships, honors, and activities
- Publications
- Volunteer work
- Proficiency in another language
- Job-related hobbies

The main function of a resumé is to get an interview. Before the writing begins, take time to study the job announcement and job description to determine what characteristics the employer is looking for in a candidate and, more importantly, to determine whether you, the candidate, are interested in this particular position. It is important to realize that the resumé should give information about what you can do in the future and not just what you have done in the past. The resumé needs to answer the following interviewer questions:

- What can this individual do for the company?
- Can this individual do the work?
- Can this individual contribute to the company beyond "just doing the work"?
- Does this individual meet the qualifications?
- What kind of individual is this particular applicant?

The style or form of writing is also of importance when developing a resumé. Once a particular style of writing is chosen, maintaining this form consistently to the end of the writing is a must. This is a sign to the reader that the individual who composed it has an organized, logical mind. It is also important to spell out most words in a resumé and use very few abbreviations. Acceptable abbreviations are used to indicate college degrees, for example B.S. (bachelor of science),

MARGARET W. SMITH

2345 Mollander Drive
Tyler, Mississippi 39000
(601) 123-4567

PROFESSIONAL OBJECTIVE	Seeking a full-time, challenging position as a medical technologist/clinical laboratory scientist in the clinical laboratory setting.
EDUCATION	Medical Technology/Clinical Laboratory Science Internship July 2002–December 2002 Superior Hospital Escatawpa, Mississippi 39992 Bachelor of Science in Medical Technology/Clinical Laboratory Science: Minor: Biology December 2002 (expected graduation date) South Mississippi University Shubuta, Mississippi 39699

WORK HISTORY	Medical Technology Intern Superior Hospital
	July 2002–December 2002 Escatawpa, Mississippi
	
	Trained in all aspects of the computerized hospital medical laboratory, consisting of approximately one hundred employees. Performed testing in all departments in the clinical laboratory and blood bank.
	
	Major instruments operated include Vitros 950 Chemistry Analyzer, Abbott AXSYM, Abbott IMX, Abbott Commander, Coulter Gen S and STKS, Microscan Walkaway 96, Bactec 9240, Beckman Array 360 System, MLA Electra 1400C and 900C Automatic Coagulation Analyzers and the Dade Behring PFA 100 Bleeding Time Analyzer. Also trained extensively on the Sunquest Information Computer System.
	
	Secretarial Assistant South Mississippi University
	    Center for Education
	    Shubuta, Mississippi
	
	Part-time employee while attending South Mississippi University. Responsibilities included answering phones, typing, preparing documents for professors, handling large sums of money per supervisor, operating and troubleshooting copying machine, and public relations.
	
	Sales Associate Accents Boutique
	February 2000–June 2000 Tyler, Mississippi
	
	Part-time employee while attending South Mississippi University. Responsibilities included sales, operating cash register, helping in opening and closing the store, and tagging and restocking merchandise.

FIGURE 3–1. Resumé #1

FIGURE 3–1. Resumé #1 (continued)

CERTIFICATION	American Society of Clinical Pathology Certification Examination Eligible January 2003
	National Credentialing Agency for Laboratory Personnel Eligible January 2003
AWARDS RECEIVED	South Mississippi University Dean's List 1999, 2000, 2001, 2002
	National Dean's List 1999, 2000, 2001, 2002
	The SMU Medical Technology/Clinical Laboratory Science Club President, 2001–2002 Member, 1999–2002
	Hugh O'Brien Youth Leadership Ambassador 1995

Ph.D. (doctor of philosophy). Use either Ph.D. (M.D.) or Dr., but not both, when writing a doctoral title. Be sure to spell out the names of states, cities, streets, avenues, and titles of persons.

The two most popular forms of writing used in the development of a resumé are the **chronological** and **functional** formats. Most new graduates will choose the chronological format, which lists the graduate's accomplishments in reverse chronological order, emphasizing the most outstanding accomplishment first. Take a look at sample resumé #1 (Figure 3-1). This resumé utilizes the chronological style of writing. Notice that the name is offset and located in the upper left margin of the paper. This will help the resumé stand out from the rest when the interviewer is shuffling through a stack of resumes to find candidates to interview. This resumé was prepared by a medical technology/clinical laboratory science intern within months of completing her baccalaureate degree requirements. Notice how nicely the internship experience has been placed in a key position so that the emphasis on education downplays the preparer's lack of work experience in the field for which she is applying. In resumé #1, the intern accentuated her willingness to assume leadership responsibilities by listing her affiliation as president of the Medical Technology club and recognition as a youth ambassador.

The functional style of writing is that which emphasizes special skills and accomplishments rather than an applicant's work experience. This style is more appropriately used when the work experience is not specific to the job for which the applicant seeks (i.e., making a career change, reentering the workforce after being self-employed, etc.). Look at sample resumé #2 (Figure 3-2). This resumé utilizes the functional style of writing and emphasizes the experience that is similar to the position sought. Notice that experience and education headings are highlighted by bold-faced lettering. The applicant's critical information is separated at the top of the first page so that it is readily seen.

Keep in mind that every line of a resumé must be carefully thought out. Be specific in describing work responsibilities and use specific examples (facts, figures) to make the point. Be careful to avoid using words that are inflated or wordy—take a more direct approach. Look at the following examples:

Too Vague	**More Specific**
Performed well under pressure.	Despite a pressing deadline, the procedure manual was available for the mock College of American Pathologist inspection two days beforehand.
Showed true signs of leadership.	Designed and implemented an employee leadership recognition program for the clinical laboratory to boost morale.

203 Fairville Drive
Hattiesburg, Mississippi 39402
Phone: 601-555-1057
E-mail: sloanejacobs@yahoo.com

Sloane W. Jacobs

Objective: To apply my experience in adult education, program design and presentation, and continuing education as a Trainer/Education Instructor for General Hospital.

Experience: **Education Program Leader, Clinical Laboratory Scientist (CLS)/Clinical Laboratory Technician (CLT) Programs**
General Hospital Clinical Laboratory
Hattiesburg, Mississippi
3/96–Present

Curriculum-Based Instruction:
- Coordinate with South Mississippi University and Leaf River Community College instructors regarding the CLS/CLT interns' coursework
- In charge of curriculum planning and implementation for the incoming CLS and CLT interns
- Instruct interns on different aspects of laboratory science including laboratory safety, phlebotomy training, specific testing, duties, and responsibilities
- Coordinate, with different departmental instructors, the instruction of CLS/CLT interns regarding the procedures and functions of the different laboratory departments
- Plan and implement course instruction for the CLS/CLT interns using case studies, research reports, literature review exams and worksheets

Program Design and Implementation:
- Coordinate the Clinical Laboratory Competency/Evaluation Design Team to appraise the effectiveness of New Employee Task List and Performance Evaluation
- Serve as Co-Coordinator of the Clinical Laboratory Community Health Fairs
- Develop Employee Recognition Program for the clinical laboratory to boost morale
- Design and provide various continuing education modules to the department's fifty-two employees
- Provide safety training and safety-related activities to the department based on Joint Commission Accreditation of Healthcare Organizations
- Update departmental employee continuing education files
- Assist in writing policies and procedures for evaluation of CLS/CLT interns in cooperation with South Mississippi University faculty and other education program leaders from affiliated hospitals

Medical Technologist
General Hospital Clinical Laboratory
Hattiesburg, Mississippi
7/93–3/96

FIGURE 3–2. Resumé #2

FIGURE 3–2. Resumé #2 (continued)

Education	**South Mississippi University**
	Hattiesburg, Mississippi
	2000–2001
	• Earning credit hours toward Masters of Adult Education
	1991–1995
	• Degree: Bachelor of Science degree in Applied Sciences
Organizations/Skills	
	• National Accrediting Agency for Clinical Laboratory Sciences volunteer and self-study paper reviewer
	• Member and board certified by American Society for Clinical Pathology
	• Author of three management case studies (in print)
	• Knowledgeable of contact hours and continuing education units
	• Microsoft proficient in Word, Power Point, and Excel

Prepare the resumé and check to be sure none of the following information is included:

- Personal information (age, weight, height, etc.)
- Date of the written resumé
- Political status
- Photos
- Salary—previous and desired
- High school data
- Religious status
- The word *resumé*

Keep the resumé to no more than one page in length (baccalaureate and most master degree candidates). A doctoral candidate may choose to write a two-page resumé, especially if pursuing an academic position. More companies are now using computers to scan for keywords, so use text that commands attention. It is still important to be conservative in choosing the type of pattern and style of print—a fancy or very creative look might not be the desired effect to land the interview.

After typing and proofreading the resumé for the final time, have an experienced reviewer look it over. This individual should proofread the resumé and provide suggestions to improve it.

The Cover Letter

To hold the reader's attention, make sure that the content of each cover letter varies from that of the resumé. A highly effective way of enhancing the cover letter is to incorporate testimonials from previous company managers, directors, or supervisors that will express how you not only proved but surpassed your responsibilities as an employee under their direction. This can be accomplished by 1) making a separate paragraph within the cover letter, 2) using the testimonial letter as the cover letter, or 3) attaching the testimonial letter to your resumé.

Cover letter essentials include the following:

- Keep the cover letter to one page with about three to five paragraphs.
- Include your name and a return address.
- Include the prospective employer's name, title, and address.
- Address the letter to a specific person.
- Include in the first paragraph the reason you are writing, the position for which you are applying, and how you heard about the position.
- Include in the second paragraph the reason you are interested in the position or the company, why you are qualified, and relate these to the employer's needs.
- Include in the last paragraph an appreciation for the employer's time in reviewing the cover letter and resumé. Request an interview or a meeting to discuss the position further. Make sure to include a contact phone number.
- In closing the letter be sure to add the word *Enclosure* two spaces below your signature.

Reply Postcard

Mailing a reply postcard with the resumé is an excellent technique used to increase the chances of receiving a response regarding a job interview. Using a standard postcard (no lines) place your name, address, and a return postage stamp on one side. Turn the card over and write several follow-up comments for the prospective employer to complete, for example:

- Ask that the employer contact you to set up an interview.
- Give the employer a comment area in which to inform you if the position is no longer available and space to provide information regarding the reason the position is no longer available.
- Include a space for the contact person's name, title, and company. A reply postcard would be prepared similar to the following example (Figure 3-3):

Dear Candidate:

I have received your resumé, and an interview date has been scheduled for _____.

The position is no longer available due to
_____.

Name: _____

Title: _____

Company: _____

FIGURE 3–3. Example Postcard

Resumé Presentation and Mailing

To effectively get the resumé in the hands of the person(s) who will actually read it, hand deliver it. When this is not possible, mail it in a 9 × 12 envelope (white). Mailing the resumé via "Priority Mail" will make a significant impact because this type of mail will likely be opened first as it appears important. Follow up by phone after allowing time for delivery of the resumé by mail. **Do not fold the resumé!** If the interviewer requests that the resumé be faxed, always follow up by mailing the original.

References

Include three personal and three professional typed references on a separate sheet of paper. Bring these to the interview. Include the reference's full name and title, address, and phone and/or fax number. Note: when selecting your references, be sure to ask individuals who will provide a positive recommendation. When you are compiling your references, you should ask the individual if he or she is willing to serve as your reference and whether they could give you a positive recommendation. If the prospective reference hesitates at all, use someone else.

BIBLIOGRAPHY

Faux, Marian. 1995. *The complete resumé guide.* 5th ed. New York: Arco Publishing, McMillan Inc.

Guterl, Gail O. 1998. Is your resumé all it can be? *ADVANCE for Medical Laboratory Professionals* 10, no. 6, 8–9.

Konecsni, John Emery. 1994. The million dollar med tech: Managing and marketing your career in the 90's. Presentation at the Louisiana/Mississippi Societies for Clinical Laboratory Science, April 13, Biloxi, Mississippi.

Massey, Laura D. 1999. Use basic marketing principles to prepare your resumé. *ADVANCE for Medical Laboratory Professionals* 11, no. 8, 6.

Prost, Marlene A. 1999. Landing that first job: Through a powerful resumé and cover letter. *ADVANCE for Medical Laboratory Professionals—Special Student Supplement*, vol. 11, no. 8, 6–7.

Reed, Jean. 1998. *Resumés that get jobs.* 9th ed. New York: Arco Publishing, McMillan Inc.

INTERNET RESOURCES

Career Development Center, University of Wisconsin, Milwaukee. <http://careerlink.cdc.uwm.edu>

College Grad.com.
<www.collegegrad.com/resumes/coverlet.html>

QUESTIONS

1. The purpose of the resumé is to (*Objective 1, Level I*)
    a. get an interview
    b. demonstrate your writing skills
    c. inform the person of your intent to apply
    d. list your entire life history

2. Two resumé format types are _____ and _____ .
   (Objective 2, Level I)

3. Discuss the appropriate use of each resumé format. *(Objective 3, Level II)*

4. Discuss the contents of the cover letter. *(Objective 4, Level II)*

EXERCISES

Completion of the exercises will enhance your knowledge of the resumé. *(Objective 5, Level III and Objective 6, Level III)*

1. Interview an individual in your organization that reviews resumés. Ask the following questions:
   - What items in the cover letter impress the reviewer?
   - What would the reviewer like to see in a cover letter?
   - What resumé format does the reviewer like?
   - What items are the reviewer seeking to find in the resume?
   - What advice would the reviewer give to you regarding the cover letter and resume?

   Summarize the information after the interview and share with others in the class.

2. Ask several experienced technologists if you might review their resumés. Study the different formats and items included. Share your information with the rest of the class.

3. Construct your resumé.

4. Construct your cover letter for a position you wish to pursue.

CASES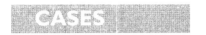

Examine each of the case studies given (Figures 3–4 and 3–5) and correct any errors in spelling, sentence structure, format, and so on to make these effective resumés. *(Objective 7, Level III)*

NANCY M. SMITH

PERMANENT ADDRESS	CAMPUS ADDRESS
P.O. Box 501	3333 Cliff View Ct.
Lucedale, MS 39452	Shubuta, MS 39999
(601) 555-5555	(601) 432-3322

EDUCATION

- (1993–1995) B.S. Degree. Medical Technology/Clinical Laboratory Science; South MS University Shubuta, MS. Graduation Date: December 1995
- (1993) Course: Breath Alcohol Technician; General Hospital–Shubuta, MS
- (1989–1991) B.S. Degree: May 1991; State University–Lucky, MS; Graduated Summa Cum Laude; G.P.A. 3.95 on 4.00 scale.

EXPERIENCE

- (1995) summer and fall: Internship; Medical Technology/Clinical Laboratory Science; Superior Hospital–Escataba, MS.
- (1995) summer: Cashier; Judy's Restaurant.
- (1993) summer: Counselor; Alliance for Minority Participation: (SMU); Dr. John Whitfield.
- (1991) summer: Medical Enrichment Program; Miracle Medical Center–Soso, MS

BACKGROUND

- HONORS: Who's Who Among Students in American Colleges and Universities, Alpha Kappa Mu National Honor Society, Award for Excellence (AHU)–1990, Dow Chemical Scholarship, Academic Scholarship (AHU), Medical Technology Scholarship (SMU), Presidential Scholar: 1989–1991, National Dean's List Scholar: 1991–1993.
- CLUBS: Medical Technology/Clinical Laboratory Science, Math, Chemistry, Baptist Student Union.
- EXTRACURRICULAR ACTIVITIES: intramural basketball and writing poetry.

PERSONAL DATA

- twenty-eight years old; married with one child; religion: Baptist faith.

FIGURE 3–4. Case 1

Resumé of Marinel Saucier

Residence: 3712 BellFountain Boulevard
Lucky, MS 39345
E-mail: www.marinels@yahoo.com

Career Objective
Seek a responsible position in the clinical laboratory. Desire opportunity for advancement.

Education
Alabama Central University, Mobile, Alabama
Bachelor of Science degree in Medical Technology/Clinical Laboratory Science
(1999–2001)

Leaf River Community College, Hattiesburg, Mississippi
Associate Degree of Science
(1994–1996)

Sigmond University, Dumaguete City, Philippines
Completed 52 credit hours toward Bachelor of Biology degree
(1989–1992)

Awards/Honors
Alabama Central, Mobile, Alabama
President's List, Spring 1999, Fall 2000
Vice-President's List, Fall 1999, 2001
High School Award—Elected "Most Likely to Succeed"

Work History
Assistant Hatchery Manager, Custom Pack Aquaculture
Pachuta, Mississippi
August 1995–April 1996

Freshwater Prawn: broodstock collection, spawning, hatching, and pond grow-out

Organizations
Member of ASCLS/MSCLS
Member of Medical Technology/Clinical Laboratory Science Club, Alabama Central University

Certification
ASCP, MLT certification #00000

References
List of references available upon request.

FIGURE 3–5. Case 2

Chapter 4

Job Description and Job Advertisement

Paula Holland, M.Ed., MT(ASCP)

OBJECTIVES

Upon completion of this chapter the learner will be able to

1. State the vital purposes of a job description. *(Level I)*
2. List the items that should be included in a job description. *(Level I)*
3. Relate a job description to the advertisement, the interview, and the hiring, orientation, and evaluation processes. *(Level II)*
4. List the items that should be included in the job advertisement. *(Level I)*
5. Prepare an advertisement for a journal. *(Level III)*
6. Prepare a job description. *(Level III)*
7. Analyze the case studies and propose solutions. *(Level III)*

TOPIC SUMMARY

A job description document not only defines and provides a baseline for the performance tasks of the employee, but it defines the employee's interactions with people and how the position is integrated into the entire organizational scheme. Job descriptions should change as the needs of the organization change. It is the basis for preparing an advertisement for the position and the basis for employee evaluation. The job description should be used in the interview process and reviewed with the employee prior to filling the position. Because it is a legal document, the employee should sign it, acknowledging receipt of the document. Careful preparation of the job description is essential.

Job descriptions also hold managers and employees in a position of accountability. It is extremely easy to get diverted with a particular task and neglect other responsibilities. Therefore, a job description serves as a tool to remind employees of the many responsibilities they have within the position for which they've been hired.

It is necessary to review job descriptions at least once a year. This review should include reviewer signature and date reviewed. Changes to the job description will depend on the changes that occur within the department and/or company. During the annual evaluation process that is based on the job description, the manager can use the job description as a means of defining goals for the next year.

The sections of a job description should include the following:

- Title of the organization
- Job title
- Position summary
- Essential functions and duties
- Authority level
- Internal/external relationships
- Working conditions
- Qualifications and experience required
- Certification and/or licensure required

A job description example developed by a medical technology management class indicating the ideal job is found in Figure 4-1.

The job advertisement should be prepared after studying the job description. Key elements of a job advertisement include the following points:

Dreamworld Health Systems
777 Always Sunny Lane
Paradise, USA

Position Description

Job Title: Medical Tech/Clin. Lab Scientist	**Department:** Clinical Laboratory
Location: X Primary _ Serene _ Other	**Reports to:** Dept. Supervisor
Job Classification: _ Exempt X Non-exempt	**Pay Range:** $16.95–27.95 plus shift diff
Status: X FT _ PT _ PRN _ Contract	**Other Compensation:** $5000 Sign-on Bonus
Hours: 0700–1700	**Required Education:** BS/BA
Schedule: Monday–Thursday	**Required Certification:** National Cert.
Date Prepared: July 7, 2002	**Prepared By:** MTC 615
Date Revised: July 8, 2002	**Revised By:** MTC 615

Position Summary:

The employee performs a full range of clinical laboratory tests (in such areas as hematology, clinical chemistry, immunohematology, microbiology, serology/immunology, coagulation, molecular, and other emerging diagnostics) and will play a role in the development and evaluation of test systems and interpretive algorithms. The MT/CLS will have diverse responsibilities in areas of analysis and clinical decision making, information management, regulatory compliance, education, and quality assurance/performance improvement wherever laboratory testing is researched, developed, or performed.

Responsibilities and Essential Functions of Position:

The essential functions of the job of Medical Technologist/Clinical Laboratory Scientist at Dreamworld include, but are not limited to, the following:

I. SPECIMEN COLLECTION, HANDLING, AND PROCESSING
  1. Consults with patients and other members of the health-care team on proper collection and submission of biological specimens.
  2. Monitors outpatient orders entered into computer, assuring strict compliance with all regulatory agencies.
  3. Troubleshoots problems related to specimens and test orders and maintains documentation of such problems and corrective action taken.
  4. Ensures that specimens are received, accessioned, and delivered to the appropriate department in a timely manner.
  5. Notifies department supervisor of significant problems related to specimens or test orders.

II. TEST PERFORMANCE
  1. Performs a variety of laboratory tests in accordance with established policies, procedures, and regulations for diagnosis and treatment of patients, quality control verification, and proficiency testing evaluation.
  2. Maintains quality/quantity standards regarding output.
  3. Prepares reagents properly, minimizes wastes, and considers cost-effectiveness in the use of supplies.
  4. Troubleshoots problems occurring during test performance and documents problems, corrective actions, and resolutions.

FIGURE 4–1. Job Description

FIGURE 4–1. Job Description (continued)

      5. Notifies department supervisor of problems occurring during the test performance that would affect patient test results.

III. TEST RESULT REPORTING
      1. Manages laboratory-generated information to enable effective, timely, accurate, and cost-effective reporting of patient data.

IV. INSTRUMENT-RELATED RESPONSIBILITIES
      1. Performs routine maintenance on instruments according to policy.
      2. Calibrates and performs method validation studies as needed.
      3. Troubleshoots instruments as necessary and maintains proper documentation of problems, corrective action, and resolutions.
      4. Ensures proper functioning of instruments before release of patient results.
      5. Notifies department supervisor of instrument malfunction.

V. PURCHASING/INVENTORY CONTROL
      1. Participates in the inventory control program to ensure appropriate levels of supplies within the department.
      2. Utilizes all supplies and equipment in an appropriate and cost-effective, efficient manner.

VI. PROFESSIONAL DEVELOPMENT
      1. Obtains a minimum of twelve hours of continuing education hours (minimum 50% PACE approved) annually as required to maintain national certification.
      2. Orients, trains new employees and provides in-service education program for laboratory staff.
      3. Performs special assignments as requested by the supervisor.
      4. Serves on hospital committees as requested, such as Infection Control, Utilization Review, Compliance, HIPAA, Safety, Performance Improvement, Outreach, Information Systems Steering or Quality Circle, as requested.
      5. Supervises subordinate employees as requested by the supervisor.
      6. Aids in maintaining technical procedure manuals to meet accreditation standards.
      7. Performs all work in accordance with the requirements of regulatory agencies, such as CLIA, CAP, JCAHO, OSHA, FDA, AABB, and so on.
      8. Abides by the Corporate Compliance plan as well as the Laboratory Compliance plan.
      9. Demonstrates ethical and moral attitudes and principles that are necessary for gaining and maintaining the confidence of patients, professional associates, and the community.

VII. OTHER JOB RELATED TASKS
      1. Demonstrates a commitment to quality patient care.
      2. Works independently as well as collaboratively.
      3. Demonstrates punctual and reliable attendance.
      4. Actively pursues ways to improve laboratory efficiency and marketing of laboratory services.
      5. Participates in maintaining a clean and orderly facility.
      6. Adheres to all laboratory and facility safety policies.
      7. Consults with members of the medical staff concerning test utilization, compliance issues such as medical necessity, and interpretation of test results.
      8. Protects patient confidentiality by abiding by hospital Confidentiality Statement.

FIGURE 4-1. Job Description (continued)

Working Conditions and Physical Requirements:

Working conditions and physical requirements may include, but are not limited to, the following:

I. WORKING CONDITIONS
   1. Exposure to blood-borne pathogens and hazardous chemicals.
   2. Required use of personal protective equipment such as gloves, lab coat, and protective eyewear.
   3. Customer service to the following age-related groups: neonates, infants, children, adolescents, adults, and geriatrics.
   4. Constant noise and vibration from equipment, computers, and printers.
   5. Works independently except where reporting is required as described by the responsibility section of this document.
   6. Internally must work with administration, supervisor, coworkers and other health-care colleagues. Externally must work with all clients of the laboratory.

II. PHYSICAL REQUIREMENTS
   1. Ability to verbally communicate and hear verbal communication and alarms.
   2. Ability to see, including such visual functions as visual acuity, far and near vision, depth perception and color vision.
   3. Ability to walk, stand, stoop, sit, and make coordinated movements of trunk and limbs.
   4. Ability to seize, hold, grasp, turn, reach, push, pull, or otherwise work with the hands and fingers.

Note: Reasonable accommodations may be made to enable individuals with disabilities to perform the essential functions of this position.

Qualifications and Experience Requirements:

1. Baccalaureate degree and graduation from a NAACLS approved school of Medical Technology/Clinical Laboratory Science
2. Current national certification
3. Experience preferred, but not required

This position description is intended to provide an overview and is not all-inclusive. The position description may be changed as deemed appropriate by Dreamworld Health Systems.

Approval Signatures:

_____   _____
Manager   Date

_____   _____
Human Resource Representative   Date

My signature below acknowledges that I have read, understand, and accept the responsibilities of the position.

_____   _____
Employee   Date

(Adapted with permission from document by RenaLab, Inc., Jackson, MS, and from document created during MTC 615 Project, Summer 2002. Authors: Tim Henry, Cyntennia Jackson, Wendy Miller, Matt Smith, David Thrash, John Ware, Beth White, and Paula Yarbrough)

- Title of job
- Location of job
- Brief description of job
- To whom, in the company/organization's chain of command, this position directly reports
- Brief description about the company/organization
- The minimum requirement regarding education, experience, training, or knowledge
- Additional comments or information related to job advancement, travel requirements, or level of responsibility
- How to apply
- Deadline for application
- Equal opportunity statement

The best advertisement is one written specific enough to attract a minimum number of qualified candidates. Advertisements that are too general will attract numerous unqualified candidates that will have to be culled from the pool. The advertisement should also present the position and the company/organization in a positive light. Information regarding the community that may make the job attractive may be included.

Be careful not to be so restrictive that you cannot consider qualified applicants. For example, if you list CLS(NCA) as the only certification, then technically you cannot consider another candidate with an equivalent certification. Also, if you list an application deadline, you cannot consider candidates that apply after that deadline. Therefore, you may want to list certification as CLS(NCA) or equivalent and candidates will be considered until the position is filled.

It is extremely necessary to market the advertisement in highly visible locations (i.e., area newspapers, Web postings, field-related journals, TV news) for effective exposure to possible job applicants. The advertisement should be attractive and proofread prior to submission. Advertisements are usually expensive items and should be done well. The Human Resource department may coordinate the advertising from all the hospital areas to maximize advertisement dollars.

An example of an advertisement for the ideal job developed by a Medical Technology management class is given in Figure 4-2.

BIBLIOGRAPHY

Varnadoe, Lionel A. 1996. *Medical laboratory management and supervision—Operations, review, and study guide.* Philadelphia: F. A. Davis Company.

Wendover, Robert W. 1991. *High performance hiring: Attracting and retaining the best.* Los Altos, Calif.: Crisp Publications, Inc.

INTERNET RESOURCES

The University of Texas Health Science Center at Houston. <www.uth.tmc.edu/ut_general/admin_fin/hr/aw/jobdescriptions.html>

Rice University Human Resources. <www.ruf.rice.edu/~humres/Training/HowToHire/Pages/4.shtml>

Alaska Department of Labor and Workforce Development. <www.labor.state.ak.us/handbook/legal11.htm>

Business Owner's Toolkit. <http://toolkit.cch.com/text/P05_0670.asp>

Get More from your career... and YOUR LIFE!

Dignity   Excellence   Respect   Responsibility   Trust

Dreamworld Health Systems, a dynamic community-owned, value-driven health-care system, has a lot to offer. Professionally, we can offer you a diversity of work in one of our five signature facilities. Personally, the quality of life in our historic region is unlike any other. Whether you choose a busy, urban hospital or a serene rural setting, rewarding opportunities await you.

MEDICAL TECHNOLOGIST/CLINICAL LABORATORY SCIENTIST
Full-time position

$5,000 Sign-On Bonus

Duties
- Perform, evaluate, develop, correlate, and ensure the accuracy of laboratory information
- Collaborate in the diagnosis and treatment of patients
- Educate staff, patients, and other health-care providers
- Comply with regulatory and accreditation agencies
- Works independently with reports to the department supervisor when specified

Requirements Baccalaureate degree and graduation from a NAACLS school of Medical Technology/Clinical Laboratory Science accredited program, current national certification

Benefits
- Competitive skill/Competency-based compensation model
- Professional clinical ladder
- Internship programs
- Team-based awards
- Flexible schedules
- Shift/Weekend/Holiday differentials
- Tuition assistance
- Flexible benefits program
- Relocation assistance
- Well & sick child care
- Retirement & 401(k) plans
- Mentorship & employee assistance
- Professional education programs
- 100% drug/smoke-free environment
- High quality of living & low cost of living
- Wellness center/Exercise facility
- Paperless state-of-the-art lab

Available July 1, 2002. Candidates considered until position filled. Enjoy the future you deserve. APPLY ONLINE TODAY. www.dreamworld.com or forward your resume to

Dreamworld Health Systems
777 Always Sunny Lane
Paradise, USA

FIGURE 4–2. Position Advertisement
(Adapted with permission from MTC 615 Project, Summer 2002. Authors: Tim Henry, Cyntennia Jackson, Wendy Miller, Matt Smith, David Thrash, John Ware, Beth White, and Paula Yarbrough)

QUESTIONS

1. Vital purposes of the job description are: *(Objective 1, Level I)*

2. The items to be included in the job description are: *(Objective 2, Level I)*
   a. _____
   b. _____
   c. _____
   d. _____
   e. _____
   f. _____
   g. _____
   h. _____
   i. _____

3. Relate the job description to the advertisement, the interview, and the hiring, orientation, and evaluation processes. *(Objective 3, Level II)*

4. The items that should be included in a job advertisement are: *(Objective 4, Level I)*
   a. Name of organization, position title, qualification/experience required, certification/licensure requirements.
   b. Name of organization, starting salary, working conditions, qualification/experience required.
   c. Name of organization, job description including essential functions, internal/external relationships.
   d. Name of organization, authority level of job, general job description, how to apply.

EXERCISES

Completion of the exercises will enhance your knowledge of the job description and the job advertisement. *(Objective 5, Level III and Objective 6, Level III)*

1. Interview the individual who prepares job advertisements in the Human Resource department to determine the advertisement requirements.

2. Prepare an advertisement for a position in the laboratory.

3. Call your local newspaper and determine job advertisement rates, then check the advertisement rates in one of your professional journals.

4. Using the job descriptions in your lab as a model, prepare a job description, being sure to address all areas.

5. Compare a job description with the performance appraisal.

6. Interview the hospital legal counsel or Human Resource personnel to determine the legal implications of the job advertisement and the job description.

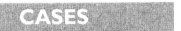

Analyze the case studies and propose solutions. *(Objective 7, Level III)*

1. The following advertisement (Figure 4-3) was prepared for a medical technology position. Critique the ad and modify as necessary.

Medical Technologist

Central Mississippi Hospital, 100-bed acute care, not-for-profit hospital, is seeking a generalist Medical Technologist. Our community is located within a one-hour drive of New Orleans, LA, Mobile, AL, the Mississippi Gulf Coast, and Jackson, MS. Within 50 miles is a comprehensive university offering courses, football games, theater shows, and so on. Many area lakes make outdoor water activities possible almost year-round.

Duties are varied and include nights and weekend shifts. Must be a registered CLS(NCA) with ten years of experience in all areas of the laboratory. Salary is $34,000 per year plus overtime.

Call by June 30, 2003. Tom.Dick@quidips.org

FIGURE 4–3. Position Advertisement

2. A new employee was given a simplified job description upon accepting the job, and the orientation to the job was hurried and very basic. After two weeks of employment, as the section supervisor, you realize that the new employee is not performing the job as you expected. Suggest how you would address this situation and prevent similar situations from happening in the future.

Chapter 5

Employment Interview and Selection Process

Paula Holland, M.Ed., MT(ASCP)

> ### OBJECTIVES
> Upon completion of this chapter the learner will be able to
>
> 1. State the employer's and candidate's purposes regarding the interview. *(Level I)*
> 2. Identify ways a candidate might prepare for the interview. *(Level I)*
> 3. Identify candidate actions that are viewed as appropriate during the interview. *(Level I)*
> 4. Identify appropriate interview dress for a candidate. *(Level I)*
> 5. Discuss methods an interviewer might use during the interview to determine if the candidate possesses technical competence and professional maturity. *(Level II)*
> 6. Identify subject areas of illegal questions. *(Level I)*
> 7. Identify components of a candidate thank-you letter. *(Level I)*
> 8. Critique personal interview skills. *(Level III)*
> 9. Compose a thank-you letter to be sent by the candidate following the interview. *(Level II)*
> 10. Propose solutions for the case studies. *(Level III)*

TOPIC SUMMARY

The employee selection process actually begins with the development of the job description and advertisement of the position. The Human Resources (HR) division of a company will play a large role in the employee selection process. Before the applications are sent to the manager, HR should have already performed background checks and verified credentials (education, certification, and license—if applicable). Once the screened HR applications are received, the laboratory manager should evaluate the candidates' qualifications in relation to the job description. Candidates for interviews are then selected. The interview is a critical step in the selection process.

The purpose of the interview process is for the employer to ensure that the written information obtained from the resumé is valid and to evaluate the candidate's skills and personality in order to select the best person for the job. The interview also provides the candidate the opportunity to disclose information not contained in the resumé, as well as provide the candidate an opportunity to learn about the people with whom he or she will possibly work, benefits, growth potential in the company, and so on.

The *candidate* may prepare for the interview by

- Reviewing the submitted resumé to be abreast of what the interviewer already knows.
- Reviewing professional and personal goals—both immediate and long-range.
- Researching the company by reading through recruitment ads, internet articles, library materials, literature from the company's public relations department, and annual reports to get an understanding of the organization's mission, services, financial status, competitors, reputation, and any recent major changes.
- Determining how one's own strengths, skills, and expertise might contribute to the company's goals. List your accomplishments and determine why you would be valuable to the company.

- Making a list of questions for the interviewer.
- Anticipating questions the interviewer might ask and preparing to answer them. Questions the interviewer might ask include:
    1. Why should we hire you?
    2. Tell me about yourself.
    3. Tell me about your background and accomplishments.
    4. What are your strengths? What are your weaknesses?
    5. How would you describe your most recent job performance?
    6. How would your previous boss or supervisor describe you?
    7. How would you describe yourself?
    8. What do you think of your present or past boss?
    9. How well do you work under pressure?
    10. Why do you want to work for this company?
    11. What are your professional goals?
    12. What motivates you and why?
    13. What position do you expect to have in two years? In five years?
    14. If you took this position, what would your goals be for the first year?
    15. Do you have a problem with working evening or night shift?
    16. Do you have a problem with working weekends and holidays?
    17. What are your preferred working hours?
    18. Do you have a reference list with you?
    19. What questions didn't I ask that you expected me to ask?
    20. Do you have any questions you would like to ask me?

For a more exhaustive list of questions and a list of the ten most commonly asked questions with answers, consult the following internet site: <www.collegegrad.com/jobsearch/16-15.shtml>.

- Identifying who is conducting the interview. This includes the name, title, background, education, and professional association of each interviewer if possible.
- Confirming where to park.
- Asking if there is anything that you should bring to the interview or any paperwork that you should complete prior to the interview.
- Asking for the approximate length of time set for the interview.

During the interview, the *candidate* should

- Be on time or a few minutes early for the interview.
- Know the exact location of the interview.
- Use the correct name (the correct pronunciation) for the interviewer and appropriate titles.
- Greet the interviewer using title and last name, smile, and employ a firm handshake exhibiting a genuine gladness to meet the interviewer.
- Provide several copies of the resumé to the interviewer.
- Make available a list of three references (not relatives) with contact numbers, titles, and addresses.
- Remember to wait until offered seating prior to sitting down. Sit up straight and do not slouch during the interview; watch for any nervous signals such as tapping fingers, leg swinging, or fidgeting.
- Look prospective employer in the eyes when speaking.
- Answer questions completely. Responding with a simple yes or no is not enough information for the interviewer. Give explanations whenever possible. Keep the length of the responses between thirty seconds and two minutes.
- Avoid making negative comments about past employers, supervisors, and coworkers.
- Act interested at all times, even if the questioning becomes difficult.
- Be honest in answering all questions—if unsure about a question, simply ask the interviewer to repeat the question.

Dressing appropriately for the interview is critical. If wearing a suit, which is usually the preferred dress, blue, black, or charcoal with dress shirt and tie is recommended for men and for women, a suit or dress using color. Both men and women should stay in the boundaries of business wear. Footwear for men should be well-shined black or brown lace or loafer style dress shoes (and socks). Women should wear leather or suede pumps and avoid sandals and open-toe or open-heel shoes. The candidate should be conservative with jewelry, hair accessories, cosmetics, and fragrances. Visible body piercing is not recommended with the exception of earrings for women. The candidate should be well-groomed. Men should be clean-shaven, or facial hair should be neat and trimmed. Both men and women should have moderate hair styles.

The *interviewer* should prepare for the interview by developing questions that will reveal how the candidate resolved problems or challenges encountered during the clinical internship or work experiences. The answer provided by the candidate can give the interviewer a sense of how this person might react to a similar situation as an employee. An effective way of accomplishing this would be to develop role-playing questions that require the candidate to reveal technical competence as well as professional maturity.

Some questions that the interviewer must avoid, due to their discriminatory and illegal nature, include questions regarding

- Race
- Age or date of birth
- Arrests
- Religious preference
- Financial status
- Height and weight
- Military discharge (type of)
- Mental or physical disabilities or any records thereof
- Asking for a photograph
- Health status or disabilities
- Pregnancy
- Birthplace or citizenship
- Sex, marital status, maiden name, and family
- Prior harassment or discrimination charges

The *interviewer* should also anticipate candidate questions such as

1. Why is this job open?
2. How often has this position been filled in the last three years? What were the reasons?
3. What are the biggest challenges in this position?
4. What would you want to see done differently by the next person filling this position?
5. What would I be expected to accomplish in this position?
6. What is most pressing? What would you like to have done in the next three months?
7. What are some of the long-term objectives you would like to see completed?
8. How do you think I fit the position?
9. What freedom would I have in determining my work objectives and deadlines?
10. Are there opportunities to advance in this position?
11. What educational resources and funding are there available for a person in this position?
12. Do you see any significant changes in the company and/or in this position in the near future?
13. How would I be evaluated?
14. What kind of benefit package does the company offer?
15. What is the salary for this position?

Psychological profiling is another tool many businesses are using to screen potential employees. A interviewer may give the candidate a series of questions related to behavior and only allows seconds for a response. The intent of the short response time is to capture a candidate's first or immediate answer to a question. Allowing the candidate less time to think about a response will give the employer a truer picture of the behavior of the candidate. The candidate's score is then compared to that of an ideal performer and is a good predictor of how similarly the candidate being screened will behave depending on how similar the candidate's score is to the ideal performer's score. Some of the proven benefits of psychological profiling include a reduction in hiring costs and turnover, increase in productivity, and better relationships between manager and staff members. The interviewer might ask the candidate to agree or disagree with psychological profiling questions such as the following:

1. Do you at times dread the thought of going to work? Yes _____ No _____
2. Do you feel that another employee doing things against company policies is none of your concern? Yes _____ No _____
3. You enjoy dreaming up new ideas to help solve problems and foster creativity. Yes _____ No _____
4. When you leave the workplace, do you try to leave work at work and not think about it? Yes _____ No _____
5. If a salesperson gave you too much money in change, would you tell that salesperson? Yes _____ No _____

At the end of the interview, the interviewer should thank the candidate for the application and provide an approximate timetable for filling the position. If the interviewer has not disclosed the timetable on filling the position, it is appropriate for the candidate to ask for this information at the end of the interview.

The candidate should not forget to thank the interviewer for the opportunity to interview and for the time spent arranging and conducting the interview. The candidate may send a thank-you letter within one to two days after the interview. This is proper etiquette and it will help the candidate stand out from other candidates trying to get the same job. Figure 5-1 presents a sample outline that may be used in composing the letter.

After the thank-you letter has been mailed, it is imperative for the candidate to stay in touch (once a week with the potential employer). This should stimulate an awareness of the interest the candidate has in employment with the company.

Selecting the appropriate employee is critical to a laboratory's success. The manager is seeking to hire

Date

Candidate's Street Address
City, State, Zip Code

Interviewer's Name, Title
Company Name
Company Street Address
City, State, Zip Code

Dear _____ :

INTRODUCTION paragraph:
- Date of interview
- Position interviewed for
- Appreciation statement
- Statement of continued interest in the position and the company

MAIN paragraph(s):
- Reemphasize skills, expertise, and the benefits candidate will offer the company
- Any information that wasn't mentioned in interview (keep brief)

CLOSING paragraph:
- Appreciation statement
- Statement regarding future contact with the interviewer

Sincerely,

Candidate's Name (signature directly above this)

FIGURE 5–1. Sample Outline for Thank-You Letter

an individual with the ability to be flexible, self-motivated, and functional in a variety of work settings. In today's health-care environment, employees are expected to use multitasking skills more than ever before, as well as be able to work as a productive team member. The manager is seeking the employee whose personality and skills best match the expectations of the institution and the job. The interview is one of the best procedures used to assess these characteristics and is very informative for the manager as well as the candidate.

BIBLIOGRAPHY

America's employers—The job seeker's home on the internet. Retrieved April 8, 2002, from <www.americasemployer.com/FAQS/successfully.html>

Career consulting corner interviewing tips. Retrieved April 8, 2002, from <www.usnews.com/usnews/edu/careers/cchome.htm>

Guterl, Gail O. 1998. What new-grad skills will land the job? Lab managers tell it like it is! *ADVANCE for Laboratory Professionals* 10, no. 6, 8–9.

Job link USA, Inc. Interview tips. Retrieved April 8, 2002, from <www.joblink-usa.com>

Ministry of education career gateway. Job search skills. Retrieved April 8, 2002, from <www.edu.gov.on.ca/eng/career/intervie.html>

Monster career center. Research before the interview. Retrieved April 8, 2002, from <http://campus.monster.com/tools/virtual/>

Online demo. Retrieved on March 19, 2003, from <http://b2secure.com/demo_interview.asp>

Preparing for a job interview. Retrieved April 8, 2002, from <www.nickelcity.com/class/employ-interview.htm>

Psychological Profiling. Retrieved March 18, 2003, from <www.abika.com/Reports/Samples/Psychologicalprofile.htm>

Simon Fraser University. Health, counseling and career centre career and employment services. Retrieved April 8, 2002, from <www.sfu.ca/employment/int_tips.html>

Spezialetti, Brian D. 1995. Do's and don'ts for winning the job interview. *Medical Laboratory Observer* (July), 51–53.

University of Wisconsin, Milwaukee homepage directory. Retrieved April 8, 2002, from <www.uwm.edu/DEPT/CDC/resdos.htm>

U.S. News online. Answer tough questions. Retrieved April 8, 2002, from <www.usnews.com/usnews/edu/careers/cchom.htm>

Wendover, Robert W. 1991. *High performance hiring: Attracting and retaining the best.* Los Altos, Calif. Crisp Publications.

INTERNET RESOURCES

Netster. <www.americasemployer.com>
U.S. News. <www.interviewcoach.com/virtual.html>
Job Link USA. <www.joblink-usa.com>
Government of Ontario, Canada, Ministry of Education, Ministry of Training, Colleges and Universities. <www.edu.gov.on.ca/eng/career/intervie.html>
Career Development Center, University of Wisconsin, Milwaukee. <http://careerlink.cdc.uwm.edu>

QUESTIONS

1. The employer's goals for the interview are to *(Objective 1, Level 1)*
   a. verify written information
   b. evaluate the candidate's skills
   c. evaluate the candidate's personality
   d. ask questions for clarification
   e. all of the above

2. Which of the following is NOT a goal of the candidate during the interview? *(Objective 1, Level 1)*
   a. Establish social contacts
   b. Provide additional information
   c. Assess the job, institution, and individuals that will be colleagues
   d. Determine the benefit package
   e. Ask questions for clarification

3. The candidate may prepare for the interview by *(Objective 2, Level 1)*
   a. placing an anonymous phone call to find out who the workers are in the laboratory
   b. researching the institution
   c. making a list of questions for the interviewer
   d. reviewing the resumé submitted and making major changes
   e. B and C

4. During the interview, the candidate should *(Objective 3, Level 1)*
   a. make available a list of three references with contact numbers, titles, and addresses
   b. refrain from negative comments about past employers
   c. make eye contact with the interviewer
   d. answer all questions completely and truthfully
   e. all of the above

5. Appropriate interview dress for a woman and man would NOT include which of the following? *(Objective 4, Level 1)*
   a. Blue or black color outfits
   b. Sandals
   c. Tongue ring
   d. B and C
   e. A, B, and C

6. On an interview, how might you, the manager, assess whether the candidate possesses the professional maturity to do the job? *(Objective 5, Level II)*

7. It is illegal to question a candidate regarding which of the following? *(Objective 6, Level I)*
   a. Date of birth
   b. Religious preference
   c. Loans
   d. Pregnancy
   e. All of the above

8. Components of the candidate thank-you letter should include *(Objective 7, Level I)*
   a. date of interview
   b. position interviewed for
   c. reemphasis of skills
   d. additional information
   e. all of the above

EXERCISES

Completion of the exercises will enhance your knowledge of the employment interview and the selection process. *(Objective 8, Level III and Objective 9, Level II)*

1. Designate one individual as the interviewer and one as the candidate. Allow the two participants to use role-playing techniques. After the role-playing activity, the participants should discuss the interview and suggest ways the interviewer and the candidate might improve.

2. Compose a thank-you letter to be sent following an interview.

3. Interview someone who has recently been a candidate for a job and someone who has served as an interviewer. Summarize the experiences of each and discuss as a group.

4. If there is a professional interviewer at your institution, ask the professional interviewer to interview you and make comments as to how you might improve your interview skills.

CASES

Four cases involving employment interviews follow. Propose answers and solutions for each case. *(Objective 10, Level III)* A group of participants may decide to work together and select the best answers as determined by group consensus.

1. You are a supervisor on the evening shift, and you are asked to prepare five interview questions for a full-time, rotating medical technologist position on your shift. Compose the questions you would consider most important and appropriate.

2. You are being interviewed for a medical technologist position, and the interviewer asks you what your strengths and limitations are.
   (1) List possible reasons for this particular question.
   (2) What is/are your best response(s) to this question?

3. You are being interviewed for a supervisory position in a 400-bed hospital laboratory, and the laboratory director poses the question "What do you want to be doing five years from now?"
   (1) List possible reasons for this particular question.
   (2) What is/are your best response(s) to this question?

4. You are a candidate being interviewed for the Laboratory Information System (LIS) manager position, and you are asked if you have any young children at home.
   (1) What bearing might this question have on your ability to perform in this position?
   (2) Is this an appropriate interview question?
   (3) What is the best way to respond to this question?

Chapter 6

Employee Evaluation

Jane Hudson, Ph.D. MT(ASCP)SM, CLS(NCA)

OBJECTIVES

Upon completion of this chapter the learner will be able to

1. Relate the evaluation instrument to the job description, performance standards, and the reward system. *(Level I)*
2. Identify the three ingredients that are necessary for motivation according to the Expectancy Theory. *(Level I)*
3. Identify four qualities of a good evaluator. *(Level I)*
4. Discuss rewards that may be available to the lab manager for use in recognizing employee accomplishments. *(Level II)*
5. Discuss how evaluation is needed in the Hersey-Blanchard model in each phase of employee development. *(Level II)*
6. Assess evaluation instruments after performing the exercises. *(Level III)*
7. Propose solutions for the case studies. *(Level III)*

TOPIC SUMMARY

Employee evaluation is one of the most critical tasks of the laboratory manager. It is as important to reward job excellence as it is to identify unacceptable behavior. Hall and O'Malley describe the competency-based and the criteria-based evaluations. The criteria-based evaluations indicate performance criteria such as the criteria found in the job description. The competency-based evaluation is used in the employee orientation process and to continuously validate competency as required by accreditation agencies. During employee orientation and validation of competency, a checklist is developed, and the manager or trainer must verify that the employee is competent to perform tasks on the checklist. The employee orientation checklist is usually more extensive because the employee is new to the job, whereas validation of the competency checklist may address only those areas that would be problematic. Education and training needs are determined as a result of the competency validation.

The evaluation instrument should be tied to the job description, performance standards, and to the reward system. Employees should understand from the beginning the basis of their evaluation. The idea is not to "catch" someone not doing their job, but to encourage all employees to do their job. In order to motivate according to the Vroom's Expectancy Theory (1975), the employee must perceive that high effort will lead to high performance, and high effort will lead to outcomes. Also the employee must have a preference for the outcomes. If the employee evaluation system is such that the employee perceives that high performance will not lead to outcomes, the employee is not motivated to do the job. Therefore, it is critical to inform the employee of the items upon which he or she will be evaluated and the rewards or lack of rewards that will result based on the evaluation.

Another important factor of the evaluation process is the evaluator. The employee must perceive that the evaluator will apply the evaluation instrument in a fair manner. According to Varnado (1996), an evaluator must 1) have knowledge of the job, 2) be close enough to the work situation to realistically be able to evaluate the employee's work, 3) have the knowledge and ability to perform evaluations, and 4) have the time to evaluate the employee. The evaluator must avoid errors caused by the tendency to mark all employees as "average" or to mark all employees with "high" marks. In addition, the evaluator must mark each job item independently of other items and evaluate the total job performance, not just the most recent performance.

The evaluation instrument must be carefully designed to indicate the level of job performance that the employer desires. A study of different types of instruments would be beneficial to the manager in preparing the instrument. Some instruments require the evaluator to select the statement that best matches the employee's performance. Other instruments use numbers that have a previously assigned definition, for example, 5 points = Excellent: Always performs job without prompting and supervision; 1 point = Poor: Never performs job even after prompting and supervision. These two instruments are probably the most commonly used in the clinical laboratory. Many instruments still measure the affective characteristics, such as initiative, enthusiasm, and soon. When using these characteristics as a measurement of performance, the characteristic needs to be carefully defined for the employee, and incidents should be cited if the employee receives a poor evaluation so that the employee will know how to improve his or her performance. Management by Objectives (MBO) may be applicable to some jobs. With the MBO method, the employer and the employee establish the objectives together, and the evaluation is based on the employee's written description of objectives accomplishment. A summary sheet is usually included with the evaluation instrument, which includes items such as total job performance score; salary adjustment, which relates to total performance score; goals; educational needs; comments and signatures of the manager and employee; and date. Figures 6–1 and 6–2 illustrate a sample part of an evaluation instrument and a corresponding summary page.

Figures 6–3 and 6–4 illustrate sample parts of an Employee Orientation form and an Employee Competency Validation form, which are components of a competency-based evaluation process.

As stated earlier, the employee must perceive that performance will lead to outcomes. The laboratory manager has several rewards that can be used to motivate. The most common reward is money; however, other rewards may include promotion, professional leave for attendance at workshops, flexible shifts, work assignment, reserved parking space, and so on. In order for the reward to motivate, however, the employee must have a preference for the reward.

Occasionally, there is the employee for which high efforts do not lead to high performance. Retraining may be the key to performance improvement. However, when retraining does not improve performance, the manager faces the difficult task of termination. Because of the financial cost to the institution and the laboratory and the emotional trauma to both the employee and employer, the interview process should be carefully designed to identify the potential employee that cannot perform the job.

The Hersey-Blanchard model indicates that the manager's role is different depending on the maturity of the employee. When the employee first starts the job, the manager is in a **telling** mode that involves detailed task instructions and not much discussion regarding the quality of performance. As the employee matures, the manager assumes a **selling** role that involves task instructions and quality of the performance discussions. The next role for the manager is the **participating** role that involves minimum task instruction and much encouragement regarding the quality of the performance. The ultimate role that the manager would like to assume with all employees is the role of **delegating,** which involves no task instruction or quality of performance discussions, because the employee is performing the job with quality and needs no instructions or encouragement. Once the employee reaches the delegating level, the manager can then focus on other employees or on other job responsibilities. The evaluation process is critical in each of the described managerial roles, even the final role of delegating, because the employee that has reached this level of job maturity occasionally needs to be assured of his or her performance through the reward system. All employees need feedback to sustain motivation. Prompt and timely feedback is necessary for it to be effective. Therefore, the evaluation process is critical to quality job performance, which is the main purpose of the evaluation process.

BIBLIOGRAPHY

Hall, Janet, and Jean O'Malley. 2003. Job analysis, work descriptions and work groups. In *Laboratory management*

Item	Performance Criteria	Rating 1-4*	Wt	Score × Wt	Comments
Maintains a safe environment	Adheres to safety procedures, recognizes & follows up on safety hazards, encourages others in proper safety techniques, and attends all safety programs.	4	.10		
	Adheres to safety procedures, attends to required safety programs.	3			
	Informal counseling has been necessary for failure to adhere to safety standards.	2			
	Formal counseling has been required for failure to adhere to safety standards.	1			
Operates clinical instruments	Performs calibration, routine maintenance, troubleshooting, operation, and documents as necessary, instructs others in these areas.	4	.40		
	Performs calibration, routine maintenance, troubleshooting, operation, and documents as necessary.	3			
	Performs calibration, routine maintenance, toubleshooting, operation, and documentation, but requires supervision.	2			
	Cannot calibrate, perform routine maintenance or troubleshoot, and has difficulty operating instruments. Requires much supervision.	1			

*4 indicates highest performance, followed by 3, 2, 1.

FIGURE 6–1. Example of a Partial Criteria-Based Evaluation Instrument

principles and processes, ed. Denise M. Harmening. Upper Saddle River, N.J.: Prentice Hall.

Hersey, P., and K. H. Blanchard. 1977. *Management of organizational behavior: Utilizing human resources.* 3d ed. Englewood Cliffs, N.J.: Prentice Hall.

Varnadoe, Lionel A. 1996. *Medical laboratory management and supervision.* Philadelphia: F. A. Davis.

Vroom, V. 1975. *Work and motivation.* New York: John Wiley & Sons.

INTERNET RESOURCES

Department of Agricultural Environment and Development Economics, Ohio State University. <www-agecon.ag.ohio-state.edu/people/erven.1/HRM/Employee_Reviews.pdf>

MindData. <www.minddata.com>

TGCI, The Grantsmanship Center. <www.tgci.com/magazine/97summer/eva/1.asp>

Note: This document corresponds to Figure 6–1.

General Hospital Annual Performance Evaluation

Employee: _____

Job Title: _____

Department: _____

Evaluation Date: _____

Job Performance Score: _____

Recommended Salary Adjustment*: _____

Goals:

_____
_____
_____
_____

Manager's Comments:

_____
_____
_____
_____

Employee's Comments:

_____
_____
_____
_____

Employee's Signature** _____   Date: _____

Manager's Signature _____   Date: _____

*Recommended salary adjustment is not effective until approved by Administration.

**Employee's signature does not necessarily mean agreement with this evaluation, but only that this evaluation was reviewed with the employee.

FIGURE 6–2. Example of a Criteria-Based Evaluation Summary Page

General Hospital Employee Orientation Checklist

Employee Name: _____

Orientation Item	Initials of Employee	Initials of Trainer	Date
GENERAL ORIENTATION			
Laboratory tour			
Attended hospital orientation			
Offered Hepatitis B vaccine			
Read and signed the Personnel Handbook			
Reviewed safety policy and procedures, had opportunity to ask questions regarding safety, and performed satisfactorily on safety training evaluation			
SPECIFIC TECHNICAL SKILLS			
Phlebotomy:			
■ Gathers materials needed			
■ Properly communicates with patient			
■ Cleans area appropriately			
■ Performs venipuncture correctly			
■ Instructs patient on proper care of site			
■ Labels tubes correctly			

FIGURE 6–3. Example of a Partial Employee Orientation Checklist—A Component of the Competency-Based Evaluation Process

General Hospital Employee Competency Validation Checklist

Employee Name: _____

Items for Competency Check	Initials of Employee	Initials of Evaluator	Date
OVA AND PARASITE PREP			
■ Reviews specimen for appropriateness			
■ Selects best portion of specimen for testing			
■ Uses proper techniques for safety			
■ Performs procedure correctly			
■ Prepares slides correctly			
■ Stains slides correctly			
■ Reviews slides correctly			
■ Identifies parasites if found			

FIGURE 6–4. Example of a Partial Employee Competency Validation Checklist— A Component of the Competency-Based Evaluation Process

QUESTIONS

1. The employee evaluation instrument should relate to *(Objective 1, Level I)*
    a. job description
    b. performance standards
    c. reward system
    d. A and C
    e. all of the above

2. Which of the following would NOT be necessary for motivation according to the Vroom's Expectancy Theory? *(Objective 2, Level I)*
    a. The employee must perceive that high effort will lead to high performance.
    b. The employee must perceive that effort will lead to outcomes.
    c. The employee must have a preference for the outcomes.
    d. The employee must be able to change the job.

3. Four qualities of a good evaluator are *(Objective 3, Level I)*

   a. _____

   b. _____

   c. _____

   d. _____

4. Discuss rewards that may be available to the laboratory manager for use in recognizing employee accomplishments. *(Objective 4, Level II)*

5. Discuss how evaluation is needed in the Hersey-Blanchard model in each phase of employee development. *(Objective 5, Level II)*

EXERCISES

Completion of the exercises will enhance your knowledge of employee evaluation. *(Objective 6, Level III)*

1. Obtain an example of an annual evaluation instrument. Assess the evaluation instrument and list the advantages and disadvantages of the instrument. This may be done as a group activity.

2. Interview technologists regarding their views about various annual evaluation instruments.

3. Interview the administrative technologist regarding his or her views about the annual evaluation process.

4. Review an employee orientation checklist and an employee competency validation checklist.

CASES

Identify the evaluation errors and list ways to improve the situation in the following cases. *(Objective 7, Level III)* This may be done as a group discussion activity.

1. A new employee starts the job. During the six-week probation period, everyone in her laboratory department was very friendly and seemed to be happy with her performance. At the end of the probation period the laboratory manager terminates her due to inability to perform the job. What happened in this situation? What are the errors? How could this situation have been corrected?

2. An employee constantly receives poor performance evaluations from his department supervisor. These evaluations are given to the laboratory manager for action, but no action ever occurs. What is the problem? What is the consequence of no action on other employees in the department? How could this situation be corrected?

3. An employee begins work in the laboratory and is given a job description and performance standards. After one month, three months, and six months, the employee is evaluated according to the job description and performance standards and is doing an excellent job. What would you do to encourage continuation of this excellent performance? Was the evaluation process handled correctly?

Chapter 7

Employee Correction and Discipline

Jane Hudson, Ph.D., MT(ASCP)SM, CLS(NCA)

OBJECTIVES

Upon completion of this chapter the learner will be able to

1. Identify the goal of correction. *(Level I)*
2. Discuss the steps of a good correction plan. *(Level II)*
3. Critique a correction plan after performing the exercises. *(Level III)*
4. Develop a correction plan for absenteeism. *(Level III)*
5. Formulate solutions for the case studies. *(Level III)*

TOPIC SUMMARY

As a manager, it would be a perfect world if everyone performed their job, and correction of employees was unnecessary. With good interview skills the manager might begin to approach this perfect world, but even good employees may occasionally act in an unprofessional manner. The interview and orientation process is very costly to the institution; therefore, the correction plan should be constructive rather than destructive. The primary goal of a good correction plan should be to salvage the employee and enhance the effectiveness of the institution. So, what comprises a good correction plan?

Once the manager becomes aware of a problem, the **first step** is to talk with the employee informally to understand the situation, identify causes, and assist the employee. *The One Minute Manager* [by Blanchard and Johnson] is a good source and describes this process effectively. At this step, no documentation is filed. Some correction systems do not include this step, but if the manager is in contact constantly with the employees, this is a step that enhances the dignity of the employee and communicates a manager's sincere concern for the employee. Also, if correction occurs after this informal talk, an excellent opportunity is created to praise the employee, thus enhancing the possibility that the problem will not occur again. If the problem persists, then the **second step** is for the manager to issue a verbal warning that involves identifying the problem, stating the performance that is needed, offering assistance, and keeping formal notes on the conference. If needed, the **third step** is a written warning that states the problem and states the performance that is needed to demonstrate that the employee has overcome the problem. The written warning is signed by the manager and the employee. If the problem persists, then the **fourth step,** a second written warning, is given. Sometimes this written warning is accompanied by a suspension period. This warning is also documented with signatures of the manager and employee, and the employee is put on notice that any further occurrences of the problem will result in dismissal. Upon occurrence of the problem again, the **fifth step** is implemented, and the employee is dismissed. For situations that pose a danger for the institution or individuals in the institution, this step-by-step process may be skipped and the employee may be immediately dismissed.

Important to the correction process is fairness and a real concern for the employee as well as the job. Getzels (1958) described the interaction of the individual with the institution and indicated that 1) the institution must match the individual, 2) the institutional role must match the individual personality, and 3) the institutional expectations must match the individual needs disposition for the institution and individual to realize the maximum benefit. Occasionally, these interactions do not match, and correction or dismissal is needed to advance not only the institution but also the individual. Correction should not occur as a result of a manager's personal issue, but rather an institutional issue that threatens the effectiveness of the institution or laboratory.

An appeal procedure must be available to the employee if the employee believes the action taken to be unfair. Usually the appeal is made to the next highest supervisor. The appeal procedure should guarantee fairness.

BIBLIOGRAPHY

Blanchard, Kenneth, and Spencer Johnson. 1982. *The one minute manager*. New York: Berkley Books.

Getzels, Jacob W. 1958. Administration as a social process. In *Administrative theory in education*, ed. Andrew W. Halpin. London, England: Macmillian Co., Collier-MacMillian Limited.

Liebler, Joan Gratto, and Charles R. McConnell. 1999. *Management principles for health professionals*. 3d ed. Gaithersburg, Md.: Aspen Publishers.

Varnadoe, Lionel A. 1996. *Medical laboratory management and supervision*. Philadelphia: F. A. Davis.

Wallace, M. Ann, and Deanna D. Klosinski. 1998. *Clinical laboratory science education and management*. Philadelphia: W. B. Saunders.

INTERNET RESOURCES

The Department of Human Resources, Southern Illinois University at Carbondale. <www.siu.edu/~humres/forms/dairf.doc>

Policy Manual, University of North Texas. <www.unt.edu/planning/UNT_Policy/volumeI/1_7_1_1.html>

University of Human Resource Services, Indiana University. <www.indiana.edu/~uhrs/training/ca/ca_index.html>

QUESTIONS

1. The goal of correction is to *(Objective 1, Level I)*
   a. salvage the employee
   b. enhance the effectiveness of the institution
   c. let the employee know that you are in control
   d. punish offenders so that others will not follow the example
   e. A and B
   f. A, B, and C

2. Discuss the steps of a good correction procedure. *(Objective 2, Level II)*

EXERCISES

Completion of the exercises will enhance your knowledge of employee correction and discipline. *(Objective 3, Level III and Objective 4, Level III)*

1. Review the corrective plan for the laboratory and interview the administrative technologist regarding the plan. Discuss as a group the advantages and disadvantages of the laboratory plan.

2. Role-play the manager and employee in a corrective situation, such as absenteeism.

3. Develop an attendance policy, define absenteeism, and develop a corrective plan for employees with an absenteeism problem.

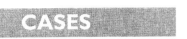

Work through the following cases individually or as a group. *(Objective 5, Level III)*

1. An employee is absent five days at the end of each month. In conversations with the employee you, the manager, find out that the employee does not have enough money to pay for child care at the end of the month, and thus misses the days to take care of children. Describe the steps you would take regarding this problem.

2. You notice an employee is not performing as well as in the past. In fact, the employee seems dazed at times and does not respond to directions. You suspect a drug problem. Discuss how you would handle this problem.

3. An employee comes in one day and gets into a verbal battle with one of his coworkers. The next day that coworker shows a weapon to another employee who reports to you that the coworker said that "if that guy ever bothers me again, I am going to shoot him." After you confront the employee about his behavior, he threatens you, the manager. What action would you take?

4. You receive a complaint from a patient regarding an employee who distributed a religious tract (literature promoting one particular religious denomination) to the patient with an intense testimony while drawing blood. Upon investigation, you find out that the employee is distributing these tracts to all the patients on her rounds to draw blood. You confront the employee regarding the requirement to respect patient privacy and the hospital policy regarding solicitations. The employee says that she will not continue her activities. However, the next week you receive information that the employee is again distributing tracts on her phlebotomy rounds. What action would you take?

5. As the laboratory manager, you receive a report from one of the evening shift technologists that another one of the evening technologists is doing the "sink test" (i.e., dumping specimens down the sink and making up the results) in urinalysis in order to get to dinner earlier. What action would you take?

Chapter 8

Celebrating Diversity

David Thrash, B.S., MT(ASCP), CLS(NCA)

OBJECTIVES

Upon completion of this chapter the learner will be able to

1. Define *diversity*. *(Level I)*
2. Discuss the advantages of a diverse workforce. *(Level II)*
3. List four diversity issues. *(Level I)*
4. Define the age categories and their impact on the workforce. *(Level I)*
5. Discuss the Glass Ceiling Commission. *(Level I)*
6. Define *culture*. *(Level I)*
7. Describe some of the special differences associated with different nationalities. *(Level II)*
8. List and discuss the areas that the Equal Employment Opportunity Commission (EEOC) addresses. *(Level I)*
9. Identify the reason for establishment of and list the areas addressed under the Age Discrimination in Employment Act. *(Level I)*
10. Describe the purpose of the Vocational Rehabilitation Act of 1973. *(Level I)*
11. Develop a policy that is EEOC compliant regarding hiring, firing, and grievances for your institution. *(Level III)*
12. Develop a philosophical statement that encourages diversity. *(Level III)*
13. Analyze the case studies and propose solutions. *(Level III)*

TOPIC SUMMARY

Diversity may be summarized as a business's response to swift sociological and cultural changes. **Internally,** it is a means of providing employees with an environment where they feel valued by and contribute to an organization. **Externally,** the organization is adaptable and perceptive about changes occurring in world markets (Becker et al. 1997).

Laboratory managers are faced each day with the task of having employees function as a cohesive team. Therefore, diversity can be addressed as a business priority to enhance effectiveness rather than just an affirmative action factor. According to Lebo (1996) diversity is needed in the workplace in order to **increase competitiveness, increase the effectiveness of quality management, decrease employee turnover, and reduce cost.** Decision making is enhanced by a more varied group because more ideas and approaches are present. Also, the diverse group reflects the consumer. If diversity is celebrated within the laboratory, employees feel comfortable in the workplace and **are empowered to do their best.** These factors reduce turnover and reduce cost. In today's workplace environment, the workforce is becoming increasingly more varied. Every employee is unique and brings a unique set of characteristics to the workplace; therefore, diversity includes everyone. However, knowledge of some of the more prominent areas of diversity should help the manager encourage an atmosphere in which diversity is celebrated, thus enhancing the productivity and efficiency of the laboratory.

One area in which diversity is increasingly apparent is **age.** Working side by side are mature workers, baby boomers, Generation X, and up-and-coming Generation Y. This can become a challenging task for managers who must promote a sense of comradeship and teamwork with employees of varying ages. Mature workers, those fifty-five and older, represent nearly sixteen million, or twenty-one percent, of today's workers.

Baby boomers, those aged thirty-nine to fifty-four, represent nearly seventy-six million, or fifty-two percent, of today's workforce. Generation X, those ages nineteen to thirty-eight, account for the fastest-growing workforce population at forty million-plus, or twenty-six percent. Generation Y, those eighteen and younger, are just beginning to enter the workforce. This group accounts for less than ten percent. With this wide-range age group, certain stumbling blocks may hinder the formation of a cohesive team. These obstacles may include the different age group's view of chain of command, a balance between work and personal life, and technology. Those workers from Generations X and Y often have an advantage over the mature and baby boomer workers in the arena of technology. With a vast knowledge of electronic technology, such as e-mail, the Internet, faxes, and videoconferences, Generations X and Y individuals will use this to their advantage as a means of communication and networking, thus making themselves more marketable to the future employer. The mature and baby boomer workers usually prefer the more "old fashioned" means of communication and networking, doing it by face-to-face meetings (Farren 1999).

Gender equality has also become a driving force in today's workplace environment. Watching an episode of "Bewitched," a throwback to the 1950's, may leave some of today's younger workers in awe. In this sitcom, the female is portrayed as someone who is married, has only a high school or moderate college education, care's for her husband and two children, does not have a job, and has to ask her husband for money to buy life's essentials. If Samantha Stephens were to have a job within an organization, it would be only in a secretarial capacity, and not one in a managerial role. In contrast, the male is also portrayed as married but has a college or moderate post-graduate education, cares for the family by making money to sustain life's essentials, and is the ultimate decision maker. Darren Stephens is portrayed as an account executive within an advertising agency, a managerial role. This cliché was used to point out that with time change would come. Women are now as educated as their male counterparts, expect equality not only in professional issues, but in personal issues as well, and comprise about forty-nine percent of professional and managerial positions (GilDeane Group 2002); therefore, in the workplace, managers must be aware of the laws regarding sexual harassment and equal pay.

Within the last decade, there have been huge strides to grant not only women but also individuals of a **minority** background the right to equal opportunity in the workplace. African Americans and Hispanics as well as women are becoming more visible in a managerial capacity. The Glass Ceiling Commission was created as a part of the Civil Rights Act of 1991. This twenty-one member body, chaired by the Secretary of Labor and appointed by the president of the United States, works to identify "glass ceiling barriers." Glass ceiling barriers are those invisible and artificial barriers that prevent qualified individuals, such as women and minorities, from advancing into positions of responsibility, whether it be within an organization or in the private sector (Catherwood Library E-Archives 2001). To further accentuate the Glass Ceiling Commission, the Equal Pay Act enacted by the Equal Employment Opportunity Commission (EEOC) states that discrimination may not be based on sex in the payment of wages or benefit if the work is of comparable effort, skill, and responsibility for the same job performed (U.S. EEOC 2001).

It has been said that America is the "melting pot" of the world, made up of individuals from different **nationalities and origins.** What makes our country so unique is its ability to accept these varied customs, values, and traditions. The combination of these elements is termed **culture,** which influences how a person may think and function and will guide their behavior and attitudes throughout life (Dunlap 2001).

As of May 2002, health-care settings are experiencing a dramatic shortage in allied health professions, such as nursing, physical therapy, respiratory therapy, and clinical laboratory science. This shortage is due to a number of reasons, such as decreased enrollment in allied health professions because of the Balanced Budget Act of 1997, Medicare reform, and low starting salaries. To alleviate this burden, professional certifying agencies, such as the National Credentialing Agency for Laboratory Personnel, Inc. (NCA), are currently trying to offer certifications to qualified individuals from around the globe. Through this certification process, persons of different origins and nationalities will more than likely be entering the field of clinical laboratory science in record numbers. Primarily, this will be seen as an influx of Asians, Latin Americans, Pacific Islanders, and Hispanic candidates into the melting pot of America. Managers must be aware of the different customs these individuals may bring into the work environment. A few examples of cultural barriers include eye contact, gestures, and personal space. Asian colleagues may never look you in the eye when talking. As Americans, we may take this as a sign of shyness or as a sign that the person does not like us. In actuality, the Asian person is showing you respect by not looking you in the eye, as this is a sign of disrespect in their native land. Also in the United States, we normally vigorously shake the hand of our colleague as a sign of goodwill and character. The Native American population may consider this a sign of aggression. Personal space should also be considered when confronting colleagues. Usually in the United States a comfort zone of about eighteen inches is expected when talking to someone else. Mexican Americans tend to stand closer, as this is a sign of importance of what is being said by the speaker (Dunlap 2001).

Other issues that might be considered under diversity issues are **sexual orientation, religion, being physically or mentally challenged**, and so on. Diversity issues are massive and may even be extended to the policies and procedures of the organization. If celebrating diversity is viewed as a way to enhance the organization, then the organization can become dynamic in an environment that is constantly changing.

A manager may be tempted to view diversity only as affirmative action issues, and indeed the manager should abide by the laws that address these issues, such as the following:

- Title VII of the Civil Rights Acts. In 1964, the EEOC, an independent federal agency, was created by the United States Congress to protect against unlawful discrimination. The manager must not discriminate regarding hiring, discharge, pay, work assignment, education opportunities, and so on because of the person's race, color, religion, national origin, sex, or age.
- The Age Discrimination in Employment Act was established in the same year to protect individuals who are forty years of age and older. This act simply states that (1) an individual may not be terminated from his or her place of employment simply for growing old, (2) the recruitment of future employees should not be limited only to younger applicants, and (3) denial of benefits to older employees is prohibited.
- The Vocational Rehabilitation Act of 1973 addresses the hiring of handicapped persons.
- Within the last few years, civil liberty unions have lobbied for sexual orientation inclusion in equal opportunity legislation.

Some of these issues are discussed in Chapter 38, Legal Considerations.

This chapter covers only a few of the many diversity issues that may challenge a future laboratory manager. There are a number of available resources, such as books and magazine articles in print, for researching diversity issues. Two books that are helpful are *The Color Code* by Taylor Hartman (Publisher: Fireside Rockefeller Center, March, 1999; ISBN: 0684848228) and *Building a House for Diversity: A Fable About a Giraffe and Elephant–A Diversity Fable* by R. Roosevelt Thomas Jr. (Publisher: AMACON, 1999; ISBN: 0814404634). Also, Internet sites may prove helpful for researching diversity as well. Direct your Web browser to your favorite search engine (Google proves most helpful) and type in one of the following: *diversity in the workplace, diversity issues, managing diversity, gender equality, sexual orientation, ageism, cultural diversity, or sexual harassment.*

BIBLIOGRAPHY

About the Glass Ceiling Commission. 2000–2001. Retrieved May 2002, from <www.ilr.cornell.edu/library/e_archive/gov_reports/GlassCeiling/derault.html?page=home>

Becker, Beverly, Erviti, Manuel, Shelly, Amelia. 2002. Retrieved May 2002, from <http://alexia.lis.uiuc.edu/~lis405/diversity/intro.htm>

Dunlap, Mary M. 2001. Understanding Cultural Differences. Personal Growth. A newsletter for ancillary and all staff. Vol. 3, no. 3.

Farren, Caela. June 1999. How to eliminate the generation gap in today's work team. Retrieved November 1999, from EBSCOhost, <www.usm.edu>

Federal Laws Prohibiting Job Discrimination, Questions and Answer. 2001. Retrieved May, 2002, from <www.eeoc.gov>

GilDeane Group, Inc. Diversity Statistics. 2002. Retrieved May 2002, from <www.diversityhotwire.com/business/diversity_statistics.html>

Leach, Joy, Bette George, Tina Jackson, and Arleen LaBella. 1995. *A practical guide to working with diversity.* New York: American Management Association.

Lebo, Fern. 1996. *Mastering the diversity challenge.* Delray Beach, Fla.: St. Lucie Press.

Managing Workplace Diversity. Retrieved May 2002, from <http://alexia.lis.uiuc.edu/~lis405/diversity/intro.htm>

Ransom, William J. Understanding cultural diversity. Retrieved June 2002, from <http://centralohio.thesource.net/Files/ran950913.html>

Sexual Harassment: Introduction. Retrieved May 2002, from <www.virginia.edu/~saeo/harassment_intro.htm>

Sexual Harassment Statistics. Retrieved May 2002, from <www.dbpargman.com/statssexual.htm>

Sexual Orientation in the Workplace. Retrieved May 2002, from <http://alexia.lis.uiuc.edu/~lis405/diversity/sexualo.htm>

Steiner, Cindy L. Cultural awareness can improve your business. Retrieved July 2002, from <www.alliancestraining.com/cultural.htm>

Steiner, Cindy L. Cultural awareness can improve your business. Retrieved July 2002, from <www.alliancestraining.com/cultural.htm>

Winfield, Liz. Myths and Facts: Sexual orientation in the workplace. Retrieved May 2002, from <www.diversityhotwire.com/business/business_case_diversity.html>

INTERNET RESOURCES

Alliance Training, Cultural Awareness Can Improve Your Business. <www.alliancestraining.com/cultural.htm>

Catherwood Library, School of Industrial & Labor Relations, Cornell University. <www.ilr.cornell.edu/library/e_archive/gov_reports/GlassCeiling/default.html?page=home>

Diversity Central. <www.diversityhotwire.com/business/diversity_statistics.html>
<www.diversityhotwire.com/business/business_case_diversity.html>

DB Pargman Diversity Training. <www.dbpargman.com/statssexual.htm>

University of Illinois, Sexual Orientation in the Workplace. <http://alexia.lis.uiuc.edu/~lis405/diversity/sexualo.htm>

The University of Southern Mississippi, search *diversity*. <www.usm.edu>

The University of Virginia, Sexual Harassment. <www.virginia.edu/~saeo.harassment_into.htm>

U.S. Equal Employment Opportunity Commission. <www.eeoc.gov/>

QUESTIONS

1. What is diversity? *(Objective 1, Level I)*

2. Discuss the advantages of a diverse workforce. *(Objective 2, Level II)*

3. List four diversity issues. *(Objective 3, Level I)*
   a. _____
   b. _____
   c. _____
   d. _____

4. a. Mature workers are ages _____ and constitute _____ percent of today's work force. *(Objective 4, Level I)*

   b. Baby boomers are ages _____ and constitute _____ percent of today's workforce. *(Objective 4, Level I)*

   c. Generation X workers are ages _____ and constitute _____ percent of today's work force. *(Objective 4, Level I)*

   d. Generation Y workers are ages _____ and constitute _____ percent of today's work force. *(Objective 4, Level I)*

5. a. The Glass Ceiling Commission is chaired by _____. *(Objective 5, Level I)*

   b. It is appointed by _____.

   c. Its purpose is to _____.

6. Culture may be defined as _____. *(Objective 6, Level I)*

7. Describe some of the special differences associated with different nationalities. *(Objective 7, Level II)*

8. Is there a provision in the EEOC protecting the employment rights of gay, lesbian, bisexual, and transgender individuals? *(Objective 8, Level I)*

9. a. Why was the Age in Discrimination Employment Act established?

   b. What are three items it states?
      (1) _____
      (2) _____
      (3) _____
   (Objective 9, Level I)

10. The purpose of the Vocational Rehabilitation Act of 1973 was to address *(Objective 10, Level I)*
    a. The hiring of handicapped persons
    b. The hiring of vocationally qualified individuals
    c. The hiring of those handicapped persons who served in the armed forces
    d. The hiring and training of persons in vocational training

EXERCISES

Completion of the exercises will enhance your knowledge of diversity. *(Objective 11, Level III and Objective 12, Level III)*

1. Interview the chief technologist to determine whether the laboratory or the hospital has a policy encouraging diversity as a business opportunity or as a legal aspect only.

2. On an individual basis, consult your current educational facility handbook and recruitment material for your allied health profession. Is there a statement concerning the EEOC? If one is not listed, is this within the boundaries of the law? What is the proper means of getting one posted in this literature? Is sexual orientation listed in the EEOC statement?

3. Call four different businesses in the local area and ask what their policy is concerning hiring and firing practices following the EEOC guidelines. Compare the findings of each company. Was each business similar? Different? Explain your findings.

4. As a group, outline a fair hiring, firing, and grievance policy, and every item in between, for your newly formed corporation "CLS on Wheels" using the following EEOC guidelines:
   (1) Federal Equal Employment Opportunity (EEO) laws
   (2) Discriminatory practices
   (3) Americans with Disabilities Act

(4) Employers and other entities covered by EEO Laws
(5) EEOC's charge processing procedures
(The current Equal Employment Opportunity Guidelines may be found at www.eoc.gov)

5. As a group, develop a philosophical statement that encourages diversity as a way of enhancing the productivity and efficiency of the laboratory.

CASES

Analyze the following case studies and propose solutions. *(Objective 13, Level III)*

1. You have just been promoted to administrative assistant chief technologist. Your job is to interview new applicants for positions posted within the Clinical Laboratory. You have recently interviewed two qualified applicants for the position of day shift microbiology assistant supervisor. Applicant 1, Laser Jett, a fifty-one- year-old black male, has been employed for the past twelve years at Brogdon Health Care Systems in Vicksburg, Mississippi. He is a graduate of the Cane Creek School of Medical Technology in Hattiesburg, Mississippi, and has excellent letters of recommendation. Applicant 2, Pine Hewlett, a thirty-one-year-old white male, has been employed by Autry Memorial Hospital in Jackson, Mississippi, for the past year, has two years of experience at Bouie River Health Systems in Hattiesburg, Mississippi, and one year of experience at Hurley Medical Clinic in Pascagoula, Mississippi. He is a graduate of Hudson School of Medical Technology in Mockingbird, Mississippi, and has mediocre letters of recommendation. You decide to hire applicant 2, even though applicant 1 is more stable and has considerably more experience. What job discrimination law may you be breaking according to the EEOC? Is this an acceptable practice according to the EEOC?

    Why do you think the assistant chief technologist decided to go with this individual?

2. You are the laboratory manager and have just hired an individual from Greece who has seven years of work experience in her country prior to coming to the United States and has completed requirements to obtain certification in this country. She is assigned as a tech in the hematology department.

    A thirteen-year-old male from Corsica comes to the laboratory for a blood test. He says he is tired, and he has prominent cheek bones and slightly slanted eyes. On the blood smear, a hematology tech notes many target cells, nucleated RBCs, and marked poikilocytosis. Your hematology techs see no abnormal pattern on the hemoglobin electrophoresis. The techs in hematology gather to discuss what should be done next. During the discussion, the newly hired tech from Greece suggests that a hemoglobin F analysis be performed by acid elution and a hemoglobin A2 analysis be done by column chromotography. Why do you think the tech from Greece suggested the additional tests? Why do you think she was able to relate to this case better than the other techs? Does having this tech from Greece increase your laboratory's effectiveness?

3. Suppose you hired a tech who was born in Mexico to work in your laboratory. Your hospital is in El Paso. What advantages does the tech from Mexico bring to your laboratory?

4. You work in a small laboratory with two other techs. One tech is just out of college and another is fifty-five years old. The Coulter Counter breaks, and you cannot get it repaired for twenty-four hours; however, a CBC on a patient is critical and must be done immediately. You discuss with the techs the situation and the fifty-five-year-old tech states that there is a hemocytometer and WBC and RBC pipettes in the drawer, and an old hemoglobinometer that still works. At the same time, a doctor requests that the laboratory assist him in reviewing the research information regarding a molecular technique on a Web site and contacting the research laboratory via e-mail. The new graduate has used the Web and e-mail extensively in school. Do you have the expertise to address both of these situations in your laboratory? How would you suggest utilization of the techs? Does the diversity in your laboratory enhance client services?

Chapter 9

Change

Jane Hudson, Ph.D., MT(ASCP)SM, CLS(NCA)

OBJECTIVES

Upon completion of this chapter the learner will be able to

1. Define *change*. *(Level I)*
2. Discuss the process that drives change. *(Level II)*
3. Implement and analyze a simple change in the laboratory according to the exercise instruction. *(Level III)*
4. Critique the case studies and propose solutions. *(Level III)*

TOPIC SUMMARY

Are you Sniff, Scurry, Hem, or Haw? If you have not read the book *Who Moved My Cheese?* by Spencer Johnson, then I encourage you to stop now, obtain a copy, and read it. Important points of this book are that change is OK, everybody is undergoing change, change can be good, and how we respond to change is up to each individual. Change is defined as anything that is different from what has been routinely done. Some important facts about change are the following:

- Change is inevitable.
- Change usually encounters resistance.
- The manager is a change agent.

Change can be instigated from many sources including new technical material, professionals or institutions, crisis, perceived need for product or organizational improvement, perception of rewards, and so on. Change occurs constantly whether we wish for it or not. In fact, if an institution, organization, or individual does not change, the outcome is that they become obsolete. If one is not going forward every day, then one is going backward. In this world, one cannot simply maintain the status quo. Change comes as a result of analysis of the environment and recognizing a need for change. The process that drives change may be diagrammed as noted in Figure 9-1:

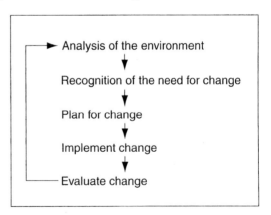

FIGURE 9-1. The Process That Drives Change

As a manager, it is important to understand change and to know how to manage it so that the change enhances organizational effectiveness. Galles (1982) provided three dimensions of change: 1) mandated or voluntary, 2) simple or complex, and 3) clear or subtle. From these dimensions the following plans of action were developed. If a change is mandated, the manager should provide information to the employees regarding the necessity of change. Informal leaders may be used if the change is mandated and complex. Clarity is needed in addition to the manager's explanation and use of the informal leaders if the change is mandated, complex, and subtle. If the change is voluntary, employees should participate in all steps of the change. In addition, informal leaders may be used and group sessions employed if the change is voluntary but complex. Individual discussions with resistant employees may be needed in addition to the informal leaders and group interactions if the change is voluntary, complex, and subtle.

For example, the laboratory manager reports to Director X, but a change is being made so that the laboratory manager will report to Director Y. This is a mandated, simple, clear change. The manager would simply provide information to the employees regarding the necessity of the change. Most employees would probably accept the change, although some employees might be concerned. The laboratory manager should try to alleviate the fears of any concerned employees, but the decision has been made and the responsibility of the manager and employees is to adapt to the change. On the other hand, consider another example of change that is voluntary, complex, and subtle: a new laboratory computer may be purchased and the hospital administration has asked the laboratory manager to make a recommendation regarding this possibility. Because this is a voluntary change, although highly complex and somewhat subtle because of the lack of details, the laboratory manager would want to include the employees and informal leaders in preparing a response for the administration. Group meetings and discussions to share information would be beneficial. Employees would be more likely to accept a change in computer systems if they were involved in the decision. Because this is a voluntary, complex, subtle change, a resistant employee might be encountered, and the manager would have to deal with this person individually so that the group process of preparing a recommendation for administration could proceed.

Understanding resistance to change is essential for the manager. You might start by asking yourself what you feel when asked to change. Galles (1982) identifies the causes for resistance as either 1) technical—related to impact of change on the job or 2) emotional—related to personal issues. The manager must recognize resistance, develop a true understanding of the basis of resistance, and deal with the resistance. Some methods of dealing with resistance to change include providing information, allowing employees to air concerns, involving informal leaders, and providing time for adjustment to the idea of change. Ultimately, if the change will enhance the institution and the owners or administrators of the institution want the change, it must be implemented, and employees must understand that to continue to be a part of the institution, the resistance to the change will have to cease.

Because change is inevitable, the leader's responsibility is to manage the change so that the group can adapt quickly and efficiently to change. If an organization is not analyzing its environment and making appropriate changes, then the organization will become obsolete. Therefore, change should be approached as a method to ensure the viability of an organization.

BIBLIOGRAPHY

Galles, Glen F. 1982. Managing change. In *Clinical laboratory management—A guide for clinical laboratory scientists,* ed. Karen R. Viskochil and Patricia A. Amos, (291–299). Boston: Little, Brown and Company.

John, Spencer. 1998. *Who moved my cheese?* New York: G. P. Putnam's Sons.

Liebler, Joan Gratto, and Charles R. McConnell. 1999. *Management principles for health professionals.* 3d ed. Gaithersburg, Md.: Aspen Publishers.

Varnadoe, Lionel A. 1996. *Medical laboratory management and supervision—Operations, review and study guide.* Philadelphia: F. A. Davis.

INTERNET RESOURCES

The Change Management Resource Library. <www.change-management.org>

State of Wisconsin, Department of Employment Relations, Reference Library. <http://der.state.wi.us/home/workplacechange-management.htm>

QUESTIONS

1. Change is *(Objective 1, Level I)*
    a. performing a task again
    b. starting at the beginning
    c. anything different
    d. a state of mind

2. Which of the following descriptions is NOT true about change? *(Objective 1, Level I)*
   a. inevitable
   b. usually enjoyable
   c. encounters resistance
   d. the change agent is the manager
3. Discuss the process that drives change. *(Objective 2, Level II)*

EXERCISES

Completion of the exercises will enhance your knowledge of change. *(Objective 3, Level III)*

1. People have established habits, such as sitting in the same place in a classroom, going to lunch at the same time and sitting at the same table, taking their coffee break at the same time each day, and so on. Find a habit that many are doing and make it impossible for them to continue the habit. Interview each person regarding the feelings that the change invoked. Write a summary of the results and present it to the employees.

2. Perform an analysis of the environment by interviewing medical technologists/clinical laboratory scientists in a lab to determine if there is something that needs to be changed, such as the furniture in the break room, the bulletin board arrangement/location, or the method for assigning phlebotomy slips, and so on. After the recognition of the need for change is done, plan the change, implement the change, and evaluate the change. This change should be done in cooperation with the employees. Write a summary of your experience.

CASES

For each of the following cases, critique the situation and indicate how you, assuming the role of laboratory manager or chief technologist, would handle the situation. *(Objective 4, Level III)*

1. Everyone in the lab has been wearing street clothes and a lab coat for work. The hospital administration decides at the Monday administrative meeting that all laboratory workers will now wear blue scrubs. This change will take effect in a week, and all of your lab employees are responsible for purchasing their own scrubs.

2. You are the chief technologist and decide to change the way the weekend scheduling of the lab is done by posting a ranked alternate list of individuals who will be available to back up any staff that have emergencies and cannot work. You decide who is on the list and the rank order. No substitutions are allowed. No one is asked for their opinion, and this is put into effect immediately.

3. The hospital administration has asked you, a laboratory director, to evaluate whether blood should be collected by the nurses on the floors instead of by the laboratory phlebotomy team. Diagram each step in the process of change in this situation.

4. The morning collection of blood is shared by all the employees on the day shift, but the "hard-to-stick cases" are being left until last, and the patients are thus not being able to get their breakfast on time. How would you as the laboratory director implement change?

Chapter 10

Stress Management

Eric Hogue, M.S., MT(ASCP), CLS(NCA)

OBJECTIVES

Upon completion of this chapter the learner will be able to

1. State four general ways that everyone can reduce stress. *(Level I)*
2. Identify the Occupational Safety and Health Act's (OSHA) position regarding job stress and the employer's responsibility. *(Level I)*
3. Discuss the use and activities of stress-related work teams as they relate to reducing stress. *(Level II)*
4. Create an outline for a stress management program based on the text. *(Level III)*
5. Analyze the results of a survey to determine stress factors in a specific laboratory as described in the exercises. *(Level III)*
6. Develop and recommend a stress management program. *(Level III)*
7. Propose solutions for the case studies. *(Level III)*

TOPIC SUMMARY

It is 12:33 A.M. at the University of Pittsburgh Medical Center Blood Bank, and the phone rings. It is the emergency room: a twelve-car pileup has occurred on I-95 due to the dense fog, and there is an instant need for blood. At this moment, the medical technologist/clinical laboratory scientist on duty is undergoing an instantaneous reaction, with a rise in blood pressure, heart rate, and skin perspiration. These are symptoms of stress. Medical laboratory personnel experience stress every day, and there will come a time when the body cannot tolerate the abuse any longer. These individuals will begin to experience fatigue, frequent infections, and an overall decline of their physical appearance. This will lead to increased time away from work because of sick days. Therefore, lab managers would benefit from implementing a stress management program in the clinical laboratory to meet the needs of a diverse group of employees (Davis 2000).

There are many techniques one can learn in order to relieve some of the stress in his or her life. A person can begin by eating balanced meals, exercising at least three times a week, and getting plenty of sleep. Also the employee should devote adequate time to some type of recreation or family activity. The lab manager should provide the employees with a variety of options to relieve some of their work-related stress. However, recent studies have shown that the majority of human resource managers believed that the responsibility of stress management is with the individual not the organization, and that stress is a personal problem (Crampton et al. 1995). Although it is the belief of many managers that the employee is responsible for the management of their stress, the government thinks otherwise. According to the Occupational Safety and Health Act of 1970, employers are held legally accountable for job-related illnesses, which have been interpreted to include stress-related problems (Crampton et al. 1995). Stress also has negative financial consequences through absenteeism, tardiness, disability claims, and decreased productivity (NIOSH 1999). Approximately forty percent of all job turnover and the majority of errors in the workplace are due to stress (Krohe 1999).

There are many options in dealing with stress, and the challenge is to match the optimal approach to each situation in the workplace (Bone 1998). The first job a manager has before implementing a successful stress management program is to identify the people or groups that are under the greatest deal of stress and implement programs designed to meet their needs. In the clinical lab, blood bankers are usually under the greatest amount of stress, because one mistake can cost a life. However, other departments in the laboratory can also be under a significant amount of stress, due to factors such as work overload or tense employee relationships. In a 300-bed hospital with twenty-five technologists, five technicians, and ten phlebotomists, everyone will need to work well together and help each other, but if there is tension between employees that leads to a stressful workplace, the barriers will need to be broken in order to meet the patient's needs (McCardle 1998).

At first, the manager might try employee-arranged work teams to reduce stress. This would allow each department to work together to resolve problems within the group, and if there are not any problems, it could allow the group to grow closer together. The group could arrange recreational activities, such as bowling or, cookouts, or form a co-ed softball or flag football team with the other groups. All of these activities could help alleviate barriers created at work, lead to better teamwork, productivity, work environment, and ultimately eliminate work-related stress for the employee (McCardle 1998).

However, many labs have deeper problems that the work team approach cannot solve. Therefore, a professional stress management program should be implemented. There are many speakers that produce videos or present seminars on-site that can aide a laboratory. The program should include the vital aspects of stress management that will allow the employee a chance to instill a portion of the ideas in their professional and personal lives. This is essential because each employee has different problems and different needs (Davis 2000).

One component that any professional stress management program should provide is an introduction to stress management, such as the definition of stress and the health consequences of stress. Stress is the nonspecific response of the body to any demand made upon it. There are two different types of stress, *eustress* and *distress*. Eustress is good stress, a motivating force that challenges employees to grow, adapt, and find creative solutions in life. Distress is bad stress, the type of stress this program is attempting to eliminate. It is the force that depletes life energy. Usually, distress is unchannelled and harms the body and mind if it is allowed to continue (McGuire 1998).

As stated earlier, stress (i.e., distress) destroys the body through hypertension, increased heart rate, and frequent infections. Therefore, a professional stress management program should include methods to alleviate these health problems. This component of the program will concentrate on the importance of nutrition, exercise, and relaxation techniques in stress management (McGuire 1998). The program encourages the employee to eat appropriate meals at least three times a day; to engage in strenuous exercise for at least thirty minutes, three days a week; and to get adequate rest every night, waking up in time to get to work without having to rush. This will eliminate many stressors in an employee's life that occur before arriving at work. Also, the implementation of relaxation techniques such as yoga in an employee's lifestyle could help eliminate stress (McGuire 1998).

In addition to nutrition, exercise, and relation techniques, the professional stress management program should provide a component that examines various personalities and identifies methods to change certain personalities to reduce stressful situations and, in turn, reduce stress. For example, a shy person will worry about certain aspects of a job such as working with new people or having to talk in front of people, which create an abundant amount of unneeded stress. On the other hand, an overbearing, perfectionist personality will create unneeded stress by constantly attempting to control the workplace environment or constantly trying to perfect a situation. In this program, the employee can attempt to build self-esteem and reduce life stressors (Davis 2000).

A successful professional stress management program will encourage the employees to set goals in the workplace that are attainable. This will reduce the stress for everyone in the workplace, because each person is moving forward at his or her own pace. This will allow the employee to manage his or her time in a manner that will produce quality results in an appropriate turnaround time. Problem solving is another skill, like time management, that will reduce stress in the employee's life once it is learned. In the clinical laboratory, the ability to problem solve is a major advantage due to the troubleshooting maintenance that needs to be performed on instruments almost daily. If a laboratorian had to call the field engineer every time a problem arose with an instrument, very little would be accomplished. With this in mind, if a tech cannot perform routine troubleshooting, this could become a very stressful situation.

Finally, the professional stress management program should have a component dedicated to improving the social skills of the medical technologists/clinical laboratory scientists. This component completes the circle by underscoring the need for employee-arranged work teams, cited earlier as the first possible technique in reducing stress (McCardle 1998). Laboratory personnel must be able to work with each other. This is a necessary skill for each department to be a success. This program will teach the importance of resolving conflicts, showing initiative, and forming good working relationships with other employees in a clinical laboratory. It will identify the various personalities of a workplace environment and encourage the technologists to learn to work together (Geber 1996).

The stress management program would be ideal for a clinical laboratory setting that is downsizing because of Medicare cutbacks or for any hospital laboratory that is developing problems within the workplace. It will help reduce stress by providing the employees with information necessary to implement changes in their lifestyle. Each component of the program will not apply to everyone; however, laboratorians may adapt applicable components of the professional stress management program to their lives, and a difference is certain to be seen.

BIBLIOGRAPHY

Bone, Susan M. 1998. *A lifestyle approach to mastering stress.* Presentation at University of Southern Mississippi, July.

Crampton, S. M., J. W. Hodge, J. M. Mishra, et al. 1995. Stress and stress management. *SAM Advanced Management Journal* 60 (summer): 10–18.

Davis, John S. 2000. Management and education. *American Society of Clinical Pathologists. Tech Sample.* No. MGM-3.

Geber, Sara Zeff. 1996. Pulling the plug on stress. *HR Focus* 73, no. 4: 12.

Inzana, Carolyn M.; Driskell, James E.; Salas, Eduardo; Johnston, Joan H. 1996. Effects of preparatory information on enhancing performance under stress. *Journal of Applied Psychology* 81: 429–435.

Krohe, J., Jr. 1999. Workplace stress. *Across the Board* 36 (February): 36–42.

McCardle, Victoria B. 1998. Self-directed work teams. *Medical Laboratory Observer* (November): 17–25.

McGuire, James. 1998. Presentation in class entitled Stress Management-CHS 436, July.

National Institute for Occupational Safety and Health. 1999. Job stress. *Risk Managing* 13 (May): 5.

INTERNET RESOURCES

The American Institute of Stress. <www.stress.org>

International Stress Management Association. <www.isma.org.uk>

Stress Management for Students, National University of Singapore. <www.med.nus.edu.sg/pcm/stress>

Wesley E. Sime, Department of Health and Human Performance, University of Nebraska, Lincoln. <www.unl.edu/stress/mgmt>

QUESTIONS

1. State four general ways that everyone can reduce stress. *(Objective 1, Level I)*

    a. _____

    b. _____

    c. _____

    d. _____

2. Identify OSHA's position regarding job stress and the employer's responsibility. *(Objective 2, Level I)*

3. Regarding stress management, discuss the use and activities of stress-related work teams. *(Objective 3, Level II)*

4. Create an outline for a stress management program based on the text. *(Objective 4, Level III)*

EXERCISES

Completion of the exercises will enhance your knowledge of stress management. *(Objective 5, Level III and Objective 6, Level III)*

1. Survey the laboratorians working in your laboratory to determine stress factors. Using this information, develop a list of all the factors. Next, survey the laboratorians to determine the importance of each factor using a Likert scale with 1 = not a stressor, 2 = minor stressor, 3 = stressor, 4 = important stressor, 5 = very important stressor. Compare the day shift, evening shift, and night shift results. Compare your results with that reported in the literature.

2. Interview the supervisor of physical therapy, occupational therapy, the X-ray department, and other allied health departments to determine whether a stress management program is used. If a program is used, describe its characteristics in a report to the other students and/or the laboratory section supervisors.

3. Interview the hospital administrators to determine whether the hospital has a stress management program or whether elements of stress management are used anywhere throughout the hospital.

4. Develop and recommend a stress management program for your laboratory by developing a program including laboratory stress management needs, timetable, resources, scheduling, cost, benefits for the laboratory, and so on. Present the proposal to the laboratory administrator.

CASES

Propose solutions for the following stress management cases. *(Objective 7, Level III)*

1. The chemistry department is not as efficient as you, the laboratory manager, would like. After reviewing the workload of the department, you note that the workload is heavy, allowing very little time for everyone to interact. In individual conversations, each tells you that no one else works in the department. When you visit the department, the tensions are evident. You decide that the tension is due to stress from the workload. You can do nothing about the workload volume. What kind of stress reduction would you use to relieve some of the stress in this situation?

2. One of the technologists in Hematology that just assumed the section supervisor role seems angry with the world, doesn't want to talk to other coworkers, sits alone in the cafeteria, and yells at nurses or doctors on the phone occasionally when reports are requested. Previously, this technologist had been one of the best employees in the

laboratory. As laboratory manager, this behavior is brought to your attention, and you ask the individual to come to your office. Upon discussion of the behavior, the technologist reveals to you that her husband has moved out of the house and filed for a divorce, the in-laws are being difficult, the financial picture is poor, and her only son is leaving in one week for college. She has not been eating or sleeping well lately. Identify the problem and what intervention strategies you would implement.

SECTION II MANAGEMENT ISSUES REGARDING COMMUNICATION

Chapter 11

Professional Writing

Mary Lux, Ph.D., MT(ASCP), CLS(NCA)

OBJECTIVES

Upon completion of this chapter the learner will be able to

1. Discuss the importance of accurate business communications. *(Level II)*
2. List parts of a letter, a memo, a report, and a proposal. *(Level I)*
3. State the specific purpose of a letter, a memo, a report, and a proposal. *(Level I)*
4. Name a journal and its publisher. *(Level I)*
5. List and briefly describe the typical sections of a journal publication. *(Level I)*
6. Discuss the importance of peer review. *(Level II)*
7. Summarize the process involved in publishing a journal article after the article manuscript is written and submitted to the publication editor. *(Level II)*
8. State the purpose of an abstract for an oral presentation or poster. *(Level I)*
9. Correct a letter, a memo, a report, and a proposal. *(Level III)*
10. Compose a letter, a memo, a report, and a proposal. *(Level III)*
11. Create an abstract. *(Level III)*
12. Create an oral presentation and/or poster. *(Level III)*
13. Propose solutions for the case studies. *(Level III)*

TOPIC SUMMARY

Professional writing skills are essential for management personnel. Written documents represent you to the professional community and serve as documentation of your communications. Business communications are an element of the official affairs of an individual or organization. When you prepare a letter, memo, or e-mail, consider that the recipient may file your document for future referral. Your signature, initials, or e-mail address signify that the document has your approval and exists as a record of your opinions, statements, ideas, or results.

All business communications should demonstrate correct grammar, spelling, punctuation, and usage. The language of a business communication should be free of colloquial terms and conversational patterns. Use of clear and concise language ensures that the reader will comprehend the writer's intended message.

It is important to take advantage of the various tools (spell check, grammar check) available in word processing programs to assist in preparation of documents. Although these tools are useful, careful proofreading is essential. Many keyboard errors result in actual words that will not be highlighted by spell-check software.

Significant types of written communications include **letters, memos, reports,** and **proposals.** The basic rules of good writing should be upheld for both conventional paper communications and for information transmitted by fax or e-mail. Word processing programs may provide formats for memos and faxed messages, or your institution may use official forms for memos and faxes. If your e-mail system does not offer check mechanisms for spelling and grammar, prepare critical documents in a word processing program to paste into an e-mail message or include the document as an attachment.

The letter is a type of formal correspondence. The letter format includes the date; sender's name, title and address (or letterhead stationery); recipient's name, title, and address; a salutation, a subject line (optional), body, complimentary close, and signature. A sample letter is shown in Figure 11-1.

The memo is a short, informal correspondence. The standard memo form includes the information for the sender (name, title, location, e-mail address, phone and fax numbers) and space for the date, name of recipient, and subject. There is no salutation, complimentary close, or signature, although the sender may initial the form near his or her name. A sample memo is illustrated in Figure 11-2.

A report gives information on a definite topic or results from a specific project. Topics for reports may include financial information, employee or client characteristics, or periodic summaries. Reports may require use of the memo format or of a specific form, such as travel vouchers or incident reports. Other reports may require the writer to use a format that includes a title, the objective(s), the data or facts, and a conclusion or recommendation.

A proposal is a plan of action submitted for acceptance by an individual or group. Proposals are frequently written to persuade an authority to fund a purchase, position, or project. Proposals should include a statement of purpose, the specific problem or situation, the solution or resolution, and a conclusion.

November 20, 2002   (Date)

Melissa Jones   (Sender's Information)
5220 South Street
Old City, PA 44400

Sam Smith   (Recipient's Information)
Lab Director
Alltown General Hospital
123 Main Street
Alltown, OH 44400

Dear Mr. Smith: (Salutation)

Thank you for granting me an interview on Tuesday, November 19, 2002. I enjoyed visiting Alltown General Hospital and meeting the laboratory personnel. I know I would enjoy the position in the chemistry department. I hope you will give my application a favorable decision.

Sincerely,   (Complimentary Close)

Melissa Jones, CLS(NCA)   (Signature)

FIGURE 11-1. Sample Letter

> Kyla Kendel
> Human Resources
> Mail Stop 15
> Oak Bluff Children's Hospital
> Phone: (800) 555-2233
> Fax: (800) 555-2244
> E-mail: KyKe@obch.org
>
> DATE: October 14, 2002
>
> TO: Department Heads
>
> SUBJECT: United Way Campaign
>
> Thank you for your cooperation during the United Way Campaign. We have reached our goal of 100% participation. Congratulate your employees on their generosity. The community of Oak Bluff will benefit as a result of their donations.

FIGURE 11-2. Sample Memo

Another aspect of professional writing is the preparation of articles for professional journals. Journal articles and professional presentations are important methods of communication among clinical laboratory scientists. Journal articles report the results of research. Research topics include new methodologies, comparisons between or among methods, case reports, and results from various surveys or educational studies. Journals are published by scientific or professional organizations. Journal submissions are reviewed by peers or persons in the same profession who share the goal of providing quality continuing education and news of discoveries for members of the organization and for readers of the journal. This process is called peer review. Two journals that address broad laboratory science issues are *Clinical Laboratory Science*, published by the American Society for Clinical Laboratory Science, and *Laboratory Medicine*, published by the American Society for Clinical Pathology. Other journals of interest to clinical laboratory scientists include publications of other professional societies such as *Journal of Clinical Microbiology* (American Society for Microbiology) and *Transfusion* (American Association of Blood Banks). *Clinical Leadership and Management Review* is a publication of Clinical Laboratory Management Association.

Each journal publishes instructions for contributors. It is important to follow the instructions for contributors and to follow rules of standard English. These instructions often are found in the January issue of the publication or on the organization's Web site. Scientific articles generally follow a format that includes the following sections:

1. Abstract. The abstract is a brief summary of the article.
2. Introduction. The introduction includes a brief review of the most recent literature on the topic to provide background for the reader.
3. Material and methods. This section delineates the type of experiments or studies done, including the methodology, the reagents, and the instrumentation.
4. Results. The data from the study is presented, often including the use of graphs, charts, or tables.
5. Discussion or conclusion. The significance of the data and outcomes is presented by the author.

6. References. Literature cited in the article is attributed to the original author(s). Publications differ in the format required for references.
7. Acknowledgments. The agency that funds the project and entities who donated time or materials for the project (at a level less than required for an author) are recognized. Many journals publish criteria for authorship requirements.

A journal article is submitted to the publication editor. The editor of the journal will send copies of the article to two or three volunteers who serve on the editorial board of the journal. These volunteer peer-reviewers assess the article and recommend acceptance or rejection of the article based on the journal's standards, purpose, and audience. Articles that are recommended for publication are frequently returned to authors with editorial recommendations for improvement. The author may make the suggested changes or explain why the change would not enhance the article. The author signs an agreement with the journal's publisher to assign copyright to the publisher. After an article is accepted for publication, the author will receive the final copy of the article page proofs. Page proofs display the article as it will appear in the journal. It is the author's responsibility to check the page proofs for accuracy. The process of submission, review, revision, and acceptance of an article for publication in a professional journal can be a lengthy process and may extend over a period of several months after the author submits the original document.

Annual or general meetings of professional organizations often issue a call for abstracts. An abstract is a short summary of original research for a proposed presentation for the meeting. The presentation may be a short talk of ten to fifteen minutes or a poster displayed on a board. An abstract usually is peer-reviewed and may be published as part of the meeting's program. An abstract should include a statement of the objective of the study, a brief account of the methods, a summary of the results, and a concise discussion of the study. Organizations publish abstract instructions, and it is important to follow the criteria concerning title, authors, and length. Typical abstracts are restricted to a brief paragraph or specific word count due to publishing costs. When an abstract is accepted for presentation, the author will be notified of the time for the presentation and given other specific instructions, such as the size of the poster board or the amount of time allotted for oral presentations. Abstracts and the subsequent presentations provide a mechanism to introduce the results of preliminary or completed research to the professional audience in a shorter time period than required for a journal article.

The abstract serves as an outline for the actual presentation. Oral presentations should include visual aids such as slides or PowerPoint programs. Take care to limit the amount of information on each slide and to consider how the use of color, diagrams, tables, charts, and so on could enhance your visual presentation. Talks should be limited to the suggested length, and remember to allow time for questions and discussions.

Poster presentations should fit the space indicated by the organization. Prepare a title board that includes the name of the presentation, the authors, and the authors' professional credentials and affiliations as allowed by the professional society that sponsors the meeting. Use the logo of your institution if possible. Display all materials in a large font so the poster can be read from a distance of four feet. Include graphs, tables, charts, or photographs to illustrate your presentation. Include judicious use of color to complement your presentation. Remember that the purpose of the abstract and the oral or visual presentation is to share your research, discoveries, or observations with the professional community. Take care to design your presentations to attract and hold the attention of meeting participants.

Contributing to journal articles and presenting ideas and discoveries at professional meetings are vital components in developing a career in management. The preparation of effective written communications is a fundamental skill for success.

BIBLIOGRAPHY

American Psychological Association. 2001. *Publication manual of the American Psychological Association*. 5th ed. Washington, D.C.: American Psychological Association.

Council of Biology Editors Style Manual Committee. 1994. *Scientific style and format: The CBE manual for authors, editors and publishers*. 6th ed. New York: Cambridge University Press.

Iverson, Cheryl, ed. 1998. *American Medical Association manual of style: A guide for authors and editors*. Baltimore, Md.: Williams & Wilkins.

Kolin, Philip C. 2000. *Successful writing at work*. 6th ed. Boston, Mass.: Houghton Mifflin.

Wians, Frank H, Jr. 2002. Guidelines for preparing scientific manuscripts. *Laboratory Medicine* 33: 77–80.

INTERNET RESOURCES

International Committee of Medical Journal Editors.
    <www.mja.com>
Online Writing Lab, Purdue University.
    <http://owl.english.purdue.edu>
Writing Solution, Inc.
    <www.writingsolution.com/services.htm>

QUESTIONS

1. Discuss why accurate business communications are essential in the professional environment. *(Objective 1, Level II)*

2. Parts of a letter include all of the following EXCEPT *(Objective 2, Level I)*
   a. date
   b. sender's name, title, and address
   c. recipient's name, title, and address
   d. salutation
   e. phone number

3. Parts of a memo include all of the following EXCEPT *(Objective 2, Level I)*
   a. name, title, location, e-mail address, phone number
   b. fax number
   c. name of recipient
   d. credentials of sender
   e. subject

4. The purpose of a report is to _____ . *(Objective 3, Level I)*

5. The purpose of a proposal is to _____ . *(Objective 3, Level I)*

6. Name one journal and its publisher. *(Objective 4, Level I)*

7. The format for scientific journal articles includes the following parts: *(Objective 5, Level I)*
   a. _____
   b. _____
   c. _____
   d. _____
   e. _____

8. Discuss the importance of peer review for a manuscript submitted to a professional publication. *(Objective 6, Level II)*

9. Summarize the process involved in publishing a journal article after the article manuscript is written and submitted to the publication editor. *(Objective 7, Level II)*

10. The purpose of an abstract is *(Objective 8, Level I)*
    a. to provide a mechanism to introduce preliminary or completed research results to the professional audience quickly
    b. to attract a journal editor so that your article will be published
    c. to showcase your institution's research opportunities
    d. to impress everyone with your writing skills
11. Rewrite the letter in Figure 11–3 making necessary corrections. Consider letter format, grammar, punctuation, spelling, capitalization, and language. *(Objective 9, Level III)*

Jody Blue
Laboratory Infromation Oficer
County Hsopital
Red Creek, MD 21900

August 13, 2002

Sandy johnson, Software specialist
SOFTWARE.com
5960 Bryson Street
Baltimore, MD 21110

Dear Ms. Blue:

SUBJECT: Visit to Red Creek

Thanks a bunch for checking out our software. What you said about our products were helpful. Maybe we can do some business later. Why don't you cum by our exhibit when ASCLS has there next convention?

cordially,

sandi

FIGURE 11–3. Letter to be Corrected

EXERCISES

Completion of the exercises will enhance your knowledge of professional writing. *(Objective 10, Level III, Objective 11, Level III, and Objective 12, Level III)*

1. Write a letter to recommend a former employee for a new position.
2. Write a memo to remind employees of a retirement party for a staff pathologist.
3. Write a report to the hospital safety committee chairman stating the outcome of the laboratory's role in the recent disaster drill.
4. Write a proposal to the hospital administration to justify the addition of a new staff technologist position for the day shift.
5. Find instructions for authors in a journal or on a Web site.
6. Prepare a 250-word abstract or summary of this chapter.
7. Prepare an oral presentation or poster presentation based on a journal article.

CASES

For the following cases, propose reasonable solutions. *(Objective 13, Level III)*

1. As manager, you wish to purchase a new hematology analyzer. You have sent a memo to your administrator simply requesting the instrument. You have received no reply. What could be the problem? How could you correct the problem?

2. The administrator requests information from all departments regarding detailed laboratory financial information. As laboratory manager, you respond with a short memo. The administrator e-mails you, indicating that your response was inadequate. Which type of written communication would have been appropriate and why?

3. As manager, you want to amend the dress code policy for laboratory employees. Your reasons for the change are sound and based on safety considerations, but the proposed change varies from the hospital's policy. What type of written communication would be the best choice to pursue this issue with administration? What should be included in your written request?

4. You have discovered a new method for staining ascospores. Four unaffiliated laboratories conduct rigorous testing of your methodology, and the personnel from each facility agree that your method is superior to the standard method. Which is the fastest means to communicate this finding to the scientific community? Which means will reach the greater audience? What is the most effective means?

5. You present a poster at a local professional meeting and are disappointed when no one stops to view your poster or discuss the results. The presentation covers the entire 4′ × 8′ board with textual information in black twelve-point font on a white background. The title board is in black fourteen-point font on a white background. You have submitted an abstract to present this same topic at a national meeting, and the abstract has been accepted. What changes could you make to the poster presentation to increase the possibility that meeting participants will be attracted to your visual presentation?

Chapter 12

Communications and Interpersonal Relationships

John Curry, M.Ed., MT(ASCP)DLM

OBJECTIVES

Upon completion of this chapter the learner will be able to

1. State five purposes of communication. *(Level I)*
2. Name the three primary routes through which communication occurs. *(Level I)*
3. Define *paraverbals*. *(Level I)*
4. Identify and discuss at least three barriers to communication. *(Level II)*
5. Identify and discuss four styles of communication. *(Level II)*
6. Define *intrapersonal* and *interpersonal* communication. *(Level I)*
7. Identify at least four sources of conflict. *(Level I)*
8. List several advantages of excellent communications and interpersonal skills. *(Level I)*
9. Critique personal communication skills and formulate a plan for improving those skills. *(Level III)*
10. Analyze the communications and formulate a solution for the case studies. *(Level III)*

TOPIC SUMMARY

It has been estimated that people spend more time communicating than in any other activity in life. This can be in the form of writing, talking with friends, speaking on the phone, and reading. Communication can be defined as the way for people to exchange feelings or ideas with one another.

We tend to forget that communication is a process. It is a series of ongoing events of processing the symbols, decoding, gathering ideas and feelings, then encoding this to another person. You must have at least two people to communicate. Figure 12-1 indicates the communication process.

People spend forty-five percent of their time listening, thirty percent speaking, and about twenty-five

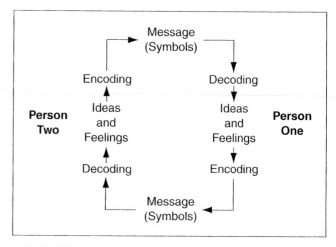

FIGURE 12-1. A Model of the Communication Process

percent reading and writing. Listening was the main way of learning until the invention of printing. However, listening has been revived in importance with the spread of radio, television, recordings, and films. When people are bored with what they hear, they tend to tune it out. Skilled listening involves both thinking and hearing. As a manager, developing listening skills is critical. A few ways to enhance listening are to paraphrase or restate what the communicator has said and ask clarifying questions while the communicator is talking. If you know that you are going to use these techniques, then you as the listener concentrate more on what the communicator is saying and not on your response. The more avenues used to communicate, the more accurate the message; therefore, development of listening, speaking, reading, and writing skills are critical to effective communications.

Communication serves five major purposes:

1. Informative communication—People sharing knowledge about the world in which they live. Informative communication is important in today's world. Nations such as the United States were once called industrial societies that manufactured products. Today these same nations are called information societies. This is due to the fact that an increasing number of jobs involve the processing of information rather than producing products. Even those who work with products rather than ideas must use job-related messages such as manuals, job descriptions, catalogs, instrument warranties, contracts, invoices, and so on in their jobs.
2. Affective communication—This is the process through which people express feelings about themselves, things, and others. Affective communication is very important in the formation of self-concept—what you think of yourself.
3. Imaginative communication—The process through which invented situations are created and shared with others. This type of communication plays a role in every person's life.
4. Persuasive communication—May be defined as the process in which people attempt to influence the beliefs or actions of others.
5. Ritualistic communication—The process through which people meet social expectations. This type of communication is important because people who violate the rules and customs of social interaction have difficulty relating well with others.

There are various mediums of communication. These are the means through which messages are encoded or transported between people. There are five possible ways that messages may enter the consciousness of people. These are sound, sight, touch, smell, and taste.

In management, communication is one of the most, if not *the* most, important skills needed. To be an effective manager you must be able to communicate well and to accept communication well. There must be communication in all directions—from the top down, from the bottom up, and from peers. With every contact with another person, you communicate something. Unfortunately, it may not always be what you want to communicate or intend to communicate.

When we think of communication we usually think of what words were said or heard (verbal). However, other ways of communicating may be through body language (nonverbal) or through the tone or pitch of your voice (paraverbal). Paraverbal is how we say what we say. Tone of voice and your words must match for effective communication.

When looking at the different types of communication, you can also recognize problems that can cause barriers to communication:

1. Nonverbal barriers include body language, eye contact, eyes rolling or shut, and so on.
2. Verbal barriers include using words that are unfamiliar to a person due to nationality or race.
3. Paraverbal barriers include things such as the tone being too high, speaking too fast, the pitch being too high, and the volume being too loud or too low.
4. Environmental barriers include temperature of the room, proper dress, proper use of cologne or perfume, neatness and cleanliness of hair, and so on.
5. Overcommunicating is a barrier in which too much communication at any one time is given.
6. Undercommunicating is not giving enough information for the person to understand what you want him or her to do or understand.
7. Communicating at inappropriate times, such as when the person is busy doing another task or talking to someone else.

Being aware of others and focusing less on self and what one is communicating will help in overcoming most of these barriers. Training sessions or counseling to enhance one's ability to focus on the other person may be helpful. Control of the environment is not always possible. In this case, one may have to adapt to the environment and strive for communications regardless of the environment. Some environmental factors may be modified to enhance communications. Environmental modification may include moving from behind the desk to sit next to an individual, rearranging the furniture in an office, meeting in a place that is not noisy, or telling the assistant to stop all phone calls while the communication is occurring. If environmental factors are inhibiting communications, they should be addressed if at all possible.

Each manager has his or her own unique style of communication. This style makes some managers more effective than others. There are four styles of communication. Managers can use one or more of these styles when communicating:

1. Concrete sequential—likes to focus on ideas or tasks, thinks methodically and predictably, slow to adjust to change.
2. Abstract sequential—prefers learning from logical presentation of ideas, relies on logical impersonal analysis, creates theoretical models from a wide range of information, is slow to decide, is less concerned with people than ideas.
3. Concrete random—prefers learning from trial and error, relies on experience-based information, makes decisions based on finding solutions, is quick to make a decision, is a risk taker, relies more on people than technical analysis for information.
4. Abstract random—prefers learning from lots of free-form ideas, is an intuitive thinker, balks at structure, likes to generate new ideas.

Communication may be intrapersonal or interpersonal. Intrapersonal communication is communication with one's self. Interpersonal communication involves one-on-one exchanges with other people.

Interpersonal relationships, along with communication, are a very important part of the manager's job and are a part of every person's job in an organization as well. These relationships range through all age groups, ethnic groups, different levels of education, and different work groups, that is, subordinates, superiors, peers, patients, visitors, and physicians. The way you interact with all groups is important because all interpersonal relationships and how they are handled ultimately impact patient care.

Interpersonal relationships from a management perspective include some conflict resolution because there is always some type of conflict occurring in the job. This can occur with any of the groups with which you interact in the job. Conflict is normal, and the causes of conflict are diverse. All conflict is not open. An open and honest environment, however, encourages a sense of safety and support within the organization. The sources of conflict can include, but are not limited to, the following:

1. Scheduling
2. Communication breakdown
3. Staffing problems or solutions
4. Costs or financial issues
5. Pressure
6. Personality
7. Inadequate interpersonal skills
8. Expectation of others
9. Administrative skills

There are five reactive ways of settling conflict:

1. Competition—someone wins and someone loses.
2. Accommodation—you lose because you accommodate someone and they win.
3. Avoidance—you both avoid or ignore the problem and you both lose.
4. Compromise—win/lose or tie. No one really wins in this situation.
5. Collaboration—win/win, both parties win.

Collaboration is the best way of handling conflict because it involves identifying agreements and differences and evaluating alternatives and solutions that have support and commitment from both parties involved. In order to achieve a win/win result, there must be a willingness to resolve the conflict, to get to the root of the problem, and to empathize with each other.

Excellent communication and interpersonal skills can work magic in an organizational culture. It helps to change an organization by getting all employees aligned. It speeds up the decision process, creates proactive behavior, and improves all working relationships. Everyone can make a difference when communication is open and used effectively at all levels of the organization.

BIBLIOGRAPHY

Cohen, Michael. 1984. *Employee handbook for on the job survival.* Oak Park, Ill.: Canoe Press.

Compton's Interactive Encyclopedia. 1994–1995. Carlsbad, Calif.: Compton's New Media.

Ford, Lisa. 1997. *Customer service excellence—It's in the details.* West Des Moines, Iowa: American Media Publishing.

Memorial Hospital Education and Research Department. 1997. *Focus on service excellence.* Gulfport, Miss.: Memorial Hospital.

INTERNET RESOURCES

Air War College and Ira C. Eaker College. Leadership, Ethics, and Command Central. Communication Skills. <www.au.af.mil/au/awc/awcgate/awc-comm.htm>

Department of Veterans Affairs. Mediator Skills. <www.va.gov/adr/medskils.htm>

University of Kansas. Department of Communication Studies. <www.ukans.edu/cwis/units/coms2/via/index.html>

QUESTIONS

1. Communication is NOT a process of *(Objective 1, Level I)*
   a. providing information
   b. expressing feelings
   c. dominating the situation
   d. persuading others
   e. meeting social expectations

2. Communication occurs through three primary routes which are *(Objective 2, Level I)*

   a. _____

   b. _____

   c. _____

3. Paraverbal is _____ we say _____ we say. *(Objective 3, Level I)*

4. List and discuss at least three barriers to communication. *(Objective 4, Level II)*

5. Identify and discuss the four styles of communication. *(Objective 5, Level II)*

6. Intrapersonal communication is with _____. Interpersonal communication is with _____. *(Objective 6, Level I)*

7. Identify at least four sources of conflict. *(Objective 7, Level I)*

   a. _____

   b. _____

   c. _____

   d. _____

8. Advantages of excellent communications and interpersonal skills include *(Objective 8, Level I)*
   a. all employees understand the direction of the organization
   b. speeds up the decision process
   c. creates proactive behavior
   d. improves all working relationships
   e. all of the above

EXERCISES

Completion of the exercises will enhance your knowledge of communications and interpersonal relationships. *(Objective 9, Level III)*

1. Practice increasing your listening skills by using the following techniques in conversations that you have: during the conversation, paraphrase what you think the person is saying, ask questions, do not plan your response until the person has completed his or her thought, and acknowledge and respond to nonverbal clues. Evaluate the effect this has on increasing your listening.

2. Observe individuals communicating and make a list of nonverbal signals over a period of a week. Does this exercise increase your awareness of nonverbal clues?

3. Observe barriers to communications for a week and make a list of those noted. Decide how you would reduce each barrier.

4. Critique your personal communication skills and formulate a plan for improving these skills.

CASES

Analyze the following cases and provide reasonable solutions. *(Objective 10, Level III)*

1. As the section supervisor, on Friday you approach one of the section techs and ask the tech to work the weekend because the weekend tech is sick. The tech says, "Well, I guess so," and quickly turns her back to you and stomps away. Discuss the tech's reaction regarding the verbal, nonverbal, and paraverbal dimensions. What actions would you now take? How could you have handled the situation better?

2. The techs in your laboratory are very busy one morning and you, the manager, walk in and explain the new policy regarding leave time. Later, several of the techs share the information with other employees over lunch, and that afternoon one of the evening shift employees that has heard the news comes into your office complaining about an erroneous concept regarding the policy. Analyze the situation and propose solutions.

Chapter 13

Motivation

Jane Hudson, Ph.D., MT(ASCP)SM, CLS(NCA)

OBJECTIVES

Upon completion of the chapter the learner will be able to

1. Define *motivation*. *(Level I)*
2. Discuss the following motivational theories: *(Level II)*
   a. Maslow's Hierarchy of Needs
   b. Herzberg's Two-Factor theory
   c. Vroom's Expectancy theory
3. Identify motivational theories used in the laboratory. *(Level II)*
4. Relate items that motivate to motivational theories. *(Level II)*
5. Choose the most appropriate motivational theory and formulate solutions in given cases. *(Level III)*

TOPIC SUMMARY

Motivation is the factor that inspires a person to act. Three major motivational theories, Maslow's Hierarchy of Needs, Herzberg's Two-Factor theory, and Vroom's Expectancy theory, are discussed briefly.

Maslow's Hierarchy of Needs

Maslow (1970) identified **physiological and safety needs** as basic physical needs that would motivate if not satisfied. Satisfaction of physical needs is required before higher level **social needs,** such as esteem and love, will motivate. If the physical and social needs are satisfied, motivation will occur as result of **growth needs,** such as self-actualization. The hierarchy of needs (physical needs, social needs, growth needs) are illustrated in Figure 13–1.

For example, an employee who does not have enough income to provide for the family (physiological need) will be motivated by money. If the physical needs of this employee are satisfied, then the employee will be motivated by higher level needs such as group membership (social need). If the physical and social needs of this individual are satisfied, then the employee will be motivated by growth needs such as self-actualization.

We may observe a senior level employee who has had the physical and social needs satisfied in the laboratory, yet the employee is unable to advance any further. Therefore, the employee seeks self-actualization satisfaction through involvement outside of the laboratory,

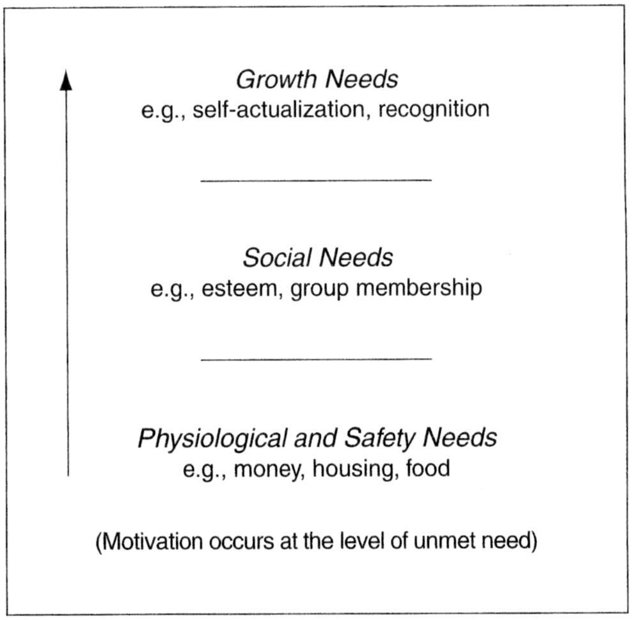

Growth Needs
e.g., self-actualization, recognition

Social Needs
e.g., esteem, group membership

Physiological and Safety Needs
e.g., money, housing, food

(Motivation occurs at the level of unmet need)

FIGURE 13–1. Maslow's Hierarchy of Needs

perhaps in a professional organization or a community group.

Herzberg's Two-Factor Theory

Herzberg et al. (1959) identified two factors: 1) the basic needs, **hygiene factors**, which correspond primarily with Maslow's physical and social needs and 2) **motivators**, which correspond primarily with Maslow's growth needs (see Figure 13–2).

Herzberg's theory differs from Maslow's theory in that Herzberg indicates that only the growth needs motivate. Hygiene factors serve only to prevent dissatisfaction with the job, not as a motivator. There is no hierarchy in that unsatisfied needs could occur in both the hygiene and motivator areas at the same time.

For example, if an employee did not have enough income to provide for the family (hygiene factors), then the employee would be dissatisfied, but money would not motivate because the employee would feel that additional money was only the fair practice of the employer. However, motivators such as self-actualization would motivate the employee. The employee could have an income need and a self-actualization need simultaneously; therefore, no hierarchy of need exists.

Vroom's Expectancy Theory

An adaptation of Vroom's (1964) Expectancy theory by Porter, Lawler, and Hackman (1975) and further adapted by Hudson and Bushardt (1987) was expressed as $E_I \times E_{II} \times$ Net Preference $=$ Motivation. The "independent variables are 1) the individual's expectation (perception) of the probability that high effort will lead to high performance (E_I); 2) the individual's expectation (perception) that high performance will lead to outcomes (E_{II}); and 3) the individual's preference for the outcome (net preference)." (See Figure 13–3.)

All the independent variables must be present in order for the employee to be motivated. For example, an

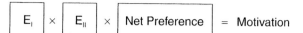

FIGURE 13–3. Modification of Vroom's Expectancy Theory

employee who does not believe he has the capability to perform the work (E_I problem) will not be motivated. On the other hand, if the employee does not believe that even if he does the work well, he will be rewarded (E_{II} problem), then the employee will not be motivated. Or if the employee does not want to do the work (net preference problem), the employee will not be motivated.

Understanding what motivates people to work is essential in getting the work done, and getting the work done is a primary task of the leader. Although no one motivational theory is applicable in all situations, a study of the different theories allows the leader to more quickly identify the motivational factors influencing a work situation. Once the factors that motivate an individual or group are identified, the group leader can seek to provide the environment that would enhance motivation.

BIBLIOGRAPHY

Hackman, J. Richard, Edward E. Lawler III, and Lyman W. Porter, eds. 1983. *Perspectives on behavior in organizations.* 2d ed. New York: McGraw-Hill.

Herzberg, Frederick, Bernard Mausner, Barbara Block Snyderman. 1959. *The motivation to work.* New York: J. Wiley and Sons.

Hudson, M. J., and S. C. Bushardt. 1987. Diagnosis and treatment of student motivational problem. *Laboratory Medicine* 18, no. 2: 107–09.

Maslow, Abraham H. 1975. *Motivation and personality.* New York: Harper and Row.

Porter, L.W., E.E. Lawler III, R. Hackman Jr. 1975. *Behavior in organizations.* New York: McGraw-Hill.

Varnadoe, Lionel A. 1996. *Medical laboratory management and supervision—Operations, review, and study guide.* Philadelphia: F. A. Davis.

Vroom, V. 1964. *Work and motivation.* New York: John Wiley and Sons.

FIGURE 13–2. Hertzberg's Two-Factor Theory

Internet Resources

Southern Illinois University, Dr. Gordon C. Bruner II. <www.siu.edu/departments/coba/mktg/courses/mktg305/lectures/motives/tsld001.htm>

Cleveland State University. <http://grail.cba.csuohio.edu/~popovich/mlr501/motivetheories.ppt>

Accel Team. <www.accel-team.com/human_relations/>

QUESTIONS

1. Define *motivation*. *(Objective 1, Level I)*

2. Discuss the following motivational theories: *(Objective 2, Level II)*
   a. Maslow's Hierarchy of Needs

   b. Herzberg's Two-Factor theory

   c. Vroom's Expectancy theory

3. An employee does not perceive that work is important. What type of problem is this according to Vroom's Expectancy theory? *(Objective 2, Level I)*
   a. E_I problem
   b. E_{II} problem
   c. Net preference problem
   d. All of the above

4. An employee is concerned that the health insurance provided by the hospital is not sufficient to protect the family. The employee would be motivated if a better insurance could be obtained according to which of the following theories? *(Objective 2, Level II)*
   a. Maslow's theory
   b. Herzberg's theory

5. An employee is unhappy with the job in the laboratory because body fluid protection precautions are not implemented. What need or factor is identified? *(Objective 2, Level II)*
   a. Hygiene factor
   b. Motivator factor
   c. Social need
   d. Physical need
   e. A and D
   f. A, B, and D

EXERCISES

Completion of the exercises will enhance your knowledge of motivation. *(Objective 3, Level I and Objective 4, Level II)*

1. Interview a hospital administrator, administrative technologist, or supervisor to determine which if any motivational theories are used in the laboratory or hospital and the advantages or disadvantages of certain theories.

2. Interview technologists in the laboratory to determine what motivates them. Relate the items that motivate to the three different motivational theories.

CASES

Using the following six motivation cases, work individually or as a group in developing solutions. *(Objective 5, Level III)*

1. A laboratorian does not make enough money to provide the essentials for his large and growing family. What would it take to motivate the laboratorian according to each of the following theories?
   a. Maslow's theory
   b. Herzberg's theory
   c. Vroom's theory

2. The manager of the laboratory receives a high salary that meets all her needs and desires. Her laboratory is a model for satisfaction of employees and productivity. She is continuously praised by the hospital administration. What would it take to motivate the director according to each of the following theories?
   a. Maslow's theory
   b. Herzberg's theory
   c. Vroom's theory

3. In examples #1 and #2, what strategy would you use to motivate the individual? (It could be another theory entirely—do you have a better one?)

4. You are the new laboratory manager, and you find that the employees are not motivated. After a few weeks you go for coffee with some of the techs and find out that they do not believe administration will reward them if they do a good job. What is the problem? What would you do to increase their motivation?

5. You are the laboratory manager and you have been told by the hospital administration that you will have no raise money this year to distribute to the employees in the laboratory. What could you do to motivate your staff?

6. A new member of the phlebotomy team comes to you and is ready to quit after only two weeks on the job after training. In discussions you can't really find out why the individual is dissatisfied, except that he keeps saying he just doesn't like the work. Upon investigation, you find out that this individual has been sent daily to the nursery and has not been successful in performing his job. What is the problem? What would you do?

Chapter 14

Leadership

Jane Hudson, Ph.D., MT(ASCP)SM, CLS(NCA)

OBJECTIVES

Upon completion of this chapter the learner will be able to

1. Define *leadership*. *(Level I)*
2. Discuss the following leadership theories: *(Level II)*
   a. Tannenbaum and Schmidt theory
   b. McGregor X and Y theory
   c. Blake and Mouton theory
   d. Hersey-Blanchard theory
   e. Fielder theory
3. Discuss factors that impact leadership. *(Level II)*
4. Evaluate leadership styles as indicated in the exercises. *(Level III)*
5. Formulate solutions for the case studies. *(Level III)*

TOPIC SUMMARY

A leader is responsible for providing the conditions necessary for employees to accomplish the work of the organization. Leadership is employing management skills, people skills, and vision to accomplish the work of the organization. Therefore, the leader must understand the **interaction of the employee and the institution, leadership approaches, the situation,** and **workplace structure and function.**

Getzels and Guba (1957) described the interaction of the individual and the institution as a social system. The individual has a personality and need-dispositions that should be matched with the institution's role and expectations as illustrated in Figure 14–1. If the match is compatible, then the social system is efficient and effective, and both the institution and individual will be satisfied. However, if there is an incompatible match, dissatisfaction will occur for either the institution or the individual or both. For example, suppose an employee does not like to interact with other people, yet the employee is hired for the supervisory position in hematology. This is not a personality-role match, and inefficiency and ineffectiveness as well as dissatisfaction may result. If the need-disposition of the employee is to be able to function independently without supervision and the institution expects the employee to report daily to a supervisor, the need-disposition of the employee does not match the role expectations of the institution, and inefficiency, ineffectiveness, and dissatisfaction may occur. Therefore, it is imperative that employees are selected to match the institution position and also that employees not accept institutional positions that do not match their personality and need-dispositions. The interaction between institution and individual, between role and personality, and between job expectations and need-dispositions are critical to production of desired

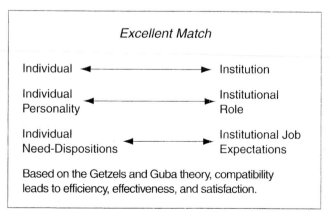

FIGURE 14–1. Matching Institution with Individual

behavior and efficiency. This interaction could be defined as the **corporate culture,** which is one of the factors that influences leadership success.

Another factor that impacts leadership success is **management style.** According to Tannenbaum and Schmidt (1973), styles can be plotted on a continuum from authoritative to democratic. McGregor's (1966) X theory relates to the authoritative leader, whereas the Y theory relates to the democratic leader (see Figure 14–2).

Blake and Mouton (1980) described five types of management situations: 1) the impoverished management characterized by a low concern for people and production, 2) the authority-compliance management characterized by a low concern for people but a high concern for production, 3) the middle-of-the-road management characterized by medium concern for people and production, 4) country club management characterized by high concern for people but low concern for production, and 5) the team management characterized by high concern for people and production. Halpin (1959), Stogdill (1974), and Hersey-Blanchard (1969) described initiating structure (task orientation) and consideration (relationship orientation) and the requirement that leaders mix these styles. If a manager is just concerned about people, then the work will not be performed. On the other hand, if the manager is just concerned about the work, people will be exploited. Therefore, both structure and consideration are required characteristics of the leader. Figure 14–3 compares the Blake and Mouton theory with the Halpin, Stogill, and Hersey-Blanchard theories.

Fiedler (1967) indicated that the style used by the leader may vary according to the **situation,** with a very favorable or very unfavorable situation requiring a task-oriented leader and a moderately favorable or moderately unfavorable situation requiring a relationship-oriented leader. Hersey and Blanchard (1969) described four leadership situations: 1) when the employee first begins the job, the employee is in the telling situation because the leader spends most of his or her time telling the employee how to do the job; 2) as the employee demonstrates job maturity, the leader moves the employee into the selling situation, because the leader is still telling the employee how to do the job, but now commenting on the job performance; 3) with continued maturity the employee is moved into the participating situation, and the leader continues to monitor the employee but no longer has to tell the employee how to do the job; and 4) when the employee has reached total job maturity, the employee is in the delegating situation, and the leader leaves the employee alone to do the work. As the employee matures, the leadership style changes (see Figure 14–4).

Corporate culture, management style, and the situation all impact the success of the leader. The corporate culture and the situation are usually preset factors. When considering a leadership position in an institution, corporate culture and the situation are two factors to investigate before deciding that a specific leadership will be effective. Leadership style does vary with the situation and the corporate culture if the leader is flexible. However, if the leader is not flexible, then serious damage can occur both to the leader and to the institution if the management style is inappropriate for the corporate culture and situation. For example, suppose a technologist assumes a position as hematology

```
Comparison of Tannenbaum and Schmidt's
Continuum and McGregor's X and Y Theory

Democratic           Continuum           Autocratic
Style                                    Style

Y Leader                                 X Leader
```

FIGURE 14–2. Management Styles

Blake and Mouton	Halpin, Stogdill, Hersey-Blanchard
Impoverished management	Low task and relationship orientation
Authority-compliance management	High task orientation, low relationship orientation
Middle-of-the-road management	Medium task and relationship orientation
Country club management	High relationship orientation, low task orientation
Team management	High task and relationship orientation

FIGURE 14–3. Comparison of Blake and Mouton Theory and Halpin, Stogdill, and Hersey-Blanchard Theories

Situation	Management Style
Situation 1: Employee new to job (very immature regarding the job)	Telling—instructions only
Situation 2: Employee has mastered some of the job, but needs supervision (somewhat immature regarding the job)	Selling—instructions and verification of good performance
Situation 3: Employee has mastered the job, but still needs verification of good performance (mature regarding the job)	Participating—verification of good performance
Situation 4: Employee has mastered the job and is confident (very mature regarding the job)	Delegating—no instructions or verification needed

FIGURE 14–4. Hersey-Blanchard Situational Management Theory

supervisor in a hematology department that is failing to reach its mission. The leader assumes an autocratic leadership style in order to correct the problems of the department. During the year, the leader hires new, motivated employees, and the department is functioning well. The leader now assumes a more democratic leadership style that allows the department employees to take part in controlling the department. If the leader had maintained the autocratic style with the motivated new employees, the employees probably would leave or revolt against the manager.

In addition to corporate culture, management style, and the situation, the leader must also recognize that the structure and function of the workplace impact leadership success. These include **authority** (empowerment to do a job), **delegation of authority** (authority transferred to another), **formal group** (those established by the organization), **informal group** (those evolving from the work group), **departmentalization** (specialization), **decentralization** (decision made close to task), **span of control** (number of people one supervises), **unity of command** (one boss), **scalar principle** (chain of command), and **exception principle** (ability to do job without checking with supervisor).

Authority empowers one to do a job and is essential for the leader to accomplish the task. Authority can be divided into position authority (that authority derived from holding the position) and personal authority (that authority derived from characteristics of the leader). The optimal situation would be for the leader to have both position and personal authority, in which case the subordinates would follow the leader very willingly. However, situations often exist in which the leader does not hold personal authority. In this case the subordinates follow, but only because of the position authority held by the leader. In addition, occasionally the leader has personal authority but no position authority, and the subordinates follow because they like the leader's characteristics. **Delegation of authority** can and should be done in some cases, but for the right reasons. Some tasks cannot be delegated. Delegation should be used as an opportunity for subordinate learning, but never as a punishment. When a task is delegated, the authority transfers to the one to whom the task was delegated. However, the responsibility for delegating the task remains with the manager. The manager should delegate wisely, because to reverse the delegation decision will cause problems in the future. **Formal and informal groups** are found in every organization; the leader must therefore recognize group structure and devise ways to work with both groups. The formal group is most influenced by the position that a leader holds, whereas the informal group is most often influenced by the personal characteristics of the leader.

Leadership is also impacted by **departmentalization,** which can influence the flexibility of a situation; however, departmentalization may also bring expertise to the situation. **Decentralization** is usually the operational style of choice unless extreme control is needed over the situation. The number of individuals one supervises (**span of control**) is also critical in making good decisions and being adequately informed. If one supervises too few subordinates, then the system is not efficient. On the other hand, if one supervises too many subordinates, attention to detail is lost. In any position it is essential to have one boss (**unity of**

command) or conflicting signals can be given and received. Also, with one boss, accountability is more powerful. The chain of command (**scalar principle**) can also influence leadership. Although it is important to respect the chain of command, it is essential that communications in the chain are adequate to provide for free information flow for making good decisions. The **exception principle** enables the subordinate to feel free to do the task without being afraid that the supervisor will disapprove.

A leader must continually evaluate all the elements that impact leadership success and relate their desirability to the particular work situation. Changes may be required in order for the work of the organization to be accomplished and thus for leadership to be a success.

BIBLIOGRAPHY

Blake, Robert R., and Jane S. Mouton. 1980. *The versatile manager: A grid profile.* Homewood, Ill.: Dow Jones-Irwin.

Fiedler, Fred E. 1967. *A theory of leadership effectiveness.* New York: McGraw-Hill.

Getzels, Jacob W., and Egon G. Guba. 1957. Social behavior and the administrative process. *School Review* 65: 423–41.

Halpin, Andrew W. 1959. *The leadership behavior of school superintendents.* Chicago: University of Chicago, Midwest Administration Center.

Hersey, Paul, and Kenneth H. Blanchard. 1969. *Management of organizational behavior—Utilizing human resources.* Englewood Cliffs, N.J.: Prentice-Hall.

McGregor, Douglas. 1966. *Leadership and motivation—Essays of Douglas McGregor.* Cambridge, Mass.: M.I.T. Press.

Stogdill, Ralph M. 1974. *Handbook of leadership—A survey of theory and research.* New York: Free Press, Macmillian.

Tannenbaum, Robert, and Warren H. Schmidt. 1973. How to choose a leadership pattern. *Harvard Business Review* 51, no. 3: 162–71. Original article in March-April 1958 issue.

This, Leslie E. 1974. *A guide to effective management—Practical applications from behavioral science.* Reading, Mass.: Addison-Wesley.

Varnadoe, Lionel A. 1996. *Medical laboratory management and supervision.* Philadelphia: F. A. Davis.

INTERNET RESOURCES

Eagle's flight. <www.eaglesflight.com/leadership/index.html>

QUESTIONS

1. Leadership is *(Objective 1, Level I)*
   a. employing management skills
   b. employing people skills
   c. providing vision
   d. assuming a position
   e. A, B, and C
   f. All of the above

2. Discuss the following leadership theories: *(Objective 2, Level II)*
   a. Tannenbaum and Schmidt theory

   b. McGregor X and Y theory

   c. Blake and Mouton theory

d. Hersey-Blanchard theory

e. Fielder theory

3. What are two types of authority? *(Objective 3, Level I)*

4. A laboratory is having difficulty organizing the work submitted to the laboratory, and the technologists are having difficulty retaining the knowledge required for all the specialized tests. The leader might employ which of the following tactics? *(Objective 3, Level II)*
   a. delegation
   b. departmentalization
   c. only one boss
   d. manager reviewing every test

5. How would the answer in #4 impact the manager? *(Objective 3, Level II)*

6. Communications in the laboratory are primarily through the gossip channel, and sometimes facts are distorted. What type of group is operating and what can be done? *(Objective 3, Level II)*

7. Discuss the leadership style that will be accepted by the group in a very good, mediocre, or very bad situation. *(Objective 3, Level II)*

EXERCISES

Completion of the exercises will enhance your knowledge of leadership. *(Objective 4, Level III)*

1. Attend hospital administration meetings and laboratory meetings and describe the leadership style of the two administrative levels. Discuss whether administrative level dictates somewhat the leadership style.

2. Survey medical technologists to determine which leadership style is preferred in your particular laboratory.

3. A project is assigned to the group. The group elects one of its members as designated leader for the project. The designated leader chooses a particular leadership style to use during the group project. After the project is completed, the group members evaluate the leadership style used by the designated leader.

CASES

For each case that follows, answer the questions and formulate solutions as appropriate.
(Objective 5, Level III)

1. Using the Hersey-Blanchard model, in what situation would you place each of the following employees?
   a. Employee has been in the job for ten years and operates independently with exceptional proficiency.
   b. Employee is new to your lab.
   c. Employee has worked independently, but recently has not produced as well as he or she is capable.
   d. Employee has been in the microbiology department one month and is still learning.

2. Given the four employees in #1, how would you, the leader, relate to each in their present situation?

3. How would you, the leader, use the Getzels and Guba theory to decide whether an employee should be moved into a supervisor position?

4. Think of a very good management situation. How would you as the leader lead? Think of a difficult management situation. How would you as the leader lead? Does your style change? Do you agree with Fielder's motivation theory?

5. Using the Blake and Mouton model, how would you describe your leadership style in a good management situation? In a difficult management situation?

6. You have the opportunity to create your own laboratory. Describe how you would organize your laboratory in regard to the following: decentralization, departmentalization, unity of command, scalar principle, span of control, exception principle, and delegation of authority.

Chapter 15

Team Building

Paula Holland, M.Ed., MT(ASCP)

OBJECTIVES

Upon completion of this chapter the learner will be able to

1. Identify the stages of team development. *(Level I)*
2. Discuss three activities that enhance team development in the early stages. *(Level II)*
3. Discuss the benefits of work teams. *(Level II)*
4. Define the meaning of quality circle. *(Level I)*
5. Discuss several characteristics of a quality circle. *(Level II)*
6. List the benefits of quality circles. *(Level I)*
7. Discuss strategies of the manager that would enhance the development of teams. *(Level II)*
8. Develop a list of activities that enhance the team environment and that a manager could use in the clinical laboratory. *(Level III)*
9. Analyze the case studies and propose solutions. *(Level III)*

TOPIC SUMMARY

Every person wants to be a part of a group or team. Within each team, each person assumes a particular role. Every person should feel comfortable in his or her particular role.

Once the team is formed, it is then ready to set goals. Every person has responsibilities that lead to the success of the team. To motivate the team to achieve its desired goals, one should take the time to determine the individual needs of each team member.

Phases of team development as identified by Tuckman (1965) include:

Forming—bringing the team members together.

Storming—members determine their roles on the team

Norming—determining standards of behavior for the team members

Performing—working together as a team for the common goals

Within the **Forming** stage, the rules, goals, and behavior of the team are established. The **Storming** stage or phase is where the conflict among team members generally occurs. It helps teams to go through this stage—challenges do not have to be counterproductive. Learning to deal with differences is extremely necessary, and the storming stage allows for differences of opinions among its members. In the **Norming** stage, team members learn to focus on the goals rather than on the differences of opinions. The last phase of team building, the **Performing** phase, is where the individuals come together as a team. There is more agreement among members to obtain results, and they learn not to take differences in opinions personally. It is within this phase that team members learn to be proud of team accomplishments.

The success of the organization, its team, and its members, depends on embracing change. Every organization has learned to function with less people. Therefore, the team members' roles have increased. Productivity depends on the trust of its team members for one another. Focusing on the team members' relationships and keeping these relationships as a top priority will result in successful operation of the organization. Team leaders should seek to drive the team in developing a stronger cohesiveness. Identifying conflicts early is key.

Constant communication between team members is a must and should be fostered by its leaders. Leaders should encourage team members to develop better listening skills, which will improve communications.

Suggestions for early stages of team development follow:

- Have the team work together on short-term challenges. This allows for the process of working together, talking to each other, and building relationships.
- Have team meetings outside the work environment. Team social events or parties are great ways to allow members the opportunity to socialize without the pressures of work-related tasks.
- Have the team research traits of successful teams. This will encourage these traits in your own team members.
- Engage in team development exercises. A team development exercise is one that focuses on developing positive images of team members. One example of a team activity to identify positive qualities of individual team members follows: Divide the entire team into groups and give each group the same number of blank cards as there are group members. Each group member is then given one card and asked to write his or her name. The cards are then rotated to other members of the group who identify positive qualities about the group member named on the card. When everyone in the group is finished, all cards are taken up, but kept as a group. The stack of cards of one group is given to another group and the exercise repeats. This can continue until several qualities are obtained on each individual or the stacks are rotated through each of the groups. All cards are then retrieved and each person is given his or her personal card with the positive characteristics listed.

Many benefits arise from implementation of work teams. Benefits include 1) team members are empowered to do the work, 2) shared responsibilities relieve individual stress of employees, 3) a sense of ownership develops when employees are involved in decision making, 4) a sense of accomplishment develops when employees learn more about the overall work process, 5) communication barriers are brought down when the employee is allowed to freely contribute ideas, 6) staff retention increases when employees are more satisfied with their jobs, and 7) productivity of staff is increased.

Team building is necessary for the best employee performance. Teamwork helps to enhance employee work performances above that which would normally be attained. Motivation to perform a particular task or function comes from the individual who is to perform the work. It is the work of an effective laboratory manager to provide the right conditions for this to occur. Relevant team building points worthy of remembering as a manager are the following:

- Develop a list of the employee motivators (e.g., recognition for outstanding work) and refer to the list regularly to ensure that all these motivators are being utilized systematically to keep the interest and enthusiasm of the employee at a high level. The list of employee motivators, other than money, might include such items as increasing the level of responsibility of the member, honoring the individual publicly or with a change in title or work space, designating a parking space for a set period of time, giving an employee of the month award, and so on.
- Verbalize performance expectations. It is also important to put these expectations in writing and relate the individual performance to the goals and objectives of the laboratory. Ensure that the staff stays informed about the successes as well as the setbacks that the laboratory is experiencing. It is important to communicate future plans or projects of the lab to all staff as these plans are developed and allow for staff input when possible. Allow staff members the control over the work they do and they will develop ownership in the organization. This will give rise to increased interest in the company as a whole, and they will try much harder to do a good job.
- Praise the staff for their hard work. A phrase that is most effective and a memorable motto is to remember to praise employees in public and discipline them in private.
- Encourage both personal and professional growth in employees.
- Have an open-door policy, and make certain that you appear approachable to staff when conflicts arise that they need to discuss. Keep in mind that a good laboratory manager will not fly off the handle or take matters too personally. A good manager will not allow a few problems to overshadow a positive outlook. It is important to consider an employee's feelings.
- Remember to hire people that are smarter than you—this truly shows that you are a wise manager.

- If you want to know what motivates your employees, simply ask them.
- Value the minds of employees as resources.
- Manage like you have no authority whatsoever. Lead by the vary quality of your ideas.
- Find the squeaky wheels and don't jump so quickly to oil them. A great idea may surface.
- When listening and collaborating with an employee, seek to understand and not just to find agreement.
- Encourage employees to bring solutions with their problems or concerns.

An example of how work teams can be effectively utilized is demonstrated in the concept of **quality circles.** Quality circles (or self-directed teams) is a term used to describe a program in which employees (team members) come together as a group to solve work issues. They do not significantly change the management structure of power but make it more acceptable to the employees. Major characteristics of a quality circle are the following:

- The program centers around management having a simple desire to build up their employees both professionally and personally.
- The program is not mandated by management but is strictly voluntary.
- All employees need to be involved—input is desired from all of the people.
- Group effort is the focus, not individual effort.
- Both the employees who participate and management should be trained in the quality circle process, and channels should be available for expressing concerns to avoid frustration.
- Each person helps other team members grow.
- A creative environment will develop when members and management encourage and support any and all ideas.
- All tasks that the teams assume must relate to their work.
- All team members need to develop an attitude of partnering for the benefit of improving the quality of their work.
- Rewards are normally not monetary, but include items such as patches, hats, T-shirts, certificates, and so on—all members of the group will be recognized.
- There are team leaders who are selected by the team members and they serve in a facilitating role to guide the team through its initial development stages.

Benefits of quality circles include the following:

- Increased productivity
- Increased communication from team member to team member and from team to management
- Decrease in the number of errors
- A more positive environment
- Increased quality of patient care
- Increased job satisfaction

Quality circles are structured so that each team member's contribution is enhanced. Figure 15–1 illustrates the quality circle structure. The quality circle is totally comprised of employees (team members), and management personnel are not given a place in the structure. Remember, quality circles are employees (team members) coming together to solve work issues.

The **steering committee** develops the policies for the quality circle program and sets the objectives and guides the program. This committee chooses the facilitator(s) and meets with the facilitator(s) on a regular basis.

The **facilitator** should have excellent people skills and will be responsible for training team leaders and members. This person should also be able to work well with management as well as the team members. This individual will be responsible for operational duties of the team, which include directing, implementing, evaluating, and recording keeping.

Teams are made up of members that identify and resolve issues. They will also select their team leaders, and this person may or may not be a supervisor.

The **team leader** is selected by the team members after the facilitator has served the function of laying guidelines for the team to build upon. The team leader directs the team through the goal-oriented process.

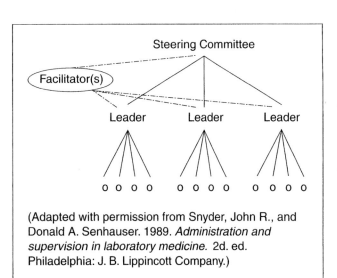

(Adapted with permission from Snyder, John R., and Donald A. Senhauser. 1989. *Administration and supervision in laboratory medicine.* 2d. ed. Philadelphia: J. B. Lippincott Company.)

FIGURE 15–1. Quality Circle Structure

The decision to choose to implement quality circles needs to be studied thoroughly by management. Factors to consider regarding cost and benefits of quality circles follow:

- Cost in time and dollars—the team will meet approximately one to two hours a week on hospital time.
- The existing management style should be able to work alongside the quality circle.
- It takes time to develop this type of atmosphere.

Effective work teams are responsible for the organization accomplishing its goals and objectives. In addition, effective work teams allow each team member to accomplish personal goals and objectives. Therefore, the manager must effectively utilize work teams for the benefit of the organization and its employees. Quality circles are an example of how one might increase employee participation. A win-win situation for the organization and the employee is produced when the work environment encourages effective work teams.

BIBLIOGRAPHY

Burdick, Ida M. 1995. Implementing work teams in the clinical laboratory. *Medical Laboratory Observer* (January): 44–47.

Dianda, Jeanne. 1995. Laboratory teambuilding: Rx for success. *Medical Laboratory Observer* (February): 40–44.

Frings, Christopher S. 1993. Setting a climate for motivating your staff. *Medical Laboratory Observer* (October): 47–50.

Synder, John R., and Donald A. Senhauser. 1989. *Administration and supervision in laboratory medicine*. 2d Ed. Philadelphia: J. B. Lippincott.

Tuckman, B. 1965. Developmental sequence in small groups. *Psychological Bulletin* 63: 384–89.

INTERNET RESOURCES

Arnold Sanow, MBA, CSP. <www.arnold-sanow.com/teambuilding.html>

College of William and Mary, Training and Technical Assistance Center. <www.wm.edu/TTAC/articles/transition/stages.html>

Martin's Rugby Coaching Archive. <www.rugbycoach.com/club/teambuild/building.htm>

The Teal Trust. <www.teams.org.uk/teambild/htm>

QUESTIONS

1. The stages of team development are *(Objective 1, Level I)*
    a. forming, talking, norming, performing
    b. planning, discussing, organizing, performing
    c. forming, storming, norming, performing
    d. planning, investigating, organizing, performing

2. Discuss three activities that enhance team development in the early stages. *(Objective 2, Level II)*

3. Discuss the benefits of work teams. *(Objective 3, Level II)*

4. A quality circle may be defined as *(Objective 4, Level I)*
    a. employees as a group solving work issues
    b. employees focusing on quality control
    c. employees organizing for benefits
    d. employers organizing for quality

5. Discuss the characteristics of a quality circle. *(Objective 5, Level II)*

6. List four benefits of quality circles. *(Objective 6, Level I)*

7. Discuss five managerial strategies that could be used to enhance teams. *(Objective 7, Level II)*

EXERCISES

Completion of the exercises will enhance your knowledge of team building. *(Objective 8, Level III)*

1. Interview a laboratory manager and determine the techniques this individual uses to enhance teams in the laboratory.
2. Observe a group solving a problem. Identify the activities of the group that enhance team building.
3. Through class discussion identify how your class/group went through the forming, storming, norming, and performing stages.
4. Create a team development exercise that could be used for a laboratory or health-care group.
5. Develop the strategies that you, as a manager, would use to enhance team building in your laboratory.
6. We have all been members of groups that worked as a team and members of groups that did not work as a team. List the activities that enhanced and destroyed the team environment. Once you have individually identified the activities, discuss as a group your list of activities and develop a list of activities that you would like to use to enhance the team environment.

CASES

Analyze the following case studies and propose solutions. *(Objective 9, Level III)*

1. You are the new manager of a laboratory. After two weeks of observation, you note the following environment in the laboratory:
   ☐ The employees are divided into department groups that don't relate well.

- When a specimen is received in the laboratory in one department that is overwhelmed with work, other techs in other departments that do not have any work to do will not volunteer to help the techs in the overwhelmed department.

As the new manager, you would like to establish a team environment. How would you encourage a team environment?

2. The hospital administrator has just informed you, the laboratory manager, that a new outreach contract will increase your laboratory workload by twenty percent for four months; however, no new positions will be given to the laboratory. You have a team approach in your laboratory. How would you handle this challenge using the team approach?

Chapter 16

Conflict Management
Jane Hudson, Ph.D., MT(ASCP)SM, CLS(NCA)

OBJECTIVES

Upon completion of this chapter the learner will be able to

1. Define *conflict management*. (Level I)
2. Name and discuss the five approaches to handling conflict. (Level II)
3. Analyze the conflict management approach used in the laboratory. (Level III)
4. Formulate solutions and choose the most appropriate conflict management approach for the case studies. (Level III)

TOPIC SUMMARY

Conflict occurs when there is disagreement between two or more parties. Conflict management is the act of handling these disagreements. When groups work, disagreements arise; therefore, the manager of the group needs to be familiar with and be able to utilize techniques regarding conflict management. Some conflict (tension) within a work group is considered valuable for progression toward the work goal. However, there comes a point at which the conflict (tension) interferes with accomplishing the goal of the work.

Five approaches to handling conflict are **avoiding, accommodating, compromising, forcing,** and **collaborating.** The appropriateness of the approach depends on the situation. A manager who is familiar with each approach can select the one best utilized in each situation addressed. A discussion of each of these approaches follows:

Avoiding—One approach to conflict would be to simply avoid the issue. This approach is defined as a lose-lose approach—neither side is satisfied. This approach would be selected by someone who believed 1) the issue is not important, 2) there is no chance of solving the issue in a self-satisfying way, 3) it is best to postpone addressing the issue to obtain more information or let the group calm down, or 4) addressing the issue is more damaging than not. This approach usually indicates low openness to and low respect for other people's ideas and an unassertive behavior.

Accommodating—This conflict approach would be to simply adapt to the circumstances of the issue. This approach is defined as a lose-win approach—one side is satisfied, but the other is not. This approach would be selected by someone who believed 1) peace in the group is more desirable than prevailing, 2) it is more important to put the other person in debt to you than to prevail, or 3) the point is lost or the point was wrong in the first place. This approach usually indicates low openness, but high respect for other people's ideas, and an unassertive behavior.

Compromising—One approach to conflict would be for each side to give up some of its demands regarding the issue. This approach is defined as a lose-lose approach—neither side is satisfied. This approach would be selected by someone who believed 1) the solution is temporary, 2) an answer is needed quickly, or 3) equal arguments are found on both sides. This approach usually indicates a moderate openness and respect for other people's ideas and a moderate assertive behavior.

Forcing—This approach to conflict would require that one party exert power over the other party, thus forcing acceptance of the issue. This approach is defined as a win-lose approach—only one side is satisfied. This approach would be selected by someone who believed 1) action is needed immediately, 2) the action to be taken is unpopular, or 3) the issue is important and not debatable. This approach usually indicates a high openness, but not much respect for ideas of others, and an assertive behavior.

Collaborating—One approach to conflict would be to work together to solve the issue. This approach is defined as a win-win approach—both sides are satisfied. This approach would be selected by someone who believed 1) the best solution will be reached by sharing and collaborating, 2) commitment is essential, and 3) both views of the issue are important. This approach usually indicates a high openness and much respect for other people's ideas and an assertive behavior.

As you will note, assertive and nonassertive behavior are mentioned when discussing the conflict management approaches. With **assertive behavior,** individual rights are expressed. Assertive behavior involves open and honest communications from the individual involved regarding what will be required in order to perform the job. Assertive behavior is required in the forcing or collaborating approaches. With **unassertive behavior,** the individual does not express his or her rights, thus this behavior is noted in the avoiding and accommodating approaches of handling conflicts.

So which is the best approach to use? Each of these approaches is appropriate in certain situations. Thus, the first and crucial step in conflict management is to gather information regarding the situation so that the appropriate approach can be employed. Once the details of the situation are fully understood, the appropriate conflict management approach can be selected and implemented.

Conflict is inevitable in work situations and some level of conflict is good for the work environment. However, when conflict causes a lack of productivity, the manager must manage the conflict. Familiarity with the different conflict management approaches will enhance the manager's ability to work with diverse work groups in diverse situations to get the work done.

BIBLIOGRAPHY

Conflict Management. *Professional issues.* (Available from the American Society for Clinical Laboratory Science, 7910 Woodmont Ave., Suite 530, Bethesda, MD 20814.)

Zuker, Elaina. *How to assert yourself for results.* Success Enhancement Series. An Audio Cassette Program. (Available from Day-Timer, Inc., One Day-Timer Plaza, Allentown, PA 18195-1551.)

INTERNET RESOURCES

Association for Conflict Resolution. <www.acresolution.org>
Conflict Management Group. <www.CMGroup.org>
Experience Based Learning, Inc. <www.ebl.org/trc.html>

QUESTIONS

1. Conflict management is the act of handling _____ between two or more parties. *(Objective 1, Level I)*

2. Name and discuss the five approaches to handling conflict. *(Objective 2, Level II)*

3. Using the list below, choose the best conflict management approach for the following situations: *(Objective 4, Level III)*

    a. Fire in the building: _____

    b. Supervisor insists that a certain action be taken: _____

    c. Both views are important in reaching the best solution and time is not a factor:
    _____

    Possible approaches:
    Avoiding
    Accommodating
    Compromising
    Forcing
    Collaborating

EXERCISES

Completion of the exercises will enhance your knowledge of conflict management. *(Objective 3, Level III)*

1. Identify and record specific situations in the laboratory that involved the use of each conflict approach. As a group, share situations and discuss the appropriateness of the approach.

2. Interview one of the laboratory managers and ask how the manager believes conflicts are best resolved. Analyze the manager's approach or approaches.

CASES

Following are five cases involving clinical laboratory conflicts. Using the information given, select the best approach for each case. A group may work together and select the best approach as determined by the group consensus. If this is a group project, you may want to choose different points of view and solve the cases using a different approach for each case, thus experiencing the feelings associated with each approach. Also, if this is a group project, the roles in each case may be acted out. The players and the group analyze the feelings of the parties involved in the case. *(Objective 4, Level III)*

1. Nurse Precise always sends the requests for two-hour blood glucose to be drawn at 3:00 P.M. This is the time that the five day-shift phlebotomists are leaving and the one evening phlebotomist, Phleb, comes in. Phleb, although working very hard, has difficulty getting all the blood collected on time. Phleb has come to you, the manager, upset because lately Nurse Precise has been telling him what a poor job he is doing. He is almost ready to quit.
    a. What is the conflict?
    b. What style is appropriate?
    c. What would you do?

2. A fire starts in Micro Lab and the fire alarm goes off. The procedure is to evacuate the building when the fire alarm rings. Rumor, Idle, and Chatter are gathered in the hall debating whether they will leave the lab or stay and catch up on the gossip while the others leave. You, the manager, pass them on your way out of the building.
   a. What is the conflict?
   b. What style is appropriate?
   c. What would you do?

3. Mr. Control, the hospital administrator, walks through the lab one day and later in the day writes you, the manager, a note requesting that the lab personnel avoid wearing jeans in the future for the professional reputation of the hospital.
   a. What is the conflict?
   b. What style is appropriate?
   c. What would you do?

4. Mr. Guy and Ms. Friendly have worked together in chemistry for five years and have been the best of pals. Recently, Mr. Handsome joined the chemistry section and you, the chemistry supervisor, noticed that Mr. Handsome and Ms. Friendly are taking coffee breaks together, leaving Mr. Guy in the lab. Mr. Guy comes to you and complains that Ms. Friendly is not carrying her workload and asks that you speak to her about it.
   a. What is the conflict?
   b. What style is appropriate? (at first)
   c. What would you do? (at first)

5. The Hematology and Chemistry departments share a technologist. Both departments must complete their quality control on the instruments at the beginning of the day shift before patient testing can begin. Both departments approach you, the manager, wanting the shared technologist to do the quality control work; however, the technologist cannot do all the quality control work within the time allotted.
   a. What is the conflict?
   b. What style is appropriate?
   c. What would you do?

Chapter 17

Telephone Etiquette

Beth Parham White, B.S., MT(ASCP), CLS(NCA)

OBJECTIVES

Upon completion of this chapter the learner will be able to

1. State why telephone etiquette is important. *(Level I)*
2. Discuss basic rules of telephone etiquette when answering a call. *(Level II)*
3. Discuss basic rules of telephone etiquette when making a call. *(Level II)*
4. Analyze your telephone etiquette. *(Level III)*
5. Plan a course of action for improvement of your telephone skills, based on data from your analysis in #4. *(Level III)*
6. Propose solutions given case studies involving telephone etiquette. *(Level III)*

TOPIC SUMMARY

For the clinical laboratory, as with almost any organization, the telephone is an important form of communication with the rest of the world. Whether it's to give a critical result to a physician, to answer a nurse's question, or to make an appointment for a patient, the laboratory relies heavily on the telephone to communicate with its customers. As a laboratory manager, it is important to make sure that all laboratory employees understand how to use the telephone in such a manner as to make a good impression on these customers. When customers call the laboratory, the type of response they get from the person who answers the phone will greatly influence their opinion of the laboratory and also the attitude they will have when dealing with the laboratory. *All* laboratory employees, not just the receptionists, must be aware of and follow some basic rules of telephone etiquette.

When answering a call

1. Be polite. Most people will respond to kindness with kindness. Sometimes it can be difficult to be polite when the person on the other end of the phone is being rude, but the best way to turn off rudeness is with kindness. A good rule to remember is to put yourself in the other person's shoes—maybe the person is in the middle of a frustrating or difficult situation. No matter what the other person's mood or attitude, being kind and polite can only improve the situation. If you must put someone on hold, be honest about approximately how long you think the wait may be and then thank the person for waiting. Avoid using a speakerphone whenever possible. When it is necessary to use one, make sure the other party is aware of it.
2. Be helpful. Listen carefully to what the caller needs and do your best to help. Remember that helping a customer on the phone is not an interruption of your job, it *is* your job. Instead of saying "I don't know," say "I'll find out for you" or "Let me check into that for you." Learn as much as possible about the laboratory and what goes on in each department. It will then be easier to connect a caller with someone who can help quickly.
3. Be interested. Make the callers feel like they are important to you and that you care about their problem or question.
4. Whenever possible, answer the phone yourself; don't rely on your voice mail unless absolutely necessary. When you do use voice mail, be sure to return your calls as quickly as possible.

When making a call

1. Again, be polite. Identify yourself and give the purpose of the call right away. Be sure to use a pleasant tone of voice. Smile—believe it or not, it will show in your voice. Respect the fact that the other person is probably very busy too. If possible, give the person being called the option of calling you back with information at a more convenient time.
2. If your call is answered by voice mail, be sure to leave complete information for the recipient so they can return your call. Give your name, phone number, and a short message stating the purpose of your call. Then, repeat your name and number for clarification.
3. If you are making a call to discuss any kind of confidential information and the person who answers the phone has you on a speakerphone, politely ask them to pick up the receiver to keep the information from being overheard by someone else.

Other rules of telephone etiquette:

1. Don't hover around a desk or office while waiting for someone to finish a phone call. The best course of action is to leave and come back at a later time.
2. If someone working with or near you is having a conversation on the phone, do your best not to eavesdrop. Again, a little politeness goes a long way when dealing with people—including coworkers.

Most hospitals today are putting a great deal of emphasis on customer satisfaction. Laboratory customers include not only patients and their families, but also coworkers in the lab, people from other departments in the hospital, and physicians. The telephone is a major link between the lab and these customers. By simply following the rules of telephone etiquette, and just using basic good manners, laboratory employees can help keep every customer as happy and satisfied as possible. If the laboratory manager makes telephone etiquette a priority in the laboratory, he or she will find that there will be fewer customer complaints and fewer conflicts to resolve.

BIBLIOGRAPHY

Rona's Telecom Tips #11. 2001. Retrieved March, 2002, from <www.andrewstel.com/tips11.html>

Telephone Etiquette. 2001. Retrieved March, 2002, from <http//cbpa.Louisville.edu/bruce/RegManagement/Mgmt325/Wed/six.htm>

Telephone Etiquette. 2001. Retrieved March 2002, from <www.iwantmymoney.com/telephon.htm>

Voice Mail Etiquette. 2001. Retrieved March, 2002, from <www.phone-srvcs.swt.edu/vmetiquette.html>

INTERNET RESOURCES

Andrews Telecommunications. <www.andrewstel.com/tips11.html>

University of Louisville College of Business and Public Administration. <http://cbpa.Louisville.edu/bruce/RegManagement/Mgmt325/Wed/six.htm>

Southwest Texas State University. <www.swt.edu/effective/upps/upps-05-03-10-att3.html>

QUESTIONS

1. Telephone etiquette is important to the laboratory operation because _____.

   (Objective 1, Level I)

2. Discuss the basic rules of telephone etiquette when answering the phone.
   (Objective 2, Level II)

3. Discuss the basic rules of telephone etiquette when making a call. *(Objective 3, Level II)*

EXERCISES

Completion of the exercises will enhance your knowledge of telephone etiquette. *(Objective 4, Level III and Objective 5, Level III)*

1. As a group, discuss some experiences that you may have had dealing with rude or uncooperative people on the telephone. Identify effective and ineffective telephone behavior.

2. Call four different businesses in the local area and ask for simple information such as
    where are you located?
    what are your hours of operation?
    do you have any job openings?

    Compare the telephone etiquette used at each place of business. Which was the best and why? Which was the worst and why?

3. Call your laboratory and ask some basic questions such as
    where are you located?
    do you perform anthrax and AIDS testing?
    what time is best to come to have my blood drawn?
    what do you do in the laboratory?

    Analyze the telephone etiquette in your laboratory and discuss as a class how the telephone etiquette skills could be improved. Discuss how you would implement change in your laboratory if you were the manager.

4. Analyze your personal telephone etiquette. Using your analysis, plan a course of action for improvement of your telephone skills.

CASES

Propose solutions for the following cases studies. *(Objective 6, Level III)*

1. You need to ask your laboratory manager a question, but when you approach her office, you see that she is on the phone. What should you do?

2. You are working in the blood bank when you receive a call from a nurse who needs a STAT potassium result. Which of the following is the best action to take and why?

    transfer her call to the Chemistry department

    transfer her call to the lab receptionist

    look up the result yourself in the lab computer

3. You make a call to the human resources department of the hospital to discuss an interview with a potential employee. When the call is answered, you suspect that you are on a speakerphone. What should you do?

Chapter 18

Customer Satisfaction/Public Relations Program

John Curry, M.Ed., MT(ASCP)DLM

OBJECTIVES

Upon completion of this chapter the learner will be able to

1. Identify the customer. *(Level I)*
2. Discuss the three *R*s of customer satisfaction. *(Level II)*
3. Formulate an argument for avoiding customer dissatisfaction using the customer service facts. *(Level III)*
4. Name seven strategies the health-care manager can use in providing an atmosphere that promotes customer satisfaction. *(Level I)*
5. Formulate a customer service policy for your laboratory. *(Level III)*
6. Formulate a plan of action for cases given in the chapter. *(Level III)*

TOPIC SUMMARY

Today the health-care industry has become more and more competitive. It has become imperative to treat customers with the utmost respect and dignity as well as to continue to provide quality care and reduce costs at the same time. In this competitive time, it is most important that the customer be satisfied with the service received during contact with the health-care institution. Every point of contact the customer has in a facility is a "moment of truth," because this is the particular moment when the customer forms a perception of the organization and its products and services. Anyone who is a recipient of an output of service should be considered a customer. In the health-care facility this includes patients, visitors, physicians and their staff, and other health-care providers within the facility.

There are three *R*s of customer satisfaction.

RESULTS: Customers expect superior results from our product or service. They expect the product or service to be the best value for their money.

RELATIONSHIP: Customers expect a relationship that is consistent with their value system.

RESOURCE: Customers expect you to be a resource to help them solve a problem.

Customer Service facts regarding satisfaction are the following:

1. Dissatisfied customers tell eight to ten people about their bad experience.
2. Satisfied customers normally will tell five people of the good service provided them.

3. It costs five times as much to attract a new customer as it does to keep an existing one.
4. Up to ninety percent of dissatisfied customers will not seek service from you again, and they normally will not tell you why.
5. The first thirty seconds of a meeting or phone call sets the tone for the remainder of the contact.
6. Ninety five percent of dissatisfied customers will become loyal customers again if their complaints are handled well and quickly.

Customer service and satisfaction begin with the employee. Employees ultimately want to do a good job, which enhances their self-concept and their satisfaction with the job. Performance recognition and feedback is essential to employees. In many industries quality of service is one of the few variables that distinguish a specific organization from its competition. Providing high quality of service can ultimately save your business money, because the same skills that lead to high customer satisfaction can also lead to increased employee productivity.

A customer is the most important person in your business, on the phone, in person, or by mail. Customers are not an interruption of the work—they are the reason for it. We are not doing a favor by servicing them; they are doing us a favor by giving us the opportunity to serve them. We are dependent on the customer. Customer service is the right people, doing the right thing, at the right time, in the right way, with the right attitude.

Ninety-eight percent of the time, businesses lose customers due to the customers' perceived indifference of the company or its employees. When things go wrong, apologize to the customer, offer fair solutions, treat them with respect, do something nice for them, and above all keep the promises you make. When dealing with a complaint, never promise anything that you cannot deliver. There is really no cost for servicing the customer; the cost lies in not doing it.

There are several strategies that can be used by the health-care manager to be sure the customer is satisfied with the service provided. These are not new strategies, and they can be used not only in the initial interview of a perspective employee but throughout every employee's and manager's career.

1. Hire service-savvy employees. This is done by using certain criteria when conducting the interview. Look for eye contact, a smile, pay attention to the tone of voice, the way the candidate speaks, their handshake, and the use of certain words such as *please* and *thank you*.
2. Establish high standards of customer service. Does your staff serve customers in a consistent manner? Establish service standards that clearly tell your staff what you expect of them when they are serving customers. Include these standards in your job description and appraisal tools.
3. Help your staff hear the voice of the customer. Give your staff the tools with which to work and allow them to hear and deal with the customer's complaints directly. They must be able to take ownership of the process.
4. Remove all barriers so that your staff can serve the customer. The first person you need to change is yourself. What is your own motive and bias against action? If you are determined to remove barriers for your staff, it is going to take work from everyone, including you.
5. If possible, reduce anxiety to increase satisfaction. Any situation can cause anxiety for the customer. This may be waiting for an appointment, finding a parking place, answering insurance questions, anticipating news on the results of tests, or worrying about being on time for the appointment. Anxiety can cause a downward spiral for the customer, which may affect the employee. As caregivers we can increase customer satisfaction by focusing on and preventing or reducing customer anxiety. Customers need to feel that we are going above and beyond our jobs to reduce their anxiety.
6. Help your staff cope better in a stressful atmosphere. Help the staff improve its workspace to reduce stress. Involve the staff in creating a space that fosters calmness, efficiency, and comfort. Help them develop coping skills that will allow them to take better care of themselves during stressful times. Try and build a supportive work team that helps each other in stressful times to avoid getting caught in the negative downward spiral of anxiety.
7. Always maintain your focus on service. Integrate your service focus into your everyday activities and routines.

All health-care facilities now have a public or customer relations program. This program is set up not only to provide education to all employees on the importance of their actions and body language in dealing with customers, but also to provide a mechanism through which customers voice their satisfaction or dissatisfaction with the service they receive. Health-care facilities spend millions of dollars each year to ensure that the customer will be satisfied and will return to the facility for care.

There are three words that are a secret to success in dealing with customers. These three words make the difference between average employees and top employees in most companies. Top people do what is expected ... *and then some;* they are thoughtful, considerate, and kind ... *and then some;* they meet their obligations and responsibilities fairly ... *and then some;* they are good friends and neighbors ... *and then some;* and they can be counted on in an emergency ... *and then some.*

One of the greatest innovative and creative challenges is to develop ways to astonish the customer and surpass expectations. The idea is intended to enhance your commitment to giving your customer the same level of service you would want; after all, both of you deserve it. In today's marketplace it is paramount for managers to hire competent, qualified, caring employees that are willing to go that extra mile and to put forth extra effort to provide exceptional customer service.

BIBLIOGRAPHY

Leebov, Wendy, Gail Scott, and Lolma Olson. 1998. *Achieving impressive customer service—7 strategies for the health care manager.* Chicago: American Hospital Publishing.

McAlindon, Harold R. 1993. *Great ideas on customer satisfaction.* Emeryville, Calif.: Parlay International.

McAlindon, Harold R. 1993/1998. *Innovating customer service.* Emeryville, Calif.: Parlay International.

Riley, Julia Balzer. 1999. *Customer service from A to Z—Making the connection.* Albuquerque, N.M.: Hartman Publications.

INTERNET RESOURCES

International Management Technologies, Inc. <www.imtc3.com/articles.html>

People Solution Strategies, Articles by Fred Martels. <www.thepeoplesolution.com/workplace_communication_feedback_articles.htm>

Quality Talk. <www.qualitytalk.com>

Shaw Resources, Customer-Inspired Management Systems. <www.shawresources.com/artind.htm>

QUESTIONS

1. Identify the customer. *(Objective 1, Level I)*

2. Discuss the three Rs of customer satisfaction. *(Objective 2, Level II)*

3. Formulate an argument for avoiding customer dissatisfaction using the customer service facts. *(Objective 3, Level III)*

4. Name seven strategies the health-care manager can use in providing an atmosphere that promotes customer satisfaction. *(Objective 4, Level I)*

   a. _____
   b. _____
   c. _____
   d. _____
   e. _____
   f. _____
   g. _____

EXERCISES

Completion of the exercises will enhance your knowledge of customer satisfaction. *(Objective 1, Level I and Objective 5, Level III)*

1. Write down a time when you were treated badly as a customer. List what the other person did to make it such a bad experience. What could the person or business have done to make things right in this situation?

2. Who are your customers? Make a list.

3. Teams develop a laboratory customer questionnaire, administer the questionnaire, and analyze the results. A report should be written with a presentation to relevant laboratory personnel. Recommendation for improvement of laboratory customer services should be formulated.

4. Interview the division responsible for assessing customer satisfaction, and prepare a report on all the activities done by the hospital regarding this area.

5. Formulate a customer service policy for your laboratory.

CASES

For the following cases, formulate a plan of action. *(Objective 6, Level III)*

1. The laboratory manager receives many complaints about the laboratory service from nurses in the neonatal unit. The complaints center around certain phlebotomists that collect the blood for PKUs. Specifically, the nurses perceive that certain phlebotomists are not proficient enough and must do multiple sticks. How would you as laboratory manager address this situation? Describe a program that you could implement that would keep this type of situation from developing.

2. A certain physician practice group constantly refuses to code the requests correctly for the laboratory testing. How would you as laboratory manager address this situation in light of the fact that the physician practice group is your customer?

3. You are seeking to obtain the laboratory testing business from a group of ten physicians. What initial questions would you ask? What customer service facts would be important to remember?

SECTION III MANAGEMENT ISSUES REGARDING THE WORK

Chapter 19

Clinical Laboratory Safety

Hermolee Thomas Barnes, M.Ed., MT(ASCP)

OBJECTIVES

Upon completion of this chapter the learner will be able to

1. Name the agency that establishes safety standards for the workplace. *(Level I)*
2. Identify important Occupational Safety and Health Administration (OSHA) mandates. *(Level I)*
3. Discuss the employer's responsibility regarding Right to Know. *(Level II)*
4. List the components of a blood-borne pathogens plan. *(Level I)*
5. State the Human Immunodeficiency Virus (HIV) and Hepatitis B Virus (HBV) needle stick risks for laboratory personnel. *(Level I)*
6. List the components of a chemical hygiene plan (CHP). *(Level I)*
7. Differentiate the responsibility of the clinical laboratory manager and the clinical laboratory safety officer regarding laboratory safety. *(Level III)*
8. Identify the five types of hazards in the clinical laboratory. *(Level I)*
9. Discuss safety precautions regarding the five types of hazards. *(Level II)*
10. Identify three major categories of barrier protection. *(Level I)*
11. Describe the National Fire Protection Association (NFPA) system of coding chemicals. *(Level II)*
12. Describe waste disposal requirements. *(Level II)*
13. Identify the requirements of record keeping. *(Level I)*
14. Evaluate the safety factors in a clinical laboratory. *(Level III)*
15. Propose solutions after examination of case studies. *(Level III)*

TOPIC SUMMARY

I. OVERVIEW

This chapter is arranged in an outline format in order to present the massive amount of safety material in a more concise and clear manner. The major sections of this chapter are Occupational Safety and Health Administration (OSHA) Requirements, General Safety, Types of Hazards in a Clinical Laboratory, Barrier Protection, First Aid, Hazard Warning Labels, Waste Disposal, and Record Keeping.

II. OSHA REQUIREMENTS

The Occupational Safety and Health Administration (OSHA) has mandated standards for employers to follow in protecting their employees from workplace hazards. These requirements are found in the Code of Federal Regulations publications. These publications address specific hazards and give stringent guidelines for protecting employees from these hazards. Some important OSHA mandates for clinical laboratories are:

A. **Hazard Communication,** standard 29 CFR 1910.1200

Employees have a "Right to Know" which hazardous substances they will encounter in the workplace and how to protect themselves from those hazards. An employer must make the information available to an employee within three working days of the employee's written request. Employers are obligated to provide training and education for employees who work with hazardous substances, upon initial assignment to the work area, and prior to a new assignment. Initial safety training and subsequent reviews must be documented in writing (at least annually) for all clinical laboratory employees.

B. **Occupational Exposure to Blood-borne Pathogens,** standard 29 CFR 1910.1030

A *blood-borne pathogens plan* should be developed and written as a safety guide for laboratory employees. The plan should describe the types of hazards employees may encounter in the workplace. It should also describe the education and training programs, workplace safeguards, barrier equipment, and medical surveillance that will be provided by the employer for protecting its employees. Blood and body fluids from any patient should be assumed to be infectious for HIV (Human Immunodeficiency Virus), HBV (Hepatitis B Virus), HCV (Hepatitis C Virus), and other blood-borne pathogens. The risk of acquiring HCV from a needle-stick injury involving an infected patient is about 1.8%, and the risk of acquiring HIV from a needle-stick injury involving an infected patient is 0.3%. In contrast, the risk of acquiring HBV infection following a needle stick from a Hepatitis B carrier is 6 to 30%. The risk may be as high as 30% if the carrier is HBeAg positive, but less than 6% if the carrier is HBeAg negative. The advent of the Hepatitis B vaccine has resulted in a 95% decrease of HBV positive health-care workers. An employer must offer the Hepatitis B vaccine to all of its employees, at no cost to the employees. An employee may decline the HBV vaccine, but should sign the employer's declination form.

C. **Occupational Exposure to Hazardous Chemicals in Laboratories,** standard 29 CFR 1910.1450

A chemical hygiene plan (CHP) should be developed and written as a safety guide for laboratory employees. The CHP should be used to teach employees about the hazards of chemicals and to instruct them in the use of personal protective equipment (PPE), safety devices, work practices, and measures to prevent or minimize exposure. The clinical laboratory safety officer or chemical safety coordinator should be designated to maintain the CHP and provide ongoing chemical safety training for laboratory personnel. This training should include policies and procedures for medical consultation and evaluation. The chemical safety instructor should be knowledgeable about chemicals used in the workplace. They must keep written records of the chemical inventory that includes 1) names, types, and amounts received; 2) types and amounts on hand; and 3) the date, type, amount, and methods of disposal.

D. **Respiratory Protection,** standard 29 CFR 1910.134 (e)(59)(916)

If a workplace task requires the use of respiratory protection, initial and ongoing training on the care, use, and hazards of respirators must be provided for the individual. When individuals are required to wear respirators in performance of their jobs, they must first be fit tested.

III. GENERAL SAFETY

The responsibility for clinical laboratory safety must be shared by everyone—employers, employees, and clinical students. Although the OSHA requirements were established to protect employees, health-care institutions have a moral responsibility to provide a safe work environment, safety training, and protective equipment for all providers and users of its facilities. The responsibility and authority vested in individuals are as follows:

A. **Safety Director**

The employer is ultimately responsible for safeguarding the health of its employees. An individual such as a laboratory director, pathologist, medical technologist/clinical laboratory scientist, or other qualified person may have the line authority to direct all or a portion of the laboratory's administration and technical operations; thus this same individual may assume responsibility for laboratory safety. The safety director has three primary responsibilities:

1. Oversee safety program and provide guidance to safety manager.
2. Provide leadership for an effective safety program.
3. Resolve problems involving employee and/or environmental safety.

B. **Clinical Laboratory Safety Officer** (an appointed position)
   1. Develop and maintain a laboratory safety training manual.
   2. Keep safety director updated on safety needs and safety conditions in the department.
   3. Conduct or coordinate safety training for supervisors. Assist with annual safety training of employees, as needed.
   4. Develop safe work methods and determine safety equipment needs.
   5. Document and maintain departmental safety training and accident investigation records. Conduct or coordinate periodic laboratory safety inspections.
   6. Represent the laboratory's interest on the facility's safety committee and/or coordinate activities for the laboratory safety committee.

C. **Clinical Laboratory Supervisor**
   1. Monitor the work habits of employees under his or her supervision.
   2. Assume responsibility for the safety of the work area and the equipment.
   3. Establish safe work practices for employees to follow.
   4. Attend safety-training programs conducted by the lab safety officer.

D. **Clinical Laboratory Employees and Students**
   1. Adhere to established safety policies and procedures.
   2. Read the material safety data sheets (MSDS) prior to using chemicals and other hazardous agents.
   3. Follow standard precautions when handling blood, tissue, and body fluids. Segregate and label all wastes that require special handling.
   4. Report injuries and safety hazards to supervisor immediately. Seek prompt attention for job injuries or incidents.
   5. Read the facility's blood-borne pathogen and chemical hygiene plans prior to working with blood specimens and chemicals.
   6. Know the location of the nearest fire safety equipment, eye wash station, and safety shower.
   7. Know the fire evacuation routes from your department and the facility.
   8. Use the required safety equipment as provided by the employer.

IV. TYPES OF HAZARDS IN A CLINICAL LABORATORY

A. **Biological Hazards**
   These are represented by exposure to an infectious agent(s). These agents may be blood borne or present in tissue and other body fluids. "Standard precautions" is a component of the blood-borne pathogens standard. It requires that all specimens and biological wastes be considered infectious. PPE should be worn when handling biohazards, and established work practices must be utilized to prevent exposure. Work practices should also be instituted to keep "clean" areas contamination free. Hand washing is the single most important method for preventing the spread of infection. Hands should be washed immediately
   - after contact with blood, body fluids, and contaminated materials
   - after removing gloves
   - before eating or smoking
   - before and after contact with patients
   - before leaving the laboratory
   - before and after using the restroom

B. **Chemical Hazards**—Types: flammable, corrosive, toxic, carcinogenic, reactive/explosive
   MSDSs must be maintained for every chemical used in the workplace. They should be immediately available for use by all employees who work with chemicals. MSDSs may be obtained from each chemical's manufacturer. The MSDSs should be made available for employees to reference prior to using the chemicals.

   PPE such as gloves, goggles, lab coats, and aprons should be worn when pouring and mixing chemicals, cleaning chemical spills, and performing other procedures where chemicals are used. Manipulations with chemicals that produce odors or fumes should be done underneath a fume hood or in a well-ventilated area.

   Containers of chemicals should be stored in a safety cabinet, below eye level. Storage containers must be compatible with the chemicals they contain. Only compatible chemicals should be stored together. Each chemical (including those in premade reagents) must be labeled with the chemical's name, specific hazard warnings, manufacturer's name and address, and an emergency telephone number. Used, outdated, and old or discolored chemicals must be promptly and properly discarded according to federal, state, and local regulations. The chemical safety/laboratory safety officer should be consulted if in doubt. When preparing acid-based solutions, the acid should always be added to its mixing base, which has been placed in the mixing flask.

C. **Physical Hazards**—(fires, cuts, punctures, bruises, falls, trips, slips, etc.) The use of approved, puncture-resistant, leak-proof, and disposable sharps containers for disposal of contaminated needles and blades may eliminate or minimize the possibility of being cut or punctured. Eliminating clutter in the work area and cleaning up spills as they occur will lessen the chance of slipping, tripping, falling, or bumping into things. All workplace accidents and incidents should be reported to the supervisor immediately!

Training in fire safety techniques should be provided for all personnel.* Flammable chemicals should be stored in a safety cabinet for flammable chemicals and away from ignition sources. Laboratory fires may be prevented through diligent awareness by laboratory employees. The first signs of fire (flames, smoke, burning smell) should be reported immediately, according to the organization's protocol.

When the fire alarm sounds or the fire emergency code is announced, evacuate the area promptly. Remove or assist patients and others to safety. Take the nearest exit leading away from the fire. Exit doors and aisles should never be blocked. Use an approved fire extinguisher as needed to provide safe passage from the hazard area. Two types of fire extinguishers are most commonly used in health care institutions. One is a combination of classes A, B, and C (Type ABC), and the other is a combination of classes B and C (Type BC). Type BC fire extinguishers are usually preferred for clinical laboratory use. Fire extinguishers are defined as

Class A (water base)—for paper and wood fires

Class B (foam or dry chemical)—for flammable liquids or gases.

Class C (foam or dry chemical)—for electrically based fires

Class D (graphite or dry chemical)—for metal fires

Fire safety and fire extinguisher training are OSHA requirements.

D. **Electrical Hazards**—(shocks, fires, burns) Electrical hazards may be lessened by using hospital-grade electrical plugs with appropriate grounding and by eliminating the use of extension cords and gang-plugs. Defective equipment (i.e., that which produces a "tingling sensation" (shock) when handled) should be unplugged immediately and labeled for maintenance (contaminated parts should be disinfected before sending out for repairs or having repair personnel come into the lab). Electrical outlets and laboratory equipment should be checked regularly and repaired or replaced as needed. Written verification of equipment maintenance and voltage checks should be maintained for certifying/accrediting agencies, for example CAP (College of American Pathologists), AABB (American Association of Blood Banks), and JCAHO (Joint Commission on Accreditation of Health Care Organizations).

E. **Radioactive Hazards**
For many clinical laboratories, radiation exposure levels are far less than required by state and federal regulators. When radionuclides are used or stored, the areas and the containers must be labeled with the radiation symbol.

V. BARRIER PROTECTION

A. **Engineering controls** are measures taken in the laboratory environment or equipment that help to eliminate or minimize exposure to laboratory hazards. These controls are the first line of defense against biological and chemical agents. Examples of engineering controls are 1) good ventilation, with regulated hourly air exchanges, 2) biological safety cabinets, for working aerosol producing or highly infections specimens, and 3) fume hoods, for mixing and pouring chemicals. Ventilation systems and hoods must be periodically checked and certified to ensure proper function. It is the responsibility of laboratory administration to implement and maintain engineering controls.

B. **PPE** worn by the laboratory worker acts as a barrier between the worker and workplace hazards. PPE should not be regarded as a primary barrier—rather, it is supplemental to engineering controls. Gloves, gowns and lab coats, masks, goggles, and face shields are all examples of PPE. Protective equipment should be provided and maintained by the employer.

C. **Work practices** are procedures established by the employer for employees to follow in order to minimize or prevent workplace injuries and exposure incidents. These practices prohibit mouth pipetting (should use mechanical devices); the recapping, breaking, and bending of needles and syringes (should use puncture-resistant containers); eating, drinking, smoking, and applying cosmetics in work areas. Enclosed, rubber-soled shoes should be worn in the workplace. All employees should be trained in safe work practices initially, upon employment, then at established intervals.

Biological spills should be contained and cleaned up as soon as possible. Appropriate PPE should be donned beforehand. Biological spills should be decontaminated with a 1:10 solution of freshly diluted household bleach (hypochlorite), a phenol solution, or other appropriate disinfectant. As a safety measure, work surfaces should be wiped daily or before and after use with a suitable disinfectant.

Chemical spills (acid and alkali) should be neutralized and absorbed with "spill kit" materials or other appropriate substances (see corresponding MSDS for details). Contaminated clean-up items should be disposed in red biohazard bags, or by other appropriate methods. Mercury poses a special hazard that must be dealt with according to EPA (Environmental Protection Agency) specifications. The facility's EPA-approved procedures for clean-up and disposal of spills should be followed. Appropriate PPE must be donned.

VI. FIRST AID

Serious injuries should be treated only by licensed medical professionals. First aid should be provided as a means of preventing further injury to the victim until professional medical care is available. First aid should be administered by an individual who has received training in first-aid and CPR (Cardiopulmonary Resuscitation) techniques. The injured individual should be directed to a medical provider immediately.

A. First aid for chemical burns of the skin or eye*
1. Remove contaminated clothing.
2. Flush with running water for at least fifteen minutes.
3. Identify the chemical(s) using the MSDS.
4. Seek prompt medical attention for the victim.
5. Document the incident for further investigation.

B. First aid for bleeding injury
1. Use a clean item to apply pressure over the cut (if cut does not contain glass or imbedded items).
2. Elevate the injured part above the victim's heart.
3. Seek prompt medical attention for the victim.
4. Document the incident for further investigation.

Eye-wash stations and safety showers should be easily accessible to areas where hazardous chemicals are used and periodically checked to document proper function.

VII. HAZARD WARNING LABELS

Hazard warning labels are required on containers of hazardous chemicals and on biological and chemical wastes containers. These labels must denote each type of hazard present. Most chemical manufacturers use the NFPA (National Fire Protection Association) system for labeling chemicals. The NFPA system consists of four small diamond-shaped symbols grouped into one larger diamond:

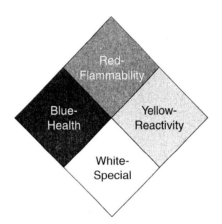

The left diamond is blue and warns of a health hazard. The top diamond is red and warns of a flammable hazard. The right diamond is yellow and warns of a reactive-stability hazard. The bottom diamond is white and is used to indicate specific properties of the chemical, for example, its incompatibility with water or radioactive properties. Areas where hazardous chemicals are stored and used should be labeled with the appropriate warning symbols.

VIII. WASTE DISPOSAL

Biohazardous wastes should be segregated from noninfectious and chemical wastes. Biohazard wastes should be discarded into red/red-orange bags in leakproof containers that have the universal biohazards symbol on them:

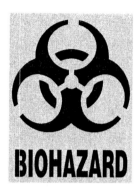

Biohazardous wastes must be incinerated or autoclaved to kill microorganisms prior to disposal. The puncture-resistant sharps containers for contaminated blades, needles, and broken glass should have the biohazards symbol affixed to the outside. In rare situations, some chemical wastes may be safely disposed of through the sewer. The chemical hygiene officer (CHO) should be consulted to make this determination. Each type of chemical waste must be collected separately. The waste container must be labeled with the chemical's name, concentration, source, method of disposal, area of use, and appropriate hazard warning labels. The containers must be leakproof and compatible with the chemical wastes. Methods of disposal must comply with federal, state, and local regulations.

IX. RECORD KEEPING

The employer should maintain records of equipment monitoring, equipment repairs, and personnel monitoring results. Job-related accidents or incidents should be thoroughly investigated and documented.

- Written records of all employee accidents and incidents must be maintained by the employer.

- Medical records must be maintained by the employer during the employee's tenure and for thirty years after the employee has left employment.

- Safety training and review records must be maintained by the employer during the employee's tenure and for three years after the employee has left employment.

The confidentiality of employees' medical records must be maintained by their employers. According to OSHA mandates, an employee may (upon request) be granted access to medical records in which he or she is the subject.

BIBLIOGRAPHY

Laboratory Safety Principles and Practices. 1995. Washington, D.C: ASM Press.

Montgomery, Lynn. 1995. *Health and Safety Guidelines for the Laboratory*. Washington, D.C.: ASCP Press.

National Committee for Clinical Laboratory Standards. September 1996. *Clinical laboratory safety*, Approved Guidelines, GP17-A, 16, 6. Wayne, Penn.: NCCLS.

National Committee for Clinical Laboratory Standards. December 2001. *Protection of laboratory workers from occupationally acquired infections*, Approved Guidelines, M29-A2, 21, 23. Wyane, Pa.: NCCLS.

National Committee for Clinical Laboratory Standards. March 2002. *Clinical laboratory waste management*, Approved Guidelines, GP5-A2, 22, 3. Wayne, Pa.: NCCLS.

Prudent Practices in the Laboratory Handling and Disposal of Chemicals National. 1995. Washington, D.C.: Academy Press.

Theriot, Betty L., and Patsy C. Jarreau. 1999. *Clinical laboratory science review: A bottom line approach*. New Orleans: Louisiana State University Medical Center Foundation.

INTERNET RESOURCES

Berkeley Lab, Biohazardous Waste Management.
<www.lbl.gov/ehs/Medical/html/biohazardous.htm>

Interactive Learning Paradigms, Inc.
<www.ilpi.com/safety/extinguishers.html#using>

The National Committee for Clinical Laboratory Standards. <www.nccls.org>

Office of Clinical & Biological Safety, Michigan State University, NSPA Chemical Hazard Labels.
<www.orcbs.msu.edu/chemical/nfpa/nfpa.html>

U.S. Department of Labor, Occupational Safety and Health Administration. <www.osha.gov/>

QUESTIONS

1. The agency that establishes safety standards for the workplace is *(Objective 1, Level I)*
    a. NCCLS
    b. OSHA
    c. NAACLS
    d. CLIA
    e. ASCLS

2. The safety mandates for clinical laboratories include all of the following EXCEPT *(Objective 2, Level I)*
   a. telephone communications
   b. hazard communications
   c. occupational exposure to blood-borne pathogens
   d. occupational exposure to chemicals
   e. respiratory protection

3. What is the employer's responsibility regarding Right-to-Know? *(Objective 3, Level II)*

4. List the components of a blood-borne pathogens plan. *(Objective 4, Level I)*
   a. _____
   b. _____
   c. _____
   d. _____
   e. _____

5. The risk of acquiring HIV from a needle-stick injury is about _____ %, whereas the risk of acquiring HBV is _____ %. *(Objective 5, Level I)*

6. A component of the blood-borne pathogen standard requires that laboratory personnel be vaccinated against the Hepatitis B Virus. True or False? *(Objective 5, Level I)*

7. List the components of a chemical hygiene plan (CHP). *(Objective 6, Level I)*
   a. _____
   b. _____

8. Differentiate the responsibilities of the safety director and the clinical laboratory safety officer. *(Objective 7, Level III)*

9. List the five types of hazards found in the clinical laboratory. *(Objective 8, Level I)*
   a. _____
   b. _____
   c. _____
   d. _____
   e. _____

10. Discuss safety precautions that could be implemented to address biological hazards. *(Objective 9, Level II)*

11. Barrier protection categories include *(Objective 10, Level I)*
    a. engineering controls
    b. PPE
    c. work practices
    d. all of the above

12. Describe the NFPA system for labeling chemicals. *(Objective 11, Level II)*

13. Describe the biological waste disposal requirements. *(Objective 12, Level II)*

14. Medical records must be kept for _____ years, and safety-training records must be kept for _____ years after an employee has left the workplace. *(Objective 13, Level I)*

EXERCISES

Completion of the exercises will enhance your knowledge of clinical laboratory safety.
(Objective 14, Level III)

1. Make a list of the safety equipment in the laboratory, review the safety manual, review the record keeping, and participate in the safety training. After completion of all, evaluate your laboratory and make recommendations for enhancing the safety of the laboratory. This may be done as a group project or as an individual.

2. Review the blood-borne pathogens and chemical hygiene plans. Describe new information that you found.

3. Either on the internet or via a hard copy, review one standard of the OSHA regulations and compare your laboratory regulations to the OSHA regulations.

4. Using either the Joint Commission or College of American Pathologist accreditation guidelines, compare the accreditation guidelines with what you find in the OSHA regulations.

5. Investigate the ergonomic situation in your laboratory and suggest whether this area should also be regulated by OSHA. Are there other areas of the laboratory that you would recommend be regulated in order to provide a safer workplace?

CASES

Analyze each of the following cases and propose solutions. *(Objective 15, Level III)*

1. Bob is a new employee who recently graduated from a medical laboratory education program. He has completed the laboratory orientation and is working alone in the urinalysis section. Bob needs to make 500 ml of ten-percent hydrochloric acid (HCL) from a gallon of concentrated HCL. Although he has made solutions during his education program, this will be the first time on his new job.
   a. What protective clothing and equipment should he use?

   b. How should HCL be handled, used, and stored?

   c. How should he handle a spill of HCL on the work surface?

2. Jeannie received a needle stick while performing a phlebotomy procedure on a five-year-old outpatient. The patient is scheduled to have a tonsillectomy performed on the following day.
   a. Should the tech be concerned about becoming infected from this patient's blood?

   b. Should all needle-stick incidents be reported? If yes, to whom?

   c. What other concerns should be addressed following a needle stick?

3. While spinning blood specimen tubes in an old, yet functional, centrifuge, Lynn (the tech) detects a burning odor. She looks up in time to see smoke and sparks coming from the rear of the old centrifuge. Lynn is the only person in the chemistry department and her immediate response is to evacuate the area.
   a. What other *immediate* actions should Lynn take?

   b. What type of fire extinguisher (if any) should be used?

   c. How should the defective equipment be handled?

Chapter 20

Marketing and Development of an Outreach Program

Gregory M. Hatten, B.S., MT(ASCP)BB

OBJECTIVES

Upon completion of this chapter the learner will be able to

1. Define *marketing*. *(Level I)*
2. Explain why hospitals have embraced marketing of their products. *(Level II)*
3. Describe actions that should be taken prior to implementing an outreach program. *(Level I)*
4. List services that should be compared with competitors when developing an outreach program. *(Level I)*
5. Define the term "anti-kickback statutes." *(Level I)*
6. Define the Stark-sponsored legislation. *(Level I)*
7. Name two groups in the laboratory that have a major impact on the outreach program. *(Level I)*
8. Create a proposal for marketing a specific test in the laboratory. *(Level III)*
9. Create a plan for development of an outreach program. *(Level III)*
10. Analyze the case studies and propose solutions. *(Level III)*

TOPIC SUMMARY

Marketing may be defined as determining what your client's needs are and providing a product and service that meets and exceeds those needs. The idea of a hospital laboratory marketing itself was once unheard of because hospitals did not sell their services, they provided them. Advertising or marketing bordered on questionable ethics. But times have changed and so have hospital laboratories' opinions on marketing and developing outreach programs. Physicians are treating patients more often on an outpatient basis, generating approximately sixty percent of the laboratories' testing volume. Hospitals can no longer assume that physicians will send their patients to the hospital laboratory for testing. National laboratories offered physician offices laboratory services well before outreach programs were implemented in hospitals. With the shift to more testing being ordered on an outpatient basis and the presence of national laboratories in hospitals' markets, it was crucial for hospitals to enter the outreach business to increase revenue and to keep the patients coming to the hospital. Because of the "we provide, not sell" philosophy, hospital laboratories have been slow entering the outreach market. With insurance reimbursement being better for outpatient testing and the increased inpatients seeking testing as outpatients, it makes good business sense to enter the outreach market.

Before a laboratory decides to implement an outreach program it must first determine the identity of the competition and what it will take to be competitive. This can be achieved by interviews with physician practices that are currently being served by another laboratory to determine the services being provided and if services are being satisfactorily received. Discovering what the physician practices like about the service and what they dislike is important. From this information an outreach program can be developed.

Knowing what value-added services are being offered by the competition and choosing the ones that are important to the physician will aid in the survival of an outreach program. Services that should be considered are the convenience of drawing stations for the patient, providing a phlebotomist for in-office collections, response time to requests for supplies, quick turnaround time of results, knowledge of staff with regard to tests, timely address and resolution of complaints or problems, and pricing of tests. A delivery system providing a quick turnaround time of results to the physician is important. Delivery system options include a courier service for hand delivery of results or electronic delivery via a dedicated printer, fax machine, or the internet.

Each of these services has value to the patient, physician, and payer. Probably the most important feature of an outreach program is pricing. The ability of physicians to bill for laboratory tests through their office is a major source of revenue. And the lower the price charged to the physician by the outreach program, the more profit the physician can realize even charging a standard price for each test. Being extremely competitive in pricing is crucial. The program may offer many services that the physician likes, but if pricing is not competitive, the physician will likely choose less in the way of services for better pricing.

Having competitive pricing is paramount for survival, but a laboratory must be careful to not offer prices below the cost of actually performing the test. This is illegal according to the Centers for Medicare and Medicaid Services (CMS), especially if the laboratory is also receiving Medicare/Medicaid business from the physician. Pricing the lab tests below cost could be construed as inducing the physician to refer his Medicare/Medicaid business to your facility. Providing incentives to physicians in exchange for their business is a thing of the past. Today those activities are prohibited by the anti-kickback statutes and Stark-sponsored legislation. Anti-kickback statutes prohibit providing inducements, such as pricing below costs, to physicians in return for their Medicare/Medicaid patient business. The Stark-sponsored legislation (Stark Law) bars physicians from referring Medicare patients to laboratories in which the physician or their family members have a financial interest. Not only do clinical laboratories have to keep up with the latest technology in order to be competitive and marketable, but they also must keep up with local and national legislation to avoid illegal and outdated practices.

Marketing laboratory services to physician offices is a major aspect of a successful outreach program, but another important aspect is marketing or selling the outreach program to the employees of the laboratory. From the technologists performing the tests to the clerical staff answering the phones, communication about the outreach program and the importance of their role is crucial in the development of a successful program. The method by which a person (customer) is greeted and treated on the phone creates a lasting impression regarding the laboratory and its services. It is important for the staff answering the phone to understand that the caller immediately forms a perception of the organization based on the conversation. Therefore, the staff's knowledge and understanding of the outreach program and its goals are important. The first impression could have an impact on the caller's desire to do future business with the lab and impact other possible clients when the impression is shared. Also, technologists performing the testing need to understand that the increase in workload will increase hospital revenues, which could translate into job stability. Marketing the outreach program to the laboratory staff makes marketing the lab's services to the customer much more effective.

Successful outreach programs provide a beneficial product for physicians, dependable laboratory services with a staff eager to help, competitive pricing, and compliance with all federal laws and regulations. Gone is the day that hospital laboratories provide services, not sell them. If that thinking still exists, those laboratories are at risk of being lost in this highly competitive marketplace.

BIBLIOGRAPHY

Kaufman, Harvey W., M.D. 1977. Don't miss the mark. *Medical Laboratory Observer*, February 27.

Kotler, Philip. 1976. *Marketing management*. Englewood Cliffs, N.J.: Prentice Hall.

Kotler, Philip, O. C. Ferrell, and Charles Lamb. 1987. *Strategic marketing for non-profit organizations—Cases and Readings*. Englewood Cliffs, N.J.: Prentice Hall.

Mardell, Christy. 1977. Hospitals as marketers: Ads gain favor. *Advertising Age*, February 21.

Rubright, Robert, and Dan MacDonald. 1981. *Marketing health & human services*. Rockville, Md.: Aspen Systems Corporation.

INTERNET RESOURCES

Boston Chapter of the American Marketing Association. <www.amaboston.org/>

Peppers & Rogers Group. <www.1to1.com>

Professional Management and Marketing. <www.practicemgmt.com/articles.html>

Chapter 20

QUESTIONS

1. Marketing could be defined as _____
   _____.
   (Objective 1, Level I)

2. Explain why hospitals have embraced marketing of their products. *(Objective 2, Level II)*

3. An action that should be taken prior to implementing an outreach program is *(Objective 3, Level I)*
   a. interview competitors
   b. interview physicians
   c. interview the laboratory personnel in your hospital
   d. interview patients

4. List services that should be compared with competitors when developing an outreach program. *(Objective 4, Level I)*
   a. _____
   b. _____
   c. _____
   d. _____
   e. _____
   f. _____
   g. _____

5. The anti-kickback statutes *(Objective 5, Level I)*
   a. prohibit providing inducements to physicians
   b. prohibit providing inducement to patients
   c. prohibit providing inducement to competitors
   d. prohibit paying higher salaries to the laboratory personnel

6. Stark legislation *(Objective 6, Level I)*
   a. prohibits physicians from making a profit from Medicare patient business
   b. prohibits the laboratory from charging more on Medicare patient business
   c. prohibits the physician from referring Medicare patients to labs in which the physician or their family members have a financial interest
   d. prohibits charging lower prices than the competitors

7. Two laboratory groups that have a major impact on the outreach program are
   _____ and _____. *(Objective 7, Level I)*

EXERCISES

Completion of the exercises will enhance your knowledge of marketing and development of an outreach program. *(Objective 8, Level III and Objective 9, Level III)*

1. Review a previous marketing proposal for a specific laboratory test that has been submitted and approved. Create a similar proposal for another laboratory test using the approved proposal as a model. This can be done individually or as a group.

2. Interview the laboratory outreach director to determine how an outreach program should be implemented. Research the literature to gain additional information. Write an outline including steps in the development of an outreach program. This can be done individually or as a group. If done as a group, one person may interview while the others perform the research. The information should be combined for the plan outline.

CASES

Analyze the following case studies and propose solutions. *(Objective 10, Level III)*

1. From your clients you get positive feedback on the turnaround time of results, timeliness of report receipts, and the professionalism of your courier staff. But when you ask the clients how they are treated when they call the lab for results or information, you are told the staff answering the phone are discourteous and the technical staff act as though they do not want to be bothered. Recommend how you would address this issue with the client and with the laboratory staff.

2. As the manager of the clinical laboratory, you develop an outreach program to increase the income of the laboratory. You note after the first six months the following:
   ☐ Physician offices are rarely using your services.
   ☐ Other hospitals are not using your services at all.
   ☐ Long-term care facilities represent your highest volume of work.

   Your laboratory is just barely breaking even on the outreach program financially. Analyze the market segments and level of participation in the program of each segment. Recommend how you might change the mix to enhance revenues. Also recommend possible additional market segments.

3. You have a successful outreach program that has been operational for five years. You don't communicate frequently with your clients because you believe they know your services. However, business has begun to drop off recently. Analyze the situation and recommend steps to rejuvenate your outreach program.

Chapter 21

Writing Procedures in the NCCLS Format

Beth Parham White, B.S., MT(ASCP), CLS(NCA)

OBJECTIVES

Upon completion of this chapter the learner will be able to

1. Name the roles that a procedure manual performs in the laboratory. *(Level I)*
2. Define NCCLS. *(Level I)*
3. Discuss the purpose of the GP2-A4 guideline. *(Level II)*
4. List the sections that should be included in a written procedure. *(Level II)*
5. Create a written procedure using a method presently in use in the laboratory. *(Level III)*
6. Compare your written procedure with the written procedure used in the laboratory. *(Level III)*
7. Analyze the case studies and propose solutions. *(Level III)*

TOPIC SUMMARY

Laboratorians rely on their procedure manuals for instructions on how to perform the many different tasks required of them on a daily basis. The procedure manual is an essential communications tool in the clinical laboratory. It is important for every procedure contained in each manual to be clear, easy to follow, and complete. Consistency between manuals is also important to avoid confusion, because one person may be required in the course of their job to refer to many different manuals. Procedure manuals are also important resource tools for laboratories; they may be used in teaching students or new employees and in providing information to inspectors from accrediting agencies.

The National Committee for Clinical Laboratory Standards (NCCLS) has published a guideline for writing laboratory procedures. The guideline was first proposed in May 1980, and the current Approved Guideline—Fourth Edition, (GP2-A4), was published in April 2002. GP2-A4 was written to be a guideline to laboratorians and can be adapted to best suit the needs of each individual institution. It is intended by NCCLS to provide a method to the clinical laboratory for producing the clear, consistent procedures it needs. The College of American Pathologists (CAP) requires that all written laboratory procedures closely follow the format set out by the NCCLS guideline.

Previous editions of GP2 focused primarily on the writing of procedures for analytic processes—actual testing procedures. GP2-A4 includes guidelines for writing all types of procedures dealing with the full scope of the laboratory's workflow. Preanalytic procedures, including order entry, patient preparation, and specimen collection and handling, are those procedures that are carried out prior to the actual analysis of the sample. Analytic procedures include the information and step-by-step instructions required for the actual testing process. Postanalytic procedures, such as reporting of critical values, turning out results—whether manually or through the laboratory information system, and storing both results and completed specimens, deal with those processes that are performed after the actual sample analysis.

According to GP2-A4, *all* procedures should contain the following "common elements":

- Title
- Purpose or principle
- Procedure instructions
- References
- Author
- Approval signatures

In addition, every procedure that deals with the handling of potentially hazardous materials, whether body fluid or chemical, should include a section on safety. For procedures that don't require any special safety requirements above and beyond those generally used in the lab, referral to the lab safety manual may be sufficient.

Analytic procedures for manual testing processes are generally the most complex type of procedures because they should provide detailed instructions for actual sample analysis. In addition to the common elements listed earlier, analytic procedure should include any of the following that would apply to each individual process:

- Specimen information—type, amount required, transport or storage instructions, cause for rejection, and so on.
- Test method—step-by-step instructions for performing the analysis
- Reagents and/or media
- Supplies—items needed to perform the analysis such as pipettes and tips
- Special safety precautions (above and beyond general requirements)
- Equipment calibration and maintenance—should only be included in a procedure for a particular assay if it is done every time the assay is performed. A separate procedure is required for maintenance and calibration that is done any time other than during actual testing—for instance daily, weekly, or monthly preventative maintenance on an automated analyzer.
- Quality control (QC)—should only be included in a procedure for a particular assay if it is done every time the assay is performed. A separate procedure is required for QC performed other than during actual patient testing—daily, at the beginning of the shift, and so on.
- Calculations—should include all necessary formulas and step-by-step instructions for using the formulas. An example should also be included.
- Expected values—should include different values for age, sex, or race
- Interpretation of results—information about possible meaning of final results should include information about possible indeterminate results and what to do in those cases and when and how to report critical results. May include educational information about certain disease states resulting in abnormal results.
- Method limitations—should include assay sensitivity and specificity, reportable range, whether or not to dilute samples with results above the reportable range and instructions on how to do so if necessary, and a list of possible interfering substances.

(Adapted with permission from NCCLS. *Clinical laboratory technical procedure manuals*, Approved Guideline 4th ed. NCCLS document GP2-A4. NCCLS. Available from 940 West Valley Road, Suite 1400, Wayne, PA 19087-1898, 2002.)

In addition to the previously discussed guidelines for writing procedures, GP2-A4 also contains information about organizing the procedure manual, archiving and managing documents, using manufacturers' procedure manuals for automated procedures, and many examples of different types of procedures.

By using the NCCLS GP2-A4 guideline and including the features listed earlier, the laboratory can be assured that its procedures are helpful tools to its personnel and that any assay or other process performed using those procedures will be done correctly with quality results turned out to the physician and good outcomes for the patient.

BIBLIOGRAPHY

National Committee for Clinical Laboratory Standards. 2002. *Clinical laboratory technical procedure manuals*, Approved Guideline. 4th ed. NCCLS document GP2-A4. Wayne, Pa.: NCCLS.

INTERNET RESOURCES

College of American Pathologists. <www.CAP.org>
National Committee for Clinical Laboratory Standards. <www.nccls.org>

QUESTIONS

1. The roles of a procedure manual in the laboratory include *(Objective 1, Level I)*
   a. instructions for daily performance
   b. communication
   c. resource
   d. teaching
   e. all of the above

2. NCCLS stands for *(Objective 2, Level I)*
   a. National Accrediting Agency for Clinical Laboratory Sciences
   b. National Committee for Clinical Laboratory Standards
   c. National Commission on Clinical Laboratory Science
   d. National Accrediting Committee on Clinical Laboratory Science

3. Discuss the purpose of the GP2-A4 guideline. *(Objective 3, Level II)*

4. List the major parts of an analytic procedure as recommended by GP2-A4. *(Objective 4, Level I)*

   a. _____   j. _____
   b. _____   k. _____
   c. _____   l. _____
   d. _____   m. _____
   e. _____   n. _____
   f. _____   o. _____
   g. _____   p. _____
   h. _____   q. _____
   i. _____

EXERCISES

Completion of the exercises will enhance your knowledge of writing procedures in the NCCLS format. *(Objective 5, Level III and Objective 6, Level III)*

1. Either individually or in groups, choose a procedure from a laboratory procedure manual. Examine the chosen procedure and identify the following parts:
   (1) Principle
   (2) Specimen requirements
   (3) List of reagents, standards, and controls
   (4) Step-by-step instructions
   (5) Expected results (normals) and panic values (if any)
   (6) Limitations of the procedure

2. Individually or in groups, create a written procedure using a method presently in use in the laboratory (e.g., ictotest, gram stain, ABO typing) that you have performed. Remember, the NCCLS format is a guideline only. Use only those sections that apply to your particular procedure.

3. Compare your written procedure with the written procedure approved and in use in the laboratory.

CASES

Analyze the following case studies and propose solutions. *(Objective 7, Level III)*

1. Given the sample procedure in Figure 21-1, analyze the following:
   a. Are all necessary elements required by the NCCLS standards present? If not, what else should be included?

   b. Assume that you are a new technologist working in hematology by yourself for the first time on the night shift, and you are referencing this procedure to perform a manual reticulocyte count. What might be the consequences if each of the following were left out of the procedure?
      (1) Cause for rejection of specimen.
      (2) Normal range for newborns
      (3) Formula for calculating final results
      (4) Requirement of filtering reagent prior to use.
      (5) Procedural step that says to let blood/stain mixture sit for fifteen minutes before making slides.
      (6) Current review signature.

   c. Why does this procedure not include steps for calibration or when to call panic results?

JOHN SMITH MEMORIAL HOSPITAL
PATHOLOGY LABORATORY

Title:	Manual Reticulocyte Count by New Methylene Blue Method
Effective Date:	April 2, 2002
Distribution:	Hematology Procedure Manual
Author:	Jane Doe, MT(ASCP), CLS(NCA)
Reviewed:	Annually
Principle:	Reticulocytes are immature non-nucleated erythrocytes that still retain some basophilic substance. Under certain conditions the basophilic substance appears as a reticulum when these cells are exposed to vital stains such as new methylene blue.
Specimen:	Anticoagulated whole blood, preferably using EDTA as the anticoagulant, stored at room temperature. Specimens containing clots will be rejected.
Reagents:	New methylene blue stain, filtered immediately before use.
Supplies:	Small glass tubes, glass slides, microscope, Miller ocular disc.
Controls:	Normal and abnormal reticulocyte controls. See package insert for current lot numbers for expected ranges. Patient results may not be released until validation of control results.
Safety Precautions:	Must follow standard precautions. See Laboratory Safety Manual.
Test Method:	1. Place equal amounts (5 drops each) of well-mixed whole blood or control material and freshly filtered new methylene blue stain in a small glass tube. 2. Mix well and let stand at room temperature for 15 minutes. 3. Make 2 good, even smears from each sample on glass slides labeled with patient's name and accession number. Smears should have good feathered edges. Let air dry. 4. Replace one microscope ocular with Miller ocular disc. Under oil immersion, count the number of RBCs in the top left (small) square of the grid. Then count the number of reticulocytes in the entire large square. Continue counting consecutive fields until 100 RBC's are counted. Be sure to count in an area of the slide where RBC's are evenly spaced and not overlapping.
Calculation of results:	Divide the number of reticulocytes counted by 10 to get the percentage of reticulocytes. (Example: 100 RCBs counted, 15 reticulocytes counted. 15/10 = 1.5%.)
Normal Ranges:	Adult: 0.5–2.0% Newborn (less than 2 weeks old): 2.5–6.5%
Interpretation of Results:	An increased reticulocyte count may be seen in cases of acute bleeding, sickle cell anemia, and other conditions resulting in blood cell loss. Decreased reticulocyte counts may be seen in cases of aplastic anemia.
Method Limitations:	Failure to allow complete staining of cells with new methylene blue stain may result in falsely decreased results. Poor staining may also occur in cases of high glucose levels. Slides that are not allowed to dry completely prior to staining may result in RBCs with a refractile appearance, which may be mistaken for cells containing reticulum causing a falsely elevated result. Also, failure to filter the stain prior to staining may cause stain precipitate to appear on the slide, which may also be mistaken for reticulum resulting in a falsely elevated count.

Reviewed by: Jane Doe
Date: 4/29/2003

FIGURE 21-1. Sample Procedure

Chapter 22

Laboratory Budgeting and Finance

Sandi Thames, B.S., MT(ASCP), CLS(NCA)

OBJECTIVES

Upon completion of this chapter the learner will be able to

1. Identify the four phases in budget preparation. *(Level I)*
2. Relate the laboratory goals to the organizational goals. *(Level I)*
3. Name areas used to develop budget assumptions for an organization. *(Level I)*
4. Name two items used by the laboratory in formulating budget assumptions. *(Level I)*
5. Differentiate capital and operational expenses. *(Level II)*
6. Name three justification categories when requesting a capital expenditure. *(Level I)*
7. Name three reasons for budget variability. *(Level II)*
8. Discuss the factors that should be considered in determining costs per test. *(Level II)*
9. Summarize the steps to be taken when requesting a new instrument. *(Level II)*
10. Calculate cost per billable test given a case study. *(Level II)*
11. Select the most cost-effective instrument arrangement given a case study. *(Level III)*

TOPIC SUMMARY

There are no hospital laboratory activities that do not incur expense, nor are there any whose expenses cannot be controlled to some extent. The challenge is to maintain a high quality service that is cost effective. A well-prepared budget that is adhered to is a vital tool in helping the laboratory become more effective and efficient.

The budget process usually begins well in advance of the implementation date and is prepared in phases.

Phase I. Development of Goals

The laboratory develops goals based on the organization's mission statement and strategic objectives. The laboratory goals must be in line with those of the organization and must be achievable. An example of a laboratory goal is that the laboratory will increase cost effectiveness.

Some examples of laboratory objectives, which are measurable and relate to the goal, follow:

1. Increase revenue by five percent through implementation of an outreach program.
2. Decrease denied claims by three percent through maintenance of charge master and review of denied claims.
3. Reduce overall cost by five percent through implementation of service standards and systems controls.

Phase II. Budget Assumptions

The organization provides a forecast of available money based on past earnings, cash flow, and changes in state or federal laws affecting reimbursement. For example, the Balanced Budget Act greatly reduced the amount of money received per Diagnostic Related Group (DRG). The outpatient prospective payment system implemented in 2000 reduces the reimbursement for outpatient procedures, including radiology, outpatient surgery, and laboratory procedures. Also included in the equation are write-off's from bad debt, changes in private payor fees, and changes in managed-care contracts. Most hospitals experience less than seventy percent payment-to-charges ratio.

The laboratory formulates budget assumptions based on annual test volume and revenue generated. For example, if the outreach program mentioned in the previous objectives was implemented, it can be assumed that the operating cost as well as the projected revenue would increase.

Phase III. Forecast of Expenses

Capital Expense: Capital expenditures are most often calculated for a three-year cycle. Items that may fall into this category include

- requests for new space or space changes
- replacement equipment
- purchase or lease of new equipment
- information technology: interfaces, hardware, licensing fees

Capital expenditure is an investment. As such, its rate of return must be evaluated and used as a criterion for budgeting decisions. Some suggested categories of capital expenditure justification and priority follow:

Justification Categories:

a. Replacement—equipment that cannot be repaired or there is excessive cost of repair.
b. New equipment—equipment required due to increased workload or improved methodology that would allow for better patient care.
c. Cost reduction—reduction of operating expenses stated primarily in terms of personnel and supplies.

Priority of Need:

a. Essential—needed immediately to maintain quality patient care.
b. Necessary—also "essential," but greater leeway with regard to time of acquisition.
c. Desirable—means of reducing cost.
d. Other—means of improving general working conditions.

Most often manufacturers and/or distributors of capital equipment offer a variety of financial options including cash purchase, equipment lease, and reagent rental. A cash purchase is advantageous for equipment you expect to keep for more than five years and is the only option for items such as microscopes, reagent storage refrigerators, and slide stainers. An equipment lease agreement is often used with an open system whereby several different manufacturers' reagents may be used. You pay a monthly fee for the "use" of the equipment but are free to shop for the most economical reagent system with no required volume to be purchased. Reagent rental agreements require the purchase of a fixed volume of a specific manufacturer's reagents. The cost for the use of the equipment is calculated into the reagent cost. Prior to any capital purchase, it is wise to do a five-year cost analysis. If you are making the purchase in order to "upgrade" to newer technology, you can compare the cost of the current system to the newer, desired upgrade.

Some items to consider in the analysis are

- equipment cost
- cost of service contract
- reagent cost
- technologist time
- cost to the patient/client
- medicare reimbursement (especially if your institution has a high percent of Medicare patients)

Some examples of cost comparisons are found in Figure 22-1 and Figure 22-2.

Operational Expenses: Operational expenses most commonly encompass a twelve-month cycle. Careful identification of all categories of expenditures and the most prudent allocation of funds for each category is required. The grouping of expense categories is often termed a "chart of accounts." A proposed hospital laboratory chart of accounts might include

- salaries including cost of benefits
- reference laboratory fees
- education and travel
- chemistry
- hematology
- microbiology
- transfusion service
    operating cost
    blood supply cost
- purchased service and maintenance
- other direct expenses
    includes inspection fees, certificate fees, CAP surveys, and so on

For every expense item in the budget, start with a budget of zero and add budget amounts to it only as far as you can justify the cost. For each item, you must be able to discuss the expected results or the expenditures and what will be lost if the money is not spent.

In this example we are evaluating the cost of the new Thin Prep Pap Smear technology. The cost of the new technology is considerably higher than that of the conventional Pap Smear method. The literature suggests that the new technology is far superior to the old method, and it is reimbursed at a higher rate. In our scenario, we are making a conservative assumption that we will achieve a 60% conversion rate, meaning the workload will be 40% conventional pap smears and 60% Thin Prep.

60% Conversion

Laboratory Profile — Anatomic Lab
Number of Paps per year — 14,547

Cost of Pap Test	Conventional Pap Smear	Thin Prep Pap Test
Screening cost[1]	$ 7.42	$ 7.42
Processing operator cost[2]	$ 2.20	$ 2.20
Supplies cost[3]	$ 0.52	$ 9.00
Total cost to lab per test	**$10.14**	**$18.62**

[1] The screening cost is indicative of the technologist's time. That dollar amount was obtained by dividing the cytotechnologists' salaries for the year by the total number of tissues screened for the year.

[2] Processing cost is reflective of the time required for the slides to be made for cytologist review. That amount can be calculated by dividing the processor annual salary by the total number of slides prepared.

[3] The supply cost is exactly that. Because this is a reagent rental agreement, the cost includes the equipment, service contract, reagent, and specimen collection supplies.

Payer Matrix	# of Paps	×40%	Reimbursement amount for Pap Smear	Revenue	×60%	Reimbursement amount for Thin Prep	Revenue
Medicare (cytotech only)	922	369	$7.15	$2,636.92	553	$17.15	$9,487.38
Medicare (cytotech + MD)	81	32	$22.15	$717.66	49	$40.90	$1,987.74
BCBS	58	23	$25.00	$580.00	35	$35.00	$1,218.00
Medicaid (cytotech only)	713	285	$7.34	$2,093.37	428	$19.40	$8,299.32
Medicaid (cytotech + MD)	58	23	$22.34	$518.29	35	$43.94	$1,529.11
Client	12,714	5,086	$7.25	$36,870.60	7,628	$25.00	$190,710.00
		5,818		$43,416.84	8,728		$213,231.55

In this example, we are assuming the laboratory has a high Medicare/Medicaid patient population. The revenue, therefore, is calculated based on the Medicare fee schedule.

Client pricing = contracted charge to a third party

	Pap Smear	Thin Prep
Actual cost of test	$10.14	$18.62
Number of Paps	5,818	8,728
Total annual cost	$58,994.52	$162,515.36
Total annual revenue	$43,416.84	$213,231.55

Total Cost	$221,509.88
Total Revenue	$256,648.39
Profit (Loss)	$35,138.51

The bottom line shows that it would be profitable to go to the new technology even though the cost per test is higher.

FIGURE 22–1. Calculating Cost of New Equipment (Methodology) Based on a Reagent Rental Plan

Chemistry Analyzer (Immunoassays)

Setting: The laboratory performs more than 18,000 immunoassays a year with the following test mix and proposed pricing:

	# Tests per Year	Reagent cost per test Lease	Purchase
Group 1 (Anemia)—B12, Folate, Ferritin	1,435	$1.40	$0.90
Group 2 (Tumor Markers)—PSA, CEA, CA 125, CA 15-3	2,172	$3.30	$2.50
Group 3 (Cardiac)—Troponin, Myoglobin, CK-MB	14,750	$2.00	$1.55
Group 4 (Fertility)—BHCG, Progesterone, Estridiol, FSH, etc.)	6,712	$1.05	$0.75
Group 5 (Thyroid Function)—T4, TSH, fT4, T3, T-uptake	8,394	$1.35	$0.85

Instrument Cost: 49,500 includes one year service
Service Agreement: 9,720 annually. Service is included in the reagent pricing on the reagent rental plan.

Based on the above information, the cost over a five-year period would be calculated as follows:

				Lease Plan[1]	Purchase Plan[2]	
Instrument Cost	included in reagent			0		49,500
Service Contract	included in reagent			0	(9,720 × 4)	38,880*
Reagent Cost	annual volume × 5 years		cost per test		cost per test	
Group 1	1,435	7,175	$1.40	$10,045.00	$0.90	$6,457.50
Group 2	2,172	10,860	$3.30	$35,838.00	$2.50	$27,150.00
Group 3	14,750	73,750	$2.00	$147,500.00	$1.55	$114,312.50
Group 4	6,712	33,560	$1.05	$35,238.00	$0.75	$25,170.00
Group 5	8,394	41,970	$1.35	$56,659.50	$0.85	$35,674.50
Total Cost				$285,280.50		$297,144.50

*the first year of service was included with purchase

Based on these calculations, it is more economical to obtain the equipment on a reagent rental plan.

[1] Reagent Rental Lease Plan
[2] Direct Purchase Plan

FIGURE 22–2. Calculating Cost of Equipment: Direct Purchase vs. Reagent Rental

Phase IV. Monitoring

Once the operational budget is implemented, expense reports are reviewed monthly for budget variances. Budget variances may be attributed to the following:

- Increased volume—the ordering and reporting of a higher volume of tests than budgeted for.
- Vendor price increases—most laboratories lock in prices for a three to five year period. However, contract pricing based on test volume will allow vendors to increase pricing if test volumes decrease.
- Changes in policy and procedure—unexpected implementation of test procedures. This is often physician driven.

Analyzing budget variances is of major importance in controlling laboratory costs.

Cost per Test/Cost per Unit of Service

Laboratory managers find it beneficial to know cost per test or cost per unit of service. In the laboratory setting these terms are synonymous. This information is often requested by administrators involved in formulating managed health agreements whereby the hospital offers service at a discount. The organization must ensure that their discount pricing is not below cost. The information may also be used in evaluating different methodologies or in calculating the amount of "free community service" that a laboratory can feasibly provide.

When calculating this cost, it is important to look beyond the mere cost of reagent, equipment, and technologist time. Many factors, such as cost of maintenance, salaries of support staff, nonmedical supplies (paper, pens, etc.), and travel and education, contribute to this bottom line. Many laboratories will even include the cost of telephone service, electricity, and water. For the sake of demonstration, a simple example is presented (see Figure 22-3).

The salary portion can also be calculated based on the amount of time required to perform the test. This method is considered much more difficult, for you have to calculate precisely the time of everyone involved in collecting, handling, and processing the sample.

Preparing and adhering to a budget requires some strategic thinking. It is often necessary to challenge the status quo in order to make processes more efficient and cost effective. Understand how other areas of your organization affect your bottom line, and establish relationships with others in a similar role with whom you can share ideas. Join professional organizations such as buying groups, which can give you cost comparison information. Most of all, keep your eye on the goal—

We want to determine the cost of performing human immunodeficiency virus (HIV) viral marker. We are given the following information:

1. The laboratory bills 3,500 HIV tests per year.
   Calculating cost is based on billable tests and compensates for controls, calibrations, CAP surveys, and repeats.
2. The reagent cost for the year is $30,000 ($500 per kit; usage is 60 kits per year).
3. The equipment used is leased with the lease price calculated into the reagent cost.
4. The laboratory pays a separate service contract for the equipment at $8,500 per year.
5. The laboratory's total test volume (billable) for the year is 800,000 tests.
6. The budget report indicates the following expenditures:
   - Salaries (including benefits) $1,925,657.00
   - Medical supplies (phlebotomy supplies, etc.) $195,113.00
   - Nonmedical supplies (paper, pens, etc.) $41,252.00
   - Other direct expense (Certification, Inspection, etc.) $47,189.00
   - Travel and education $17,685.00

Our cost per test for HIV would be calculated as follows:

Reagent cost	HIV reagent cost / HIV billable tests ($30,000 / 3,500)	$8.57
Service contract	Cost of service contract / HIV billables ($8,500 / 3,500)	$2.43
Salaries	Salaries / total billable tests ($1,925,657 / 800,000)	$2.41
Medical supplies	Medical supplies / total billable tests ($195,113 / 800,000)	$0.24
Nonmedical supplies	Nonmedical supplies / total billable tests ($41,252 / 800,000)	$0.05
Other direct exp.	Other direct expense / total billable tests ($47,189 / 800,000)	$0.06
Travel & edu.	Travel & education / total billable tests ($17,685 / 800,000)	$0.02
	Cost per test	**$13.78**

FIGURE 22–3. Cost Per Test

maintaining a high quality laboratory that is cost effective.

Bibliography

Davis, Brian L., Carol J. Skube, Lowell W. Hellervik, Susan H. Gebelein, and James L. Sheard. 1996. *Successful manager's handbook:* 5th ed. Minneapolis, Minn.: Personnel Decisions International.

Laboratory Industry Report. September 2000. Washington G2 Reports. Washington, D.C.: Dennis W. Weissman.

Shuffstall, R. M. 1979. *Modern concepts of management, operations, and finance.* St. Louis, Mo.: C. V. Mosby Company.

Vantage Point. September 2000. Wayne, Pa.: Clinical Laboratory Management Association.

Internet Resources

About, Inc., Financial Planning. <http://financialplan.about.com>
Solucient. <www.solucient.com>
Managed Care On-Line. <www.mcol.com/>
University of Pittsburgh, Guide to Budgets and Budgeting. <www.pitt.edu/~offres/proposal/budget.html>
Health Department of Western Australia. <www.health.wa.gov.au/publications/budrefor.html#FOREWORD>
Clinical Laboratory Management Association. <www.clma.org>
VHA. <www.vha.com/public/>

QUESTIONS

1. The four phases in budget preparation are *(Objective 1, Level I)*
   a. development of goals, budget assumption, forecast of expenses, and monitoring
   b. development of goals, calculation of income, calculation of expenses, and reviewing
   c. development of financial statement, calculation of income, estimation of taxes, and reviewing
   d. develop of financial statement, determining investment portfolio options, estimation of taxes, and accounting

2. How do the laboratory goals relate to the organizational goals? *(Objective 2, Level I)*

3. Name three areas used to develop budget assumptions for the organization. *(Objective 3, Level I)*
   a. _____
   b. _____
   c. _____

4. Name two items the laboratory uses to formulate budget assumption. *(Objective 4, Level I)*
   a. _____
   b. _____

5. Differentiate capital and operational expenses. *(Objective 5, Level II)*

6. Name three justification categories when requesting a capital expenditure. *(Objective 6, Level I)*
   a. _____
   b. _____
   c. _____

7. Name three reasons budgets may vary. *(Objective 7, Level II)*

   a. _____

   b. _____

   c. _____

8. Discuss the factors that should be considered in determining cost per test. *(Objective 8, Level II)*

EXERCISES

Completion of the exercises will enhance your knowledge of laboratory budgeting and finance. *(Objective 2, Level I and Objective 9, Level II)*

1. Interview a laboratory section supervisor who is considering or has considered requesting the purchase of a new instrument. Summarize the steps in the process.

2. Review the laboratory and organizational goals and interview the administrative technologist to determine how the laboratory goals relate to the organization goals.

3. Interview a hospital administrator and ask what key questions would be asked if you wanted to purchase a new piece of equipment.

CASES

For case study #1, calculate cost per billable test *(Objective 10, Level II)*, and for case study #2, select the most cost-effective instrument arrangement *(Objective 11, Level III)*.

1. Given the following information, calculate the cost per billable test for a drug screen.
   - The drug screen is composed of five independently measurable assays: Amphetamines, Barbiturates, Cannabinoids, Cocaine, and Benzodiazepines.
   - The instrument was purchased for a price of $116,000. *Equipment is depreciated over a period of five years.*
   - The service contract for the instrument is $9,212 per year.
   - The laboratory reports 539 drug screens per month.
   - The reagent cost for the year follows:

Reagent	Cost per Kit	Annual Usage
Amphetamines	$135.00	128 kits
Barbiturates	$130.00	125 kits
Benzodiazepines	$130.00	133 kits
Cocaine	$145.00	129 kits
Cannabinoids	$115.00	146 kits

- From the budget report you have spent the following:

Medical supplies	$205,874.00
Nonmedical supplies	$51,722.00
Other direct expense	$47,892.00
Travel & education	$22,171.00
Salaries	$1,892,364.00

- Total billable tests for the year = 789,352

2. Your institution is considering the purchase of a new cell counter for hematology. You have evaluated many models from several manufacturers and have narrowed your choice down to two. Both companies offer reagent rental agreements as one purchasing option. Based on the following information, which instrument and which option is the most economical?

	Instrument 1		Instrument 2	
	Purchase	Lease	Purchase	Lease
Purchase Price	$87,750.00	$0.00	$78,000.00	$0.00
Service Agreement (annual cost) (assume that the service contract will be in place for four years)	$15,150.00	$0.00	$16,310.00	$0.00
Reagent Cost (Calculate reagent pricing for a five-year period)	$0.85	$1.10	$0.90	$1.14

The rental reagent pricing is based on a daily test volume of 265 samples per day.

Chapter 23

Fraud and Abuse

Hassan Aziz, Ph.D., CLS(NCA)

OBJECTIVES

Upon completion of this chapter the learner will be able to

1. Identify the purpose of a compliance program. *(Level I)*
2. List the common elements of a compliance plan. *(Level I)*
3. Discuss responsibilities of the lab manager regarding compliance. *(Level II)*
4. Critique the laboratory compliance plan and formulate suggestions for improvement. *(Level III)*
5. Propose solutions for the case studies. *(Level III)*

TOPIC SUMMARY

Today's clinical laboratories are facing yet another financial challenge. In the nationwide crackdown on fraudulent coding and billing of laboratory testing services reimbursed under federally financed programs, government authorities expect laboratories to develop an effective compliance program that corrects and prevents fraud and abuse (the frequent, intentional, and purposeful billing for services that were never provided). The compliance program should be customized according to the laboratory needs and financial demands, such as client and payer mix. In addition, the program should comply with the federal, state, and local laws and regulations applicable to the laboratory's scope of operation. Such a program should be implemented, updated regularly, communicated, and enforced.

The Department of Health and Human Services Office of the Inspector General (OIG; 2002) issued a model compliance plan (MCP) to assist clinical laboratories in voluntarily reducing fraud and abuse. The zero tolerance plan serves as a framework and should be implemented and enforced. All laboratories regardless of size, location, or corporate structure can use the common elements of the compliance plan. The OIG suggests that a compliance plan should include the following elements:

1. Development of written policies, procedures, and standards of conduct that promote the laboratory's commitment to compliance.
2. Compliance with all OIG fraud alerts.
3. Appointment of a compliance officer and other appropriate bodies.
4. Development of effective training and education programs for all employees.
5. Development and maintenance of effective lines of open communications (hotline) with the compliance officer to receive complaints while maintaining the anonymity of complainants.
6. Periodic laboratory compliance audits and other evaluation techniques.
7. Enforcement of standards through well-publicized disciplinary directives.
8. Development of procedures to respond to detected offenses and to initiate corrective actions.

Adherence to the compliance plan is expected for a laboratory to hold and maintain licensure, accreditation, and/or certification. A noncompliant laboratory may be fined, suspended, or even shut down.

Laboratories should designate a chief compliance officer (CCO) or equivalent (e.g., committee) to serve as the focal point for compliance activities. Depending on the circumstances of the laboratory (size, resources, etc.), this responsibility can be the individual's sole duty or added to other management responsibilities. The CCO should oversee the day-to-day operations of the compliance program and must be readily accessible to staff to discuss and resolve compliance issues. Implementation of the compliance plan is monitored by laboratory managers through performance of periodic audits of laboratory operations. Standards of conduct must be developed for all employees clearly delineating the laboratory's policies regarding fraud and abuse.

One of the substantive goals of any compliance plan is to ensure the medical necessity of laboratory services and the accuracy of billing. In order to meet the standard on medical necessity, the OIG recommended the implementation of several mechanisms. For example, requisition forms must be revamped to assist physicians in obtaining their test orders from code-specific test lists while maintaining their freedom of choice. Also, annual notices setting forth the medical necessity policy and components of each laboratory profile should be sent to physicians and other individuals authorized by law to order tests. Although laboratories can offer customized profiles including tests in logical subgroups to their physician clients, these clients must sign an acknowledgment form stating their understanding of the potential implications of ordering customized profiles. For instance, a physician may request that the laboratory construct a profile that includes a basic metabolic panel, total protein, albumin, and total cholesterol. Laboratories agreeing to create these customized profiles should request that the physicians sign an acknowledgment form affirming that only those tests that are medically necessary for the patient will be ordered. The form should also include an advisory to the physician that using customized profiles may result in the ordering of tests that are not financially reimbursable according to regulations established by Medicare or other federally funded health-care programs. The physician should be advised to order individual tests (total protein or albumin) or less inclusive profiles (basic metabolic panel) when all of the tests included in the customized profile do not meet the medical necessity criteria. Test utilization monitoring of the most frequent tests will provide the laboratory with valuable investigative data. Excessive utilization of laboratory services may prompt the compliance officer to address the issue to ensure that fraud is not being committed.

A laboratory should also ensure that all claims for testing services submitted for reimbursement accurately and correctly identify the services ordered by the physician *and* performed by the laboratory. Only medically necessary laboratory tests ordered and performed should be billed and only in accordance with government billing rules. When billing federal healthcare programs, laboratories are expected to select the most appropriate current procedural terminology (CPT) code to describe the service that was ordered and performed and to submit the International Classification of Diseases, 9th revision: Clinical Modifications (ICD-9-CM) diagnostic codes obtained only from the ordering physician or other authorized individuals. Advanced beneficiary notice (ABN) should be made available to Medicare patients when there is a likelihood that an ordered service will not be paid. The notice provides documentation that a test may not be reimbursed and that the patient may be financially responsible for it. Standing orders (specific laboratory protocols generated by a health-care provider and used as guidelines in execution of medical and surgical procedure) are allowed in connection with extended courses of treatment, but they should be monitored to verify their validity. Calculated tests (LDL, indices, etc.) may not be billed when the calculation is derived from underlying laboratory tests. This is considered double billing for the same service. Overpayment can also occur when laboratories bill for individual tests that should have been grouped together (i.e., bundled) for payment purposes and billed at a lower rate (e.g., charging separately for WBC count and CBC count when the WBC count is part of CBC count). Therefore, chemistry panels, CBC, and routine urinalysis may not be "unbundled" and each test billed separately. Similarly, claims for tests that were not performed due to laboratory accidents or insufficient specimens should not be submitted for payment. Software editing capabilities for medical necessity and billing accuracy are critical to maintaining billing compliance. Such products should be examined for accuracy and reviewed periodically to implement any changes. Correct application of coding and billing activities and review of claims may determine if billing edits, bundling edits, and information system interfaces are functioning properly.

Periodically, the OIG issues fraud alerts to identify fraudulent and abusive practices within the health-care industry. They are designed to educate the laboratory community about potential violations. Over the past years, fraud alerts covered a broad spectrum of activities, from blatant actions intended to defraud Medicare to subtle efforts that mix legitimate claim information with false information. Fraud alerts describe practices that appear to violate the law such as unbundling clinical laboratory tests, billing for tests not performed, using false diagnostic codes to obtain payment, and billing for laboratory tests that were not ordered and medically unnecessary. If applicable, the laboratory is required to cease and to correct any conduct criticized in such alerts and to prevent it from reoccurring in the future. The compliance programs encourage the laboratory to adopt honest and nondeceptive marketing strategies for its services.

Moreover, managers carry the responsibility of educating and training all their employees (individuals authorized by state law to order lab tests, phlebotomists, testing personnel, and coding/billing staff) on fraud and abuse issues. Training sessions are to be conducted for new employees and on a periodic basis thereafter. All training and education should be documented and certified. Compliance practices should also be part of all employees' evaluations. Disciplinary actions should be taken against employees failing to adhere to compliance practices.

The goal is to achieve a 100% compliance to avoid fraud and abuse. Adopting and implementing an effective compliance program requires substantial commitment of time, energy, and resources. After all, the plan should not only correct a fraud but also prevent it from happening in the first place, whether by intent, by mistake, or by inadvertence.

BIBLIOGRAPHY

Lavanty, Don. 1997. Model compliance plan for clinical laboratories. *Clinical Laboratory Science* 10, no. 4: 178–179.

U.S. Department of Health and Human Services. August 24, 1998. Department of Health and Human Services—Office of Inspector General—Publication of IOG Compliance Program Guidance for Clinical Laboratories. *Federal Register* 63, p. 163.

U.S. Department of Health and Human Services Office of Inspector General. 2002. *Model compliance plan for clinical laboratories.* Retrieved January 24, 2002, from http://oig.hhs.gov/modcomp/cpcl.html

Voorhees, Diana. 1999. Uncle Sam still pursuing lab fraud and abuse. *Advance for Medical Laboratory Professionals* 11, no. 14: 12–15.

Wallace, M. A., and D. D. Klosinski. 1998. *Clinical laboratory science education and management.* Philadelphia: W. B. Saunders.

INTERNET RESOURCES

American Association for Clinical Chemistry, Clinical Laboratory News. <www.aacc.org/cln/features/97features/sep97feat.html>

American Society for Clinical Laboratory Science. <www.ascls.org/position/health.asp>

Centers for Medicare & Medicaid Services. <http://cms.hhs.gov/providers/fraud/default.asp>

Health and Human Services, Office of Inspector General. <www.oig.hhs.gov/fraud/docs/complianceguidance/cpcl.html>

SNA Counsulting. <www.snaconsulting.com/newsroom/8-98_vol.6.htm>

QUESTIONS

1. A compliance program _____ and _____ fraud and abuse. *(Objective 1, Level I)*

2. List the common elements of a compliance plan. *(Objective 2, Level I)*

   a. _____
   b. _____
   c. _____
   d. _____
   e. _____
   f. _____
   g. _____
   h. _____

3. Discuss responsibilities of the lab manager regarding compliance. *(Objective 3, Level II)*

EXERCISES

Completion of the exercises will enhance your knowledge of fraud and abuse. *(Objective 3, Level II and Objective 4, Level III)*

1. Interview technologists and their laboratory manager (or compliance officer), and list the duties performed by each that pertain to controlling fraud and abuse.

2. Review and summarize the Joint Commission or College of American Pathologists (CAP) accreditation guidelines regarding compliance plans.

3. Review the compliance plan in a laboratory and the model compliance plan produced by the OIG. Suggest how the laboratory compliance plan might be improved.

CASES

Evaluate each of the following cases and propose answers to each question. *(Objective 5, Level III)*

1. Cosmo Kramer Hospital is a small hospital with limited supplies. The emergency room physicians order a variety of laboratory tests including urinalysis. The nurses usually order all laboratory testing on one requisition. Most of the time when the blood is collected, the urine is not available. The urine sample is usually sent to the laboratory later or when the patient is admitted, along with a new requisition, without canceling the first requisition. The laboratory manager is not comfortable with the situation.
   a. Can you identify the problem?

   b. Can you suggest any reasonable solutions?

2. George Kastanza, the laboratory manager and the CCO, is very friendly. To keep all clinicians in his area satisfied with the laboratory services, he designed custom panels for each one. He also provided them with the information necessary for making informed choices.
   a. Is this practice legal?

b. What parameters need to be taken for such a practice?

3. Dr. Newman orders all chemistry tests individually. The medical technologist/clinical laboratory scientist grouped those tests into the appropriate panel and believes he did the right thing. The physician, however, is afraid that the laboratory is scrutinizing his orders.
   a. Who is right?

   b. What can be done to avoid such misunderstanding?

Chapter 24

Workload Recording

Dixie Daniels, B.S., MT(ASCP)

OBJECTIVES

Upon completion of this chapter the learner will be able to

1. Define the primary use of workload recording. *(Level I)*
2. Identify the components of the College of American Pathologists (CAP) workload recording system. *(Level I)*
3. Identify how the ratio is calculated for the adjusted patient days workload recording method. *(Level I)*
4. Identify a commonly used workload recording method. *(Level I)*
5. Discuss the advantages of the Laboratory Management Index Program (LMIP) for workload recording. *(Level II)*
6. Calculate staffing productivity. *(Level II)*
7. Analyze staffing using the workload recording information. *(Level III)*
8. Analyze the case studies and propose solutions. *(Level III)*

TOPIC SUMMARY

Workload recording for measuring employee productivity is an essential responsibility of today's laboratory manager. In the business-oriented health-care world of today, it is increasingly important for a laboratory manager to not only be able to manage his/her expenses for reagents and supplies but also be adept in utilizing the appropriate number of employees necessary for the volume of work the lab is processing. The mission of many laboratories that are either independent or for-profit hospital labs is to be successful financially as well as to provide high quality laboratory testing. Without proper staffing, quality laboratory testing can be compromised. Workload recording provides the manager with a tool to validate the staffing he or she decides is needed, based on particular variables that are determined by the method used.

There are several systems currently in use for workload recording. Laboratories may be directed by their finance department as to which instrument should be used for their lab in measuring the workload. The results obtained by each method will not necessarily provide comparable conclusions, so it is crucial that the lab manager be knowledgeable of the instrument being used and of the others that are available. This chapter addresses three of the more commonly used workload recording methods used today: The College of American Pathologists (CAP) method, the adjusted patient days method, and the billable procedures method.

CAP developed a method of workload recording more than two decades ago that is still in use today in some form by a number of laboratories. This system determines the amount of time required to perform a test by using the variables of test method, instrumentation, and specimen processing. It also figures in time for paperwork, phone calls, and so on in formulating the total amount of time necessary to complete the test from the time the specimen arrives in the lab to the reported result. This is called the CAP Workload Recording Unit. For example, a blood glucose level performed on a Beckman Synchron CX3 was given a CAP unit value of 2.6 minutes to complete. This was based on the actual hands-on time required by the testing personnel to process the specimen, put the sample on the analyzer, program the analyzer, and report the result. The 2.6 minutes was broken down into 2.5 minutes to process and report and 0.1 minute to place the specimen on the instrument and program. If the test ordered was a profile, such as the commonly ordered four-test electrolyte panel, the time allowed would have been 2.9 minutes: 2.6 for the first test and 0.1 for each additional test in the panel. The more hands-on time required in performing a test, the more time was given to the CAP unit. Thus, a totally automated chemistry test was given a much lower value than compatibility testing in the blood bank. An example of CAP workload recording calculations is found in Figure 24-1.

Laboratories would typically separate their workload reports into three sections for each test:

1. Ordered tests performed.
2. Repeat tests performed.
3. Quality control tests performed.

This method, although more realistic as to what is actually being done in the lab, can be quite laborious to record and easily manipulated if recorded manually. Many laboratory information systems now support this method, making it easier and more reliable to report.

The second system utilizes **adjusted patient days** as a standard by which to measure staff productivity. Adjusted patient days is a value that is determined by taking the number of inpatients and applying a ratio to that number to account for the outpatient testing that is occurring at the same time. This ratio is determined by historical statistics indicating that, based on a certain in-house census, one should be encountering a set number of outpatient visits or tests. This approach is flawed in that it assigns a greater weight on outpatient procedures than on the same tests ordered for an inpatient due to reimbursement values. Outpatient procedures are generally reimbursed per test, whereas inpatients are reimbursed by diagnosis. For example, if there were 300 outpatient procedures ordered and 200 inpatient tests ordered, your standard would be higher, allowing you more hours to do the same amount of work than if there were 300 inpatient procedures ordered and 200 outpatient tests ordered. The calculations use revenue, rather than number of tests, in determining the number of hours needed. This makes the adjusted patient day method invalid in its assumptions and inaccurate in its conclusions. Calculations for adjusted patient days are shown in Figure 24-2.

The method of using **billable procedures** as a standard is currently a commonly used method of recording workload. This process uses the number of procedures, both inpatient and outpatient, that are billed on a daily basis to determine the number of hours required to do that volume of work. A standard is assigned to the lab, based on historical statistics or national benchmarks, to use in a calculation against the number of billed tests that were performed for the day or the interval of time being measured.

Using billable procedures, a weekly staffing performance report can be generated as illustrated in Table 24-1. In the illustration, the staffing index is more than 100, thus indicating that the staff is being highly productive. The justification for the overproductivity is that one full-time equivalent (FTE) is out on sick leave. If this was a continuous situation, a part-time position could be justified.

Unfortunately, this method does not weigh the tests for complexity or hands on time, so each procedure is counted strictly on a one-to-one basis. This means that a laboratory would receive the same amount of time allowed for a compatibility test in the blood bank as a dipstick-urine test. As a result, a laboratory doing many automated chemistry tests might look much more efficient than a lab that has numerous blood bank or microbiology procedures.

CAP has taken this type of measuring system and weighted the procedures to provide a more accurate process in determining the productivity of a laboratory. This process is part of their more extensive program, the **Laboratory Management Index Program,** (LMIP) which involves not only workload recording for labor per billable procedure, but also other expenses per billable tests and expenses for nonbillable tests. In addition, this program will compare the lab with peer groups based on size and complexity.

The laboratory manager's role in providing appropriate staffing is essential in providing quality laboratory testing, and the methods discussed previously can assist in that process.

BIBLIOGRAPHY

Varnadoe, Lionel A. 1996. *Medical laboratory management and supervision, operations, review and study guide.* Philadelphia: F. A. Davis.

Travers, Eleanor M. 1997. *Clinical laboratory management.* Baltimore, Md. Williams and Wilkins.

INTERNET RESOURCES

College of American Pathologists. <www.cap.org/HTML/capsearchminussecure.html> (enter workload recording in search box)

Date	CMP/Unit Value 3.3				Elec/Unit Value 2.8				K/Unit Value 2.5				GLU/Unit Value 2.5				Totals/Column Points
	Patient Volume	Q.C. Cal	Repeat Tests	Totals/ Points	Patient Volume	Q.C. Cal	Repeat Volume	Totals/ Points	Patient Volume	Q.C. Cal	Repeat Tests	Totals/ Points	Patient Volume	Q.C. Cal	Repeat Volume	Totals/ Points	
1/1/03	25	3	2	30/99	10	0	0	10/28	5	0	1	6/15	7	0	2	9/22.5	
1/2/03	40	3	0	43/141.9	20	0	1	21/58.8	10	0	0	10/25	20	0	3	23/57.5	
1/3/03	45	3	1	49/161.7	25	0	1	26/72.8	15	0	1	16/40	25	0	2	27/67.5	
Totals Row Points	110	9	3	122/402.6	55	0	2	57/159.6	30	0	2	32/80	52	0	7	59/130	

Total Cap Points = 772.2
Totals for Each Analyte calculated by addition of patient volume number + Q.C./Cal number + Repeat Tests.
Example CMP: 25 + 3 + 2 = 30
Points for Each Analyte calculated by multiplying totals for each analyte by CAP value.
Example CMP: 30 × 3.3 = 99
Total Cap Points calculated by adding total row points.
Example: 402.6 + 159.6 + 80 + 130 = 772.2

To calculate hours allowed for performance of the work in the example, divide 772.2 total CAP points by 60 min/hr = 12.87 hrs. Therefore, in this CAP workload recording example, 12.87 hours are needed to perform the work presented in the table.

CMP = comprehensive metabolic profile
Elec = electrolyte
K = potassium
Glu = glucose
CAP = College of American Pathologists
Unit value = CAP unit assigned value
Q.C. = quality control test
Cal = calibration test

FIGURE 24–1. CAP Workload Recording Calculations

Productive Hours Earned =

$$\frac{\text{Total Laboratory Revenue}}{\text{Inpatient Laboratory Revenue}} \times \text{Patient Days}$$

(Assume inpatient tests have the same monetary charge as outpatient tests.)

Example 1:   **Given:** Inpatient Laboratory Revenue = $33,604
                    Outpatient Laboratory Revenue = $26,104
                    Total Laboratory Revenue = $59,708
                    Patient Days =   75

            Calculation: Productive Hours Earned = $\frac{\$59,708}{\$33,604} \times 75 = 133.26$

Analysis: If the actual worked hours were 146.67, then the laboratory would not have budgeted successfully to accomplish the workload within the budget. Inpatient revenue is greater than outpatient revenue in this example.

Example 2:   **Given:** Inpatient Laboratory Revenue = $23,500
                    Outpatient Laboratory Revenue = $36,208
                    Total Laboratory Revenue = $59,708
                    Patient Days =   75

            Calculation: Productive Hours Earned = $\frac{\$59,708}{\$23,500} \times 75 = 190.56$

Analysis: If the actual worked hours were 146.67, then the laboratory would have budgeted successfully to accomplish the workload. Outpatient revenue was greater than inpatient revenue in this example.

FIGURE 24–2. Adjusted Patient Days Calculations

TABLE 24-1 Weekly Staffing Performance Report

Dept: Laboratory
Week ending: 12/8/01
Dept #: 7060
Standard: 0.21

DAY	UNIT VOL.	EARNED HOURS	ACTUAL HOURS	DAILY VAR.	CUMMULATIVE VAR.	STAFFING INDEX
Sun.	282	59.22	54.25	4.97	4.97	109.1613
Mon.	628	131.88	108.25	23.63	28.6	121.8291
Tues.	550	115.50	119.25	-.75	24.85	96.8553
Wed.	541	113.61	110.50	3.11	27.96	102.8145
Thurs.	527	110.67	95.00	15.67	43.63	116.4947
Fri.	572	120.12	114.50	5.62	49.25	104.9083
Sat.	367	77.07	56.25	20.82	70.07	137.0133
Total	3,467	728.07	658.00	70.07		110.6489

Comments/Justification: We continue to have one FTE out on sick leave.

Definitions:
Unit volume—the number of billable procedures.
Earned hours—the number of billable procedures multiplied by the standard (0.21).
Actual hours—the number of actual hours worked.
Daily variance—the variance between earned hours and actual hours.
Cummulative variance—the variance as it accumulates through the week.
Staffing index—productivity index by percentage with 100% or greater as your goal. Calculated by dividing earned hours by actual hours.
FTE—full-time equivalent

QUESTIONS

1. The primary use of workload recording is. *(Objective 1, Level I)*

2. The CAP workload unit *(Objective 2, Level I)*
   a. determines the amount of time required to perform a test
   b. includes the time for paperwork, phone calls, and so on.
   c. separates workload reports into three sections of ordered test, repeat tests, and quality control test
   d. A and C
   e. all of the above

3. The adjusted patient days method for analyzing workload is dependent on a ratio of inpatients to outpatients. *(Objective 3, Level I)*

   True or False?

4. Identify a commonly used workload recording method that considers the number of procedures billed on a daily basis. *(Objective 4, Level I)*

5. Discuss the advantages of the Laboratory Management Index Program (LMIP) for workload recording. *(Objective 5, Level II)*

EXERCISES

Completion of the exercises will enhance your knowledge of workload recording. *(Objective 6, Level II and Objective 7, Level III)*

1. Interview the administrative technologist to determine how employee productivity is determined and what level of productivity is expected.

2. Working with one of the department supervisors, calculate the staffing productivity of that department for the last three months. Analyze whether the department is under, over, or adequately staffed.

3. Consider a department that is understaffed. Prepare a case to convince the hospital administration to hire additional personnel based on the productivity level.

CASES

Analyze the following case studies and propose solutions. *(Objective 8, Level III)*

1. Your workload volume has been averaging 4,000 tests per week, and with a standard 0.21 to determine your weekly productivity using the billable procedure method, your percent productivity has been running eighty-five percent. You increase your staffing to accommodate the additional training and paperwork involved in the new perpetual inventory system that you are about to implement. A month later your CEO tells you that you must let someone go in order to get your staffing down. What are the errors in this situation? How might you correct this?

2. Your hospital's physician recruitment team successfully recruited two internal medicine doctors, one family practice doctor, and two OB-GYN doctors six months ago. Your monthly volumes have increased by an average of 1,000 procedures, placing your staffing productivity at 120–135%. You know your CAP biannual inspection will be coming up in another three months, and your techs are already getting short tempered and very stressed. What should you do?

Chapter 25

Purchasing

Eric Reed, B.S., MT(ASCP)

OBJECTIVES

Upon completion of this chapter the learner will be able to

1. Define *purchasing*. *(Level I)*
2. Name the ordering categories. *(Level I)*
3. State the advantages of using a central storeroom or warehouse. *(Level I)*
4. Name important factors to consider when evaluating a capital purchase. *(Level I)*
5. Explain the difference between a contract agreement and a time and material arrangement. *(Level II)*
6. Differentiate the use of a requisition versus a purchase order. *(Level I)*
7. Develop a flow diagram of the ordering process. *(Level III)*
8. Evaluate a laboratory's materials management program and make suggestions for improvements. *(Level III)*
9. Analyze the case studies and propose solutions. *(Level III)*

TOPIC SUMMARY

Purchasing—the word alone implies the buying of something. In its purest sense, that may be true. But in a more practical sense, it is much more complex than that. Purchasing involves the determination of what is needed, evaluation of which product meets the need, where the needed product can be most efficiently obtained, which supplier offers the best value, and what restrictions or guidelines are applicable to the "buyer" relative to the purchase of that product.

Although not usually the case in health care, supplies and equipment can account for more dollars spent annually than those spent on salaries. This usually occurs in individual functional areas of the organization that have excessive supplies and equipment cost. Therefore, it is imperative that managers exercise diligence in selecting products. Likewise, employees must be fiscally responsible and accountable for the proper and conservative use of those products.

When one thinks of the items that must be purchased by an organization, those items can generally be placed into three categories: **operational supplies, capital,** and **services.** Each of these has its own unique characteristics. Therefore, each category will be discussed separately in the following sections.

Operational Supplies

Each department of any health-care facility uses items daily that are unique to its service line. Each department also uses items that are common to the organization. Because of this, those products that are common are usually managed and purchased by a central storeroom or warehouse for the organization and distributed from that point. This provides for greater efficiency in inventory control, stock rotation, and "buying power" of the organization. Products can certainly be obtained at a lower price when purchased in bulk from a central point. Bulk purchasing can often give the buyer negotiating power for purchasing contracts for long periods of time and for certain "perks" associated with large purchases.

For example, a hospital uses a lot of copier/printer paper annually and foresees an increase in that use in the immediate future. Hospital management determines how much has been purchased in the past five years and projects usage for the next five years. Several suppliers are contacted, given expected usage volumes, and asked to submit a bid price for the paper with the understanding that the hospital is committed to buying a certain amount annually. Because the bidder knows that there will be a "guaranteed sale" each year, it can agree to sell the paper at a price that is usually much less per case than when there is no assurance of what sales will be. The bidder may also offer other incentives, such as even greater discounts if purchases exceed a certain amount. This type of purchasing requires more work than just simply submitting a weekly order to "Dead Tree Paper Company," but that extra work results in savings that can be applied elsewhere.

This same type of strategy can be applied by individual department managers for those items that are unique to the department. Although the volume of these purchases may not be as big as for the central point of the hospital, because of the nature of the product relative to how it has to be manufactured, better pricing can be given by the supplier when it is known how much will be used annually. The savvy manager will continuously review applicable supplier literature to look for "deals" relative to his unique supplies. In the interest of curbing rising health-care costs, it is not just prudent for the manager to do this, but is also his or her fiscal responsibility. Knowledge is power. And being knowledgeable of the market empowers the manager to negotiate agreements that not only make his or her operation run more smoothly but allow his or her department, and thus the organization, to be more economically efficient.

For example, the clinical chemistry supervisor in a laboratory reports to his manager that the chemistry/immunochemistry quality control material from Company "S" has shown excellent performance. And the technical support provided by that company has been superb. The manager then contacts the sales representative, relays the thoughts of the supervisor, and inquires about incentives and pricing for a long-term purchasing agreement. He discovers that he can save thirty percent off the price he is currently paying *and* receive the same lot number of product for each eighteen-month period if he is willing to sign a three-year agreement. This type of agreement proves to be a bonanza operationally for the laboratory and economically for the laboratory and the hospital.

Bear in mind that this example is not theoretical—the benefits are real, and there are many more types of opportunities available to those managers and staff employees who are willing to search for them.

Capital

Up until the early to mid 1990s, the word *capital* was always associated with equipment. However, since computer technology became so widespread and software has become so expensive, capital applies to more than just equipment. Therefore it has become necessary for most health-care agencies to define what is classified as capital. Generally, it may be defined as any item equal to or exceeding a certain dollar amount and having a specified useful life expectancy. These definitions are important for department managers to be able to project what "capital" costs will be. In larger facilities, capital costs are usually separated from operational supplies and services for budgeting purposes. There are well-founded reasons for this because some capital acquisitions can be extremely expensive. But, more importantly, capital items, because they have a defined life expectancy, can be depreciated over that period of time, which is important to the fixed asset list of the organization. Depreciation as discussed here means measuring the loss in value, over time, of an asset. Straight-line depreciation, presented in this chapter, simply means that an item is assigned a life expectancy, then the initial value of the item is divided by the number of years of life expectancy, thus providing the amount of depreciation per year. As the capital items of an institution are depreciated in value, the assets of the institution are therefore less. A lower value of assets is not always good, but it is often the case. Certainly it is an advantage relative to the amount of casualty insurance that must be owned, as the lower the value of assets, the less the amount of insurance needed. Diligence must be exercised in the evaluation and acquisition of capital items because these types of items are usually expensive and are expected to last several years. One should always consider the following when evaluating capital: **applicability, quality,** and **value.**

- Applicability: It may seem unimaginable, but people will buy things that do not meet their needs. That's why it is very important to consider what it is that you want an item to do and be sure that you only consider items that will do what is needed. Also, realize that you do not have to have more than is needed. Try to evaluate your needs at work in the same prudent manner you would for personal or home use. A good way to evaluate applicability is with this analogy: you need a truck to haul things on the farm—not a car. But, you don't need a luxury truck just to perform a task. Make a decision based upon need, not want.

- **Quality:** There's a lot of truth to the statement "You get what you pay for." Once a decision has been made as to the item that is needed, be sure to carefully look at the quality of craftsmanship on all available items. Remember that most new knives are sharp, but good quality steel will hold a sharp edge for a long time and can be easily resharpened. Pick a product that will do the job and is so well made that it will last a long time. Also, be sure to consider how easily the product is to maintain and repair. There is no substitute for quality.
- **Value:** Value doesn't mean just the price you pay for something. Value applies to how much you get for that price. It relates a lot to the item's quality, other components such as length of use or warranty, availability of service, cost of service and parts, and cooperation of the manufacturer or vendor when difficulties arise.

Acquisition of capital, to serve the institution best, requires a lot of effort. It should be as important to the manager as buying a house or a car. Give it plenty of thought! And remember, capital doesn't have to be acquired by purchase. There is always the option of capital lease. Leases are usually more costly when annualized, compared to purchases, but often have some advantages. One needs to always consider the "pros and cons" of purchase *and* lease.

Purchased Services

You may not think of the many services provided by others to your institution as something that you "buy," but they are. After all, these services are usually not free. However, we tend to think of "buying" resulting in a product that can be seen and felt. As in our personal day-to-day lives, services account for many of the purchases in a business. Just as we buy electricity and telephone service at home, we buy maintenance, repairs, consultation, and so on in business. Simply put, purchased services are those services provided to our business by others for which we pay fees. Believe it or not, these services can constitute a large part of the overall purchasing dollar. Therefore, we must be financially prudent in our selection of regular services and in our selection of random services. Services are usually purchased in two ways—**contractual agreement** and **time and materials.** Each of these is important in its own way and must be well thought out prior to making a decision.

- **Contractual Agreement:** For those services that we know are always going to be needed on a regular basis, it is good to consider a contract for the provision of those services. A contract usually allows for negotiating a fixed rate for the service over an extended period and *may* (not always) be less expensive than a noncontract arrangement. Contracts also place the burden on the vendor, not the owner, to meet certain time schedules for the work and to ensure satisfaction to the customer that service will meet expectations. After all, if satisfaction is not met, then the contract can be canceled. This results in a negative impact on the vendor. Consider the following example of the word *may* as used in the discussion of a contract.

    Suppose your laboratory has an expensive, complex instrument on which you are highly dependent for providing day-to-day patient testing. When you purchased the instrument, it came with a one-year warranty; however, you expect to have the instrument five years. Although the instrument was well proven operationally, via historical data from other users when you purchased it, you knew that if it were to fail, it would need to be repaired quickly. Therefore you negotiated with the supplier to provide service for years two through five via a service contract. This contract, although seemingly expensive, allows for peace of mind during "down times" because you know the vendor will respond promptly and provide repairs quickly. And, regardless of what or how many parts have to be replaced or how much time it takes, it's all "covered" by the contract cost. That's a great feeling, and it makes budgeting for purchased services easy. At the end of the five-year period, you decide that it will be at least two more years before you can get a new replacement for the instrument. So you must decide if you will or will not renew the service contract. At this point, you determine how much the contract has cost you for the previous four years versus how much repairs would have cost if you had not had the contract. It is during this analysis that you will determine if you overpaid by having the contract or if you realized considerable savings by having the contract. Either way, you will have to make a decision about which way to proceed for the next two years. A proven recipe for how to make that decision is not possible. There are too many factors to consider before you can make that decision. That's why *you* are the manager! Just remember, always make a decision you can defend and one in which you are confident.
- **Time and Materials:** This simply means that when you need service, you call a reliable vendor to perform the service and then you pay for his travel, labor, and the parts he has to use to complete repairs or preventive maintenance. Rates for travel and labor often seem very expensive but paying for this

service on an infrequent basis may be less expensive than a service contract. An example follows:

Suppose you have an instrument on which you have had a service contract for several years. The vendor has notified you of the impending expiration of the contract. Now you must decide to either renew the contract or not. You have the service provider give you an audit of the repair records on the instrument for those years for which it has been under contract along with what repair costs would have been if there had not been a contract. After analysis you determine that annual repair and preventive maintenance costs would have been, on average, $2,000 less than the contract cost. Therefore you decide that you will not renew the contract. This is a decision based on best available information, and only time will show whether that decision proves to be beneficial financially.

The two previous examples have been relevant to instrumentation. However, purchased services are not applicable to instrumentation only. Some other types of purchased services are air quality analysis, reference lab testing services, clinical and anatomic pathology consultative services, annual review of billing practices and procedures, fees for on-site physical facility and practice inspections, and so on. There are many types of purchased services that do not result in a tangible product but which are vital to the ongoing operation of the facility.

Buying power can often be enhanced by being a member/participant in a group purchasing organization (G.P.O.). G.P.O.s are entities developed as a consortium of member facilities. The management of the G.P.O. negotiates, on behalf of the members as a whole, contracts for goods and services with various vendors. As stated previously, when vendors are aware that many facilities will be buying from them, they are more likely to lower prices to reap the rewards of volume sales. Obviously the best advantage of being part of a G.P.O. is the positive effect on the financial bottom line. However, there are at least two potential disadvantages:

1. The G.P.O. management may negotiate "best pricing" with a vendor whose product(s) do not meet the expectations or needs of your facility. When this is the case, you are then faced with a management decision—either make a purchase based solely on price or consider the quality of the testing your facility does to be of utmost importance and then negotiate pricing with the vendor of your choice.

2. Oftentimes, if a manager is willing to put forth the effort to negotiate better pricing, more value and more perks can be obtained than by "just going with the contract." G.P.O. contracts have a tendency to make managers lazy. Don't become one who falls into that trap.

Consortia can definitely work to your advantage most of the time. Participation in such an arrangement is a good business practice, but one must not forget to explore all options.

The mechanics of purchasing involve two tools: the **requisition** (Figure 25–1) and the **purchase order** (Figure 25–2). The requisition is used to request the purchase of a product and is completed by the requesting department and sent to the purchasing department. In the purchasing department, the purchase order is prepared after review of the budget and, if needed, consultation with the vendor. The purchase order authorizes payment from the institution to the vendor for delivery of the product.

Do not be misled into believing that purchasing is only as complex as this chapter has presented it. But perhaps this overview and examples have been educational and shown you that a lot of effort and thought must be exercised before "just buying something." Never forget that there is no substitute for experience. Therefore as you purchase more, you will become a more savvy buyer. In times of doubt consult with someone with more or different experience. Remember that information results in knowledge, which only benefits the decision-making process.

BIBLIOGRAPHY

Travers, Eleanor M. 1997. *Clinical laboratory management.* Baltimore: Williams & Wilkins.

Varnadoe, Lionel A. 1996. *Medical laboratory management and supervision—Operations, review, and study guide.* Philadelphia: F. A. Davis.

INTERNET RESOURCES

Advance for Administrators of the Laboratory. <www.advanceforal.com/common/contenttools/pastarticles.aspx>

Advance for Medical Laboratory Professionals. <www.advanceformlp.com>

Coalition for Healthcare eStandards, Inc. <www.chestandards.org>

Healthcare Publishing News, Nelson Publishing, Inc. <www.hpnonline.com/inside>

Medical Laboratory Observer. <www.mlo-online.com>

Virtual Hospital, University of Iowa. <www.vh.org>

Virtual Hospital, University of Iowa. <www.vh.org/adult/provider/pathology/CLIA/KitInstrumentSelection/index.html>

Requisition No. 0001

General Hospital and Clinics
Purchase Requisition
(Not to be used as a purchase order)
To be filled in by department

Department _Clinical Laboratory_ Date _3/28/03_

Deliver to _Clinical Laboratory_ / _200_
               Bldg.   Room

Name and Address of Vendor(s) suggested (if any):
1. _Scientific Company_ 2. _____
   7788 Street
   Detroit, MI   50112

Quantity	Unit	Description	Unit Price	Total Price
5	kits	B2000 Enteric Kits	$20.00	$100.00
6	cases	A7700 100 × 15 mm Petri Plates	$40.00	$240.00
TOTAL				$340.00

Requested by: _____   _____
                    Signature   Date

Department Director approval: _____   _____
                    Signature   Date

Administration approval: _____   _____
                    Signature   Date

To be filled in by purchaser

Purchase Order No. _____   Date Ordered _____
Order to _____ of _____
          (representative)   (company)

Quoted by _____ to _____
        (vendor representative)   (hospital representative)

Expected Delivery Date _____

Freight to be paid by _____vendor _____hospital   Not to exceed _____

Comments: _____

FIGURE 25-1. Purchase Requisition.

General Hospital & Clinics
Purchase Order

Purchase Order: 7000
Department: Clinical Laboratory
Date: 3/28/03

Vendor: 00077224
Scientific Company
7788 Street
Detroit, MI   50112

Please ship the following items noting the terms, prices, and conditions given below:

Payment terms: 30 days
Freight terms: FOB: Destination
Ship by: Trucking Company
Department ID: Clinical Lab
Requisition ID: 0001
Requestor: Clinical Lab
Buyer: General Hospital & Clinics

Item #	Quan	Unit	Description	Unit Price	Total Price
1.	5	kits	B2000 Enteric Kits	$20.00	$100.00
2.	6	cases	A7700 100 × 15 mm Petri Plates	$40.00	$240.00
			Total PO Amount		$340.00

Bill to: General Hospital & Clinics   Ship to: General Hospital & Clinics
          Financial Services   Receiving Department
          1000 Long Street   1000 Long Street
          Hattiesburg, MS 70020   Hattiesburg, MS 70020

FIGURE 25–2. Purchase Order.

QUESTIONS

1. Purchasing is *(Objective 1, Level I)*
   a. determining need, justifying need, and ordering
   b. determining need, evaluating product, locating product, and determining best value
   c. determining need, evaluating product, abiding by guidelines of state, and ordering
   d. buying product

2. Items to be purchased can be categorized into *(Objective 2, Level I)*
   a. operational supplies
   b. capital equipment
   c. services
   d. salaries
   e. a, b, and c
   f. all of the above

3. Discuss the advantages of using a central storeroom or warehouse. *(Objective 3, Level I)*

4. When evaluating a capital purchase, consideration should be given to *(Objective 4, Level I)*
   a. _____
   b. _____
   c. _____

5. Explain the difference in a contract agreement and a time-and-material arrangement. *(Objective 5, Level II)*

6. The requisition is *(Objective 6, Level I)*
   a. used to request supplies and so on
   b. completed by the requesting department
   c. sent directly to the company to order supplies and so on
   d. a & b
   e. all of the above

7. The purchase order *(Objective 6, Level I)*
   a. is sent by the requesting department to purchasing
   b. authorizes payment from the institution
   c. never leaves the requesting institution
   d. a & b
   e. all of the above

EXERCISES

Completion of the exercises will enhance your knowledge of purchasing. *(Objective 7, Level III and Objective 8, Level III)*

1. Follow a requisition from preparation in the department to the purchasing department and observe the processing of the order from initial implementation through mailing of the order. List the steps in the process and prepare a flow diagram of the process.

2. Interview the administrator of materials management or purchasing and determine the administrator's view of the laboratory's role in the process. Discuss ways that the administrator believes the laboratory could improve the process.

3. Evaluate the materials management program for the laboratory. Are there ways the program could be improved? Survey the supervisors and determine how they view the program, and make recommendations for change if needed.

CASES

Analyze the following case studies and propose solutions. *(Objective 9, Level III)*

1. You are the supervisor of microbiology and have the blood agar plates on a drop shipment arrangement every month; however, every month you run out of blood agar plates because some of the plates are outdated and cannot be used. Analyze this situation and suggest how you could solve the problem, while keeping the solution cost effective.

2. You have a $50,000 autoclave in your laboratory that is ten years old. It still operates properly and you have it presently under a contractual agreement that costs $2,400 per year. There are certain parts not covered under the agreement including the compressor, which the service technician has told you may fail at any time. The new compressor will cost you approximately $4,000. Everything else on the autoclave seems to be in working condition. You have had to call the service technician an average of two times per year in the past, and he has spent approximately five hours on each service call. Your in-house biomedical department has never worked on the autoclave because it is under a contractual agreement and your service is done regularly by the service technician. You are discussing the possibility of nonrenewal of the contractual agreement in favor of a time-and-materials arrangement with the autoclave company. The labor is quoted as $100 per hour and includes travel time, which is five hours round-trip, thus the travel by automobile from the company to your laboratory would be approximately $500 round-trip. Hotel cost per night ranges from fifty dollars to sixty-five dollars.

    Analyze this situation and develop a proposal for your administrator indicating your recommendation as to whether to continue the service contract or implement the time-and-materials arrangement.

Chapter 26

Employee Scheduling

Kathy Shields, M.H.S., MT(ASCP)

OBJECTIVES

Upon completion of this chapter the learner will be able to

1. List factors that impact scheduling. *(Level I)*
2. Identify factors that impact salary budget. *(Level I)*
3. Calculate number of full-time equivalents (FTEs) required for a specific work volume. *(Level II)*
4. Explain how the scheduled staff mix would impact salary dollars. *(Level II)*
5. Relate productivity and efficiency to salary dollars and scheduling. *(Level II)*
6. Calculate productivity. *(Level II)*
7. Illustrate the impact that education and experience would have on scheduling, budget, and staff mix. *(Level II)*
8. Identify the scheduling factors that must be considered for employee morale and retention. *(Level I)*
9. Describe the impact of test menu and staff skills/training on scheduling. *(Level II)*
10. Identify the minimum number of weeks a schedule should be posted in advance. *(Level I)*
11. List three shift scheduling options. *(Level I)*
12. Relate overtime pay to scheduling. *(Level II)*
13. Name advantages of PRN (pro re nata-as needed) personnel in scheduling. *(Level I)*
14. Describe how changes in the schedule should be handled by the manager. *(Level I)*
15. Construct a schedule. *(Level III)*
16. Propose solutions for the case studies. *(Level III)*

TOPIC SUMMARY

A well-managed laboratory is like a puzzle with many individual pieces that should fit together smoothly to create the perfect picture. Employee scheduling is one piece of the puzzle that is bordered on each side by other areas of the manager's responsibilities, including budgeting, monitoring of productivity and efficiency, recruitment of new employees, and retention of current employees. The combination of the test menu, education and experience level of staff members, number of employees needed for the anticipated test volume, number of emergency areas served, turn-around time expectations, and level of complexity of testing will determine the staffing needs of the department and the scheduling of employees. It is important to understand the relationship of each of these areas as they relate to employee scheduling.

Dollars spent on employee salaries compose the majority of the departmental budget; therefore, the proper use of human resources through efficient scheduling is critical to a manager's success. The salary budget is dependent on several factors: number of employees, number of hours worked by each one, and educational and experience level of each. The number of employees needed is determined by a combination of elements, so a method of calculating this estimate can be useful. A standard unit is assigned to each billable test and multiplied by the number of tests performed to calculate the number of worked hours needed. For example, if the standard unit of measure applied is 0.25 and the billable test volume for a fourteen-day period is 12,000, then the number of worked hours earned is 3,000 hours. When 3,000 hours is divided by 80 (the number of hours worked by a full-time employee in a fourteen-day period), the suggested number of employees is 37.5 full-time equivalents (FTEs). Another approach could be to divide the 3,000 hours among several part-time and PRN (pro re nata, which means "as needed") employees in addition to the full-time staff members. Keep in mind that this method is a tool to be adapted to the individual needs of the laboratory. Lastly, the education level of employees as well as their number of years of experience also affects the amount spent on salaries. Of course, medical technologists/clinical laboratory scientists will be paid at a higher rate than medical laboratory technicians/clinical laboratory technicians, phlebotomists, and assistants. Staff members with more years of experience will be paid more than those with fewer years. The manager needs to determine the staff mix that will satisfy testing requirements while considering the impact on the budget.

Scheduling is also dependent on the productivity and efficiency of the department. Productivity measurement is a financial indicator that is closely monitored by an effective manager. If the testing volume is below average, the productivity and efficiency of the department is lower. With less revenue coming in, fewer salary dollars need to be spent. When the productivity decreases below the established level, scheduling should be adjusted accordingly by working fewer hours. A calculation to determine departmental productivity is to divide the earned hours by the number of actual worked hours and multiply by 100. In the earlier example, 3,000 hours were earned based on the workload of 12,000 billable tests. If 3,200 hours had actually been worked during this period, the laboratory was operating at 93.8% productivity. A productivity index of greater than 100% while still achieving high quality is ideal.

When considering the recruitment of new employees, the employee schedule must be consulted to determine the educational and experience levels required for the vacant positions. For example, if the vacancy on the schedule is on the night shift in a small facility where the technologist will work alone, the manager might select a technologist with several years of experience rather than a technician with no experience. In contrast, if the vacancy is on the day shift in a busy automated department with several technologists, the technician with no prior experience might be the better choice. Again, the employee schedule, budget, and staff mix are intertwined.

The laboratory work schedule has a major impact on employee morale and, therefore, retention of employees. The goal of the scheduler should be that of a win-win situation: adequate staffing to care for patient needs balanced with a work schedule that satisfies the personal needs of the employee. When a manager hires an employee, the employee's family has also entered the picture—the manager who attempts to meet the needs of the family will maintain a high level of morale. The schedule should be analyzed by reviewing it in one direction for adequate coverage in each section and then by careful review of each employee's individual schedule for fairness, personal preferences, and opportunities for rewards. For example, if Monday is the busiest day of the week for testing, the majority of staff members should be scheduled to work that day; however, if Monday is also a day that an employee needs to be off to take a college class, perhaps a PRN employee could be scheduled instead. If an attractive pattern can be found in the schedule such as three- or four-day weekends, this can be a reward to boost morale and promote retention. Also, employees should be asked for their preferences in their schedules—one may prefer to have Wednesdays off for church activities, whereas another asks for Thursdays for piano lessons. If the manager tries to work with the employee, employee satisfaction and retention should remain at a high level.

The test menu determines which lab section will need employees. A wide range of services on the menu would constitute a larger number of employees; for example, some laboratories may need technologists in microbiology, immunohematology, hematology, chemistry, immunology/serology, virology, immunochemistry, toxicology, and urinalysis. On the other hand, a laboratory in a small hospital facility with a narrow range of in-house services provided would not need a different employee to be scheduled in each section.

Next, knowledge of the skills and training of the staff and the needs of the section is required in order to determine the expertise of the individuals to be scheduled. For instance, the microbiology department always needs at least one experienced microbiologist on duty, and the blood bank needs at least one technologist experienced with antibody identification on the schedule. Automated sections of the laboratory, on the other hand, may need larger numbers of bench techs with one or more experienced techs to offer supervision. Test complexity also determines the schedule assignments.

A thorough analysis of the work flow in each section is necessary to decide the number of employees to be assigned to each duty shift. The number should be directly related to the number of procedures performed, and the staffing level can be determined using the same formula as mentioned previously. A factor that may affect the calculation, however, is the number of emergency areas served by the laboratory. A large hospital facility with a central laboratory servicing an emergency department, Intensive Care Unit, Coronary Care Unit, Neonatal Intensive Care Unit, cardiovascular surgery, trauma center, plus medical and surgical nursing units may not fit the formula, and additional staff may need to be scheduled to provide for the expected turnaround times to the critical areas.

One person may prepare the schedule for the entire laboratory or, in the case of large laboratories, several supervisors may prepare schedules for individual sections. The scheduler should begin early enough so that the finished product can be posted in advance, preferably three to four weeks. A deadline should be posted for vacation and holiday requests to be submitted. Also, a deadline should be established for the posting of the schedule to allow employees to plan ahead.

A schedule starts with a blank template. The names are listed on the schedule along with the dates of the month as shown in Figure 26–1.

Some facilities prepare a schedule for shorter or longer periods of time than a month. For labs that require twenty-four-hour coverage seven days per week, it is easier to cover the weekends and then the night shift sections first. Unless other employees have been hired specifically for weekend coverage, all bench techs should fairly rotate weekend coverage. Weekends are normally staffed with a smaller number of employees due to an anticipated reduction in workload. Fewer number of employees working on the weekend also allows employees to work a fewer number of weekends.

After weekends and nights are covered, employees with regularly established schedules (i.e., 6 A.M., 7 A.M., 8 A.M., 1 P.M., 3 P.M., 11 P.M., etc.) are filled in next. Traditional shifts once were 7 A.M.–3 P.M., 3 P.M.–11 P.M., and 11 P.M.–7 A.M.; however, nontraditional schedules have emerged, and new ones are being created for individuals as needed. Attractive options such as seven days on and seven days off work best for some employees, whereas full-time students who also have to work full time find extended weekend shifts suitable.

When scheduling, consideration must be given to the prevention or minimization of overtime hours. When an employee works a weekend shift, another day off during the week should be scheduled so that he will not accumulate overtime during the week and will obtain a rest day. Different facilities use different payroll options, such as a forty-hour week or the "eight and eighty" option available to hospitals. The choice of payroll option determines at what point an employee begins getting paid at an overtime rate. Overtime rate is paid when the employee on the forty-hour week works more than forty hours in a week. With the eight and eighty option, the employee receives overtime pay when he works more than eighty hours in a pay period or more than the eight hours in a workday. The manager must understand the guidelines and schedule employees so that overtime is not necessary.

In order to provide coverage for the employees' scheduled days off, the use of part-time or PRN personnel is invaluable. PRN personnel help to eliminate the need for overtime by full-time staff and allow for greater flexibility in the schedule. They are helpful when scheduling around requested vacations and holidays as well. After scheduling the full-time employees, the PRN and part-time personnel are added to the schedule.

Once the schedule is complete, it should be reviewed carefully and objectively for completeness and fairness to all employees. It should then be posted in a visible location. Adjustments to the schedule should be made only with permission of the scheduler.

The time spent on the schedule after it is posted should be minimal, but in times of shortages or emergencies, scheduling may become a daily activity. When there are not enough employees to cover the departments and shifts, the schedule can become a daunting task. Changes are sometimes made at the last minute to provide coverage, and employees may have to be scheduled to work in areas or on shifts that they do not normally work. Good communication by the manager becomes critical at this stage, and it must always be known that changes may be necessary to take care of patients. Changes to the routine schedule or previously posted schedule should always be discussed with the employee by the scheduler. Also, any denial of requested paid time off should be discussed with the employee.

This summary on scheduling is based on a somewhat traditional method. Self-scheduling by the employees has also been successful for some laboratories. Also, computer programs for scheduling are available commercially. Regardless of the method used for scheduling, the manager must look at the entire picture when making decisions related to the schedule. The needs of each patient, physician, and employee must be considered prior to the posting of the final product to guarantee that the number one mission is always accomplished: excellence in patient care.

Employee Scheduling

Name	Sun	Mon	Tues	Wed	Thurs	Fri	Sat	Sun	Mon	Tues	Wed	Thurs	Fri	Sat
Tech 1		7a-3:30p	7a-3:30p	7a-3:30p	7a-3:30p	7a-3:30p			7a-3:30p	7a-3:30p	7a-3:30p	7a-3:30p	7a-3:30p	
Tech 2	7a-7p	6a-2:30p	6a-2:30p	6a-2:30p	7a-7p				6a-2:30p	6a-2:30p	6a-2:30p	6a-2:30p	6a-2:30p	
Tech 3		6a-2:30p	6a-2:30p	6a-2:30p	6a-2:30p	6a-2:30p		7a-7p	6a-2:30p	6a-2:30p	6a-2:30p	6a-2:30p	6a-2:30p	
Tech 4			5a-11a	5a-11a	5a-11a					5a-11a	5a-11a	5a-11a		
Tech 5					7p-7a	7p-7a	7p-7a						7a-5:30p	
Tech 6		7:30a-4p	7:30a-4p	7:30a-4p	7:30a-4p	7:30a-4p			7:30a-4p	7:30a-4p	7:30a-4p	7:30a-4p	7:30a-4p	
Tech 7		7a-7p	7a-7p				7a-7p		7a-7p	7a-7p				
Tech 8		9a-5:30p	9a-5:30p	9a-5:30p	9a-5:30p	9a-5:30p			9a-5:30p	9a-5:30p	9a-5:30p	9a-5:30p	9a-5:30p	
Tech 9		7a-3:30p	7a-3:30p	7a-3:30p	7a-3:30p	7a-3:30p			7a-3:30p	7a-3:30p	7a-3:30p	7a-3:30p	7a-3:30p	
Tech 10		6a-2:30p	6a-2:30p				7a-7p	7a-7p	6a-2:30p	6a-2:30p				
Tech 11		1p-9:30p	1p-9:30p	1p-9:30p	1p-9:30p	1p-9:30p			1p-9:30p	1p-9:30p	1p-9:30p	1p-9:30p	1p-9:30p	
Tech 12		1p-9:30p							1p-9:30p					
Tech 13				5p-9:30p							5p-9:30p		5p-9:30p	
Tech 14	7a-7p													7a-7p
Tech 15		6:30a-3p	6:30a-3p	6:30a-3p	6:30a-3p	6:30a-3p			6:30a-3p	6:30a-3p	6:30a-3p	6:30a-3p	6:30a-3p	
Tech 16		1p-9:30p	1p-9:30p	1p-9:30p	1p-9:30p	1p-9:30p				1p-9:30p	1p-9:30p	1p-9:30p		7a-7p
Tech 17				4p-9p	4p-9p						4p-9p	4p-9p		
Tech 18	9p-7:30a	9p-7:30a	9p-7:30a	9p-7:30a				9p-7:30a	9p-7:30a	9p-7:30a	9p-7:30a			7p-7a
Tech 19	7p-7a	7p-7a	7p-7a	7p-7a	7p-7a	7p-7a	7p-7a		7p-7a	7p-7a	7p-7a	7p-7a	7p-7a	
Tech 20						5p-9p							5p-9p	
Tech 21														
Manager		8a-4:30p	8a-4:30p	8a-4:30p	8a-4:30p	8a-4:30p			8a-4:30p	8a-4:30p	8a-4:30p	8a-4:30p	8a-4:30p	
Manager		8a-4:30p	8a-4:30p	8a-4:30p	8a-4:30p	8a-4:30p			8a-4:30p	8a-4:30p	8a-4:30p	8a-4:30p	8a-4:30p	

FIGURE 26–1. Work Schedule

Bibliography

Dessler, Gary. 1997. *Human resource management.* 7th ed. Upper Saddle River, N.J.: Prentice Hall.

Frings, Christopher, ed. 2001. Management q&a. *Medical Laboratory Observer* 33, 12: 36–37.

Rakich, Jonathon, J. Longest, B. Beaufort, and K. Darr. 1992. *Managing health services organizations.* 3d ed. Baltimore: Health Professions Press.

Internet Resources

Find Articles, The Web's first Free Article Search. <www.findarticles.com/cf_0/m3230/12_33/81582437/p2/article.jhtml?term=scheduling>

QUESTIONS

1. List six factors that impact scheduling. *(Objective 1, Level I)*
   a. _____
   b. _____
   c. _____
   d. _____
   e. _____
   f. _____

2. Factors that impact a laboratory salary budget include all of the following EXCEPT *(Objective 2, Level I)*
   a. number of employees
   b. number of hours worked by each employee
   c. excess profit for the institution
   d. education and experience level of each employee

3. The number of FTEs required if the fourteen-day billable test volume was 5,000 and the standard unit was 0.5 is *(Objective 3, Level II)*
   a. 21.25
   b. 26.15
   c. 31.25
   d. 41.25

4. Explain how the scheduled staff mix would impact salary dollars. *(Objective 4, Level II)*

5. Relate productivity to salary dollars and scheduling. *(Objective 5, Level II)*

6. The productivity is _____, given that 2,500 hours were earned and 2,750 hours were actually worked. *(Objective 6, Level II)*
   a. 80.8%
   b. 82.5%
   c. 85.6%
   d. 90.9%

7. Illustrate the impact that staff education and experience would have on scheduling, budget, and staff mix. *(Objective 7, Level II)*

8. Which of the following scheduling factors must be considered for employee morale and retention? *(Objective 8, Level I)*
    a. adequate coverage
    b. fairness
    c. personal preference
    d. opportunities for rewards
    e. all of the above

9. Describe the impact of test menu and staff skills/training on scheduling. *(Objective 9, Level II)*

10. The minimum number of weeks a schedule should be posted in advance is _____. *(Objective 10, Level I)*

11. List three shift options. *(Objective 11, Level I)*
    a. _____
    b. _____
    c. _____

12. Relate overtime pay to scheduling. *(Objective 12, Level II)*

13. State three advantages of using PRN personnel. *(Objective 13, Level I)*
    a. _____
    b. _____
    c. _____

14. Describe how the manager should handle schedule changes. *(Objective 14, Level I)*

EXERCISES

Completion of the exercises will enhance your knowledge of employee scheduling. *(Objective 15, Level III)*

1. Examine a laboratory schedule. Propose a plan to cover the same workload if one of the full-time employees needs a six-week leave of absence.

2. Plan a fourteen-day schedule for a chemistry section that performs 24,000 tests during this time frame. The schedule should be covered twenty-four hours per day for each day of the week.

3. Interview several laboratory managers for innovative and attractive scheduling options that have been useful to them. Determine pros and cons of each one.

CASES

Analyze the following cases and propose solutions. *(Objective 16, Level III)*

1. The laboratory outreach representative informs you, the laboratory manager, that she has just recruited a new physician's office. The workload from this account will be approximately 60 samples per day or 140 tests per day; most of the tests will be routine hematology and chemistry. The majority of the samples will arrive after 3:00 P.M. You need to evaluate your current staffing and schedule to make sure that the department is ready. Include items to investigate in the areas of appropriate staffing level, staff mix, and productivity.

2. The surgery department manager reports that she has noticed an increasing number of 7:30 A.M. surgeries being delayed due to lab results being late in getting to the patient's chart. What details on the schedule should you review in order to investigate this problem?

3. You are the manager of a hospital-based laboratory that is facing a salary budget cut. How could you use various scheduling options to reach a solution?

4. A long-term employee approaches you about a family member's illness and tells you that she needs more time at home to take care of things. However, she needs to continue to work because her family will need the money and insurance benefits. What are some scheduling options that you could suggest?

Chapter 27

Evaluation of New Test Methods—The Comparison Study

David Thrash, B.S., MT(ASCP), CLS(NCA)
Margot Hall, Ph.D., F.A.I.C., CChem MRSC

OBJECTIVES

Upon completion of this chapter the learner will be able to

1. Define *comparison study*. *(Level I)*
2. State the purpose of a comparison study. *(Level I)*
3. Identify the criteria used to justify changing to a different methodology. *(Level I)*
4. List feasibility factors that must be considered prior to changing methodologies. *(Level I)*
5. Discuss why new analytical methods are developed. *(Level II)*
6. Identify the federal agency that grants approval for use of new test methods. *(Level I)*
7. Identify what is required for submission for approval of a new test method. *(Level I)*
8. Identify the function of precision, accuracy, analytical sensitivity, analytical specificity, and diagnostic validity. *(Level I)*
9. Identify contents of the letter to physicians prior to implementation of a new method. *(Level I)*
10. Analyze the data of a comparison study and determine whether the new test can be used. *(Level III)*
11. Develop a proposal to justify a comparison study for a new procedure. *(Level III)*
12. Analyze the case studies and formulate solutions. *(Level III)*

TOPIC SUMMARY

What is a laboratory comparison study? In current literature a laboratory **comparison study** is referred to as a **method validation.** Both the practical aspects and the statistical analysis must be addressed in the comparative study. The purpose of a comparison study is to demonstrate any differences there may be in results due to differences in reagents and methodology from one system to the next. In addition, laboratory comparison studies will also point out any differences there may be in therapeutic ranges as well as expected values due to differences in the sensitivities of reagents being compared (Coulter Corporation 1997). This evaluation may include any test as simple as one-step hCG testing to a more complex test such as comparing the WBC counts from two different hematology analyzers that currently may be in use in your laboratory.

Before a comparison study is performed in your laboratory, certain practical criteria must be met in order to justify switching to a different methodology. These may include the following:

- A need has been determined for this new methodology (i.e., will the addition of this new test benefit patients by providing a diagnosis more quickly?).
- Requirements have been determined for this new methodology (i.e., physicians and other members of the health-care team have been involved in the decision process of adding a particular test;

preanalytical, analytical, and postanalytical requirements as outlined by the National Committee for Clinical Laboratory Standards (NCCLS) have also been discussed).

- A review of the current literature available on this new methodology has been solicited (i.e., documents supplied by the manufacturer as to the validity of said method; researching the said method on your own by reviewing articles appearing in professional journals, contacting professionals at other health-care institutions who currently have this test in use, and using internet search engines may also be prudent).
- The manufacturer has provided training with the new methodology (i.e., the capital equipment contract between the manufacturer and health-care institution should stipulate whether the manufacturer will train an individual(s) off site or if in-house training will be offered).

In addition, questions must also be asked to determine if it is feasible to switch methodologies. These may include the following:

- What is the cost per test?
- What is the turnaround time?
- What is the materials management required?
- What is the availability and skill of laboratory staff needed?

Normally, new analytical methods come into being to increase precision or accuracy over current methods, to reduce reagent costs, or to measure a new analyte. When the manufacturer develops a new method, it is required by the Food and Drug Administration (FDA) to submit claims and extensive experimental data about the accuracy and precision of said method. Once FDA approval is granted based on the required data, the new method is then marketed by the manufacturer for use in either a hospital setting or commercial laboratory (Kaplan and Pesce 1996).

Once all of these criteria are satisfied, one may proceed with performing a comparison study. Personnel within a hospital or commercial setting will perform the majority of method validations. Comparison studies are performed to determine whether the proposed method will reduce technologist workload or decrease the turnaround time required to perform and return the result to the physician. The comparison study will also determine if any errors, either systematic or routine, exist using patient samples and if diagnostic criteria are being met. Both the reference method and the test method are used to analyze the patient samples. The reference method will serve as the "gold standard" because of its known accuracy and precision (Kaplan and Pesce 1996).

For instance, your institution is currently using PT and APTT reagents produced by Metamyelocyte Corporation. This same corporation has just received FDA approval to market its synthetic version of both reagents, which offers more sensitivity, precision, and accuracy over the previous reagents marketed. Before you may place these new reagents into use, you must collect data from both the old (reference) and new (test) reagents so that normal ranges may either be adjusted or new ones formatted. A description of the statistical aspects of a method evaluation follows.

METHOD EVALUATION STATISTICS

(Coleman 2003; Cembrowski 2000; Garber and Carey 2003; Koch and Peters 1996; Solberg 1996; and Shultz 1996)

A method evaluation involves the comparison of a new method (test method) to an established method (reference method). Algorithms for method evaluation, protocols for reference methods, and chemical standards for these methods have been developed by such agencies as the National Bureau of Standards (NBS), NCCLS, FDA, the Scandinavian Society for Clinical Chemistry and Clinical Physiology (SCCCP), and the American Association for Clinical Chemistry (AACC). Ideally one would compare any new method to such a reference method because its performance has been very well documented, and it is believed to be the most accurate method. In common practice, one frequently compares a new method to the in-house method in an effort to determine if the new method is at least as reliable as the one currently in use.

In order to compare two different assay methods, one must first evaluate and then compare their analytical performances and their diagnostic performances. The analytical performance characteristics describe how well a test is able to measure a specific analyte (e.g., concentration of glucose), whereas the clinical (diagnostic) performance studies describe the ability of the test to correctly discriminate between health and disease in a patient (e.g., diabetes mellitus vs. healthy). Analytical performance characteristics typically measured include linearity, precision, accuracy, analytical sensitivity, and analytical specificity. Diagnostic or clinical performance studies typically include diagnostic sensitivity, diagnostic specificity, diagnostic efficiency, positive and negative predictive values, and normal or healthy reference intervals. The following is a description of some simple tests that can be performed to evaluate both analytical and clinical (diagnostic) performances.

Linearity

Linearity is a measurement of how well a test method can discriminate between low and high assay results (i.e., different concentrations of an analyte). Linearity is determined by assaying in replicate a series of standards (calibrators) or dilutions of an elevated patient sample and then plotting the results, calculating a percent recovery, and/or performing regression analysis. The standards should be selected to cover the medically important range and to bracket the expected patient results. Replicate results are averaged and then plotted on the y-axis against the expected concentrations (known concentrations of the standards) on the x-axis. The plot is considered to be linear if a line can be drawn through the data points that has a forty-five degree angle to the x-axis and the line does not deviate from that angle at either end. Linear regression will mathematically describe how close to a perfect curve (perfect correlation between the expected values and the observed values) one has obtained. A curve with a R^2 value (multiple correlation squared) of 1.0 is considered to have perfect linearity, and one that is 0.95 is acceptable. R^2 measures the proportion of shared variability. That is to say, R^2 is a measure of the extent to which two variables (observed values vs. expected values) increase together or the extent to which one increases as the other decreases. R^2 is always a positive value (square of a term) and an R^2 of 1.0 represents 100% shared variability. Alternatively, one can calculate a percent recovery for each standard and determine if it is within the acceptable range (95–105% recovery) or not. To calculate the percent recovery for a standard, one divides the value recovered (mean of the replicates) by the expected value (known concentration) and then multiplies this by 100%.

$$\% \text{ recovery} = \frac{\text{value recovered}}{\text{value expected}} \times 100\%$$

Precision

Precision tests the reproducibility of an assay method. That is to say it measures how closely replicate test results on a given sample agree with each other. One should measure both within-run and between-run assay precision. Within-run precision assesses the ability of an assay method to repeat a value for a sample no matter where the sample is placed within an assay run, whereas between-run precision assesses the ability of the assay method to repeat a value on different runs (performed on different days). The method precision should be determined for low, normal (healthy), and elevated concentration levels using aliquots of control sera or patient samples that are treated so they will not change in value over time (frozen, lyophilized, or treated with a preservative).

Coefficient of Variation (%CV)

For each set of replicate values, one calculates the mean, standard deviation (SD), and coefficient of variation (%CV). The %CV can then be compared with the manufacturer's reported results, the in-house method's %CV, or the %CV of the reference method. The lower the %CV, the better the precision. Values less than ten percent are generally considered acceptable, and values less than five percent are often found using automated instruments. To calculate a %CV, one should divide the standard deviation for a set of replicates by their mean and then multiply the quotient by 100.

$$\bar{x} = \frac{\Sigma x_i}{n}$$

where: $\bar{x}$ = mean
Σ = sum of
x_i = individual value
n = number of values or data points

$$SD = \sqrt{\frac{\Sigma(x_i - \bar{x})^2}{(n-1)}}$$

where: SD = standard deviation
$\sqrt{}$ = square root of
Σ = sum of
x_i = individual value
$\bar{x}$ = mean
n = number of values or data points

$$\%CV = \frac{(SD)}{\bar{x}}(100\%)$$

where: %CV = coefficient of variation
SD = standard deviation
$\bar{x}$ = mean

One advantage of calculating the %CV's for methods is that one can use the results to compare two assay methods that have very different mean values (e.g.,

Tietz enzyme units vs. *Système international* (SI) enzyme units or kinetic assay results [U/L] vs. immunologic assay results [ng/mL] for an enzyme). By contrast, note that a direct comparison of standard deviations (SDs) can be misleading. For example an SD of 10 Tietz U/L is large relative to a mean of 1.0 Tietz U/L, whereas the same standard deviation (10 U/L) is relatively small compared to a mean of 100 U/L for the SI system.

F Test

If the %CV for a new method is slightly higher than that claimed by the manufacturer, one can use the results of the F-test to determine if the difference in the precision values is statistically significant or not. The F-test is a quotient of the variance obtained by your lab to that claimed by the manufacturer (or of a new method to that of a reference method). The F-test result is then compared to values found in a table of statistical probabilities, which will indicate if there is a statistically significant difference between the laboratory's precision results and those claimed by the manufacturer.

$$\text{F test} = \frac{\text{larger variance}}{\text{smaller variance}}$$

where: variance = $(SD)^2$

A table of significance for the F-test will have cutoff points listed for different degrees of freedom for both the numerator and the denominator of the F-test. The degrees of freedom (n−1) reflect the number of data points (assay values) that were included in the calculation of the variances (SD^2). If the calculated result for the F-test is greater than the cutoff point, it suggests that the two sets of precision data are statistically significantly different. If the F-test result is less than the cutoff value, there is no significant difference between the two sets of data. Tables of significance exist for different levels of probability, and in the clinical lab one usually uses a 0.05 probability level. This implies that ninety-five percent of the time there would be a statistically significant difference between the variances used to calculate an F-test result that was more than the cutoff value and five percent of the time there would be no difference between them.

Accuracy

Accuracy tests the agreement between the mean estimate of a quantity (measured by a new method) and its true value (measured by a reference method). To determine the accuracy of a method, one splits patient samples and compares the results obtained on these samples by the new method and the reference method. Ideally, one should use a recognized reference method for comparison purposes, but frequently one uses the existing in-house method. For a patient comparison study, 1) one should use at least forty patient samples; 2) the samples should have analyte concentrations in the low, medium, and high ranges; 3) the analyses should be performed in duplicate by each method; 4) the duplicate values should agree within five percent of each other; and 5) the analyses should be performed at approximately the same time. Method bias is calculated by subtracting the mean of the results of the reference method from the mean of the results of the new method. A positive bias implies that the results of the method will generally be higher than those of the reference method, whereas a negative bias implies the opposite (i.e., the new method will have lower results). Ideally the bias should be zero. To determine the statistical accuracy of a new method one can use a paired t-test or perform linear regression analysis.

Paired t-test

The paired t-test uses coupled data points (from the new and reference methods) and measures the statistical difference (bias) between the methods. This result can be compared with cutoff values found in a two-tailed table for significance of paired t-test to determine if there is statistically significant difference between the means. This is a measure of the accuracy of the new test. To calculate the paired t-test result, (t), one must first calculate the bias, the standard deviation of the differences (SDd), and the standard error of the mean (SEM) for the paired samples in the comparison study. The t-test result is then equal to the bias divided by the SEM. The SDd is the average deviation of the individual differences (for each split) from the overall difference or bias. The SEM for the SDd adjusts for any error in the calculation due to the number of data points from which the average was calculated.

$$\text{Bias} = \bar{x} \text{ (new method or Y method)} - \bar{x} \text{ (reference method or X method)}$$

$$SDd = \sqrt{\frac{[\Sigma(Y-X) - \text{Bias}]^2}{n-1}}$$

where: Y−X is the difference between each pair value on the new method minus the value on the reference method.

n−1 = degrees of freedom or n−1 pairs

$$SEM = \frac{SDd}{\sqrt{n}}$$

where: SDd = standard deviation of the differences
n = number of data points (pairs)
SEM = standard error of the mean
$\sqrt{}$ = square root of

$$t = \frac{Bias}{SEM}$$

where: SEM = standard error of the mean
t = paired t-test value
Bias = $\bar{x}$ (of new method) − $\bar{x}$ (of reference method)

The two-tailed table for the significance of paired t-test values involves the use of cutoff points (+ and − values) for different degrees of freedom (based on different numbers of paired data points or patient samples). Again, tables exist for different levels of probability, and in the clinical laboratory we typically test at the 0.05 probability level.

Slope/Linear Regression

Another approach to measuring the correlation between a new method and a reference method is to plot the results of the patient sample splits (new method value on the y-axis vs. reference method value on the x-axis) and determine if the curve (line) passes through zero and makes a forty-five degree angle with the x-axis. Such a curve has a slope of 1.0, which implies that the values measured by the new method are exactly identical to those obtained by the reference method. The slope is actually a measure of the angle of the curve (line) relative to the x-axis and is calculated by dividing the change of Y by the change of X ($\Delta Y/\Delta X$). One can calculate the best fit line (regression line) for this curve using linear regression by the least squares method. Traditionally, one calculates the slope of the line (b), the y-intercept (a), and the least squares regression line equation ($\hat{Y}$).

$$b = \frac{(n)(\Sigma XY) - (\Sigma X)(\Sigma Y)}{(n)(\Sigma X^2) - (\Sigma X)^2}$$

where: b = slope
ΣXY = sum of each X value times each Y value
ΣX = sum of all the X values
ΣY = sum of all the Y values
ΣX^2 = sum of all the squared X values
$(\Sigma X)^2$ = the squared sum of all the X values
n = the number of data pairs

$$a = \bar{Y} - b\bar{X}$$

where: a = y-intercept   b = slope of the line
$\bar{Y}$ = mean of the values from the Y method (new method)
$\bar{X}$ = mean of the values from the X method (reference method)

$$\hat{Y} = a + bX$$

where: $\hat{Y}$ = the value of Y on the regression line
a = y-intercept
b = slope of the line
X = specific X value

Some laboratories will also perform recovery studies that essentially give the same information as the y-intercept. They are done by spiking aliquots of a patient sample with known concentrations of analyte and calculating the percent recovered. A percent recovery of 95–105% is acceptable.

$$\% \text{ recovery} = \frac{\text{concentration recovered}}{\text{concentration added}} \times 100\%$$

where: concentration recovered = measured concentration
concentration added = known concentration

Analytical Sensitivity

Analytical sensitivity (minimal detectable concentration) is a measure of the lowest concentration of analyte in a sample that can be accurately measured. It is determined by assaying twenty or more replicates of a sample that has zero amount of the analyte of interest (diluent or zero calibrator) and calculating the mean plus two standard deviations ($\bar{x} + 2SD$). Patient values that fall below this cutoff are considered to be negative for the analyte, whereas values in excess of the cutoff are positive for the analyte.

Analytical Specificity

The analytical specificity (interference) represents the degree of assay interference from drugs or other chemicals (e.g., bilirubin, hemoglobin, lipids) present in the specimen. This can be determined by splitting patient samples and spiking the different aliquots with varying concentrations of the suspected interfering substances (drugs or chemicals). The samples are then assayed, and differences in the results obtained are noted.

Statistical Parameters and the Type of Error Identified

Analytical studies identify two types of error: random error and systematic error. Random error is unpredictable, and systematic error occurs consistently and has direction (positive or negative). Systematic error can be either constant or proportional. Constant systematic error affects the measured concentration identically over the entire analytical range, whereas proportional systematic error increases as the concentration of the analyte increases. Random error is measured by the %CV and the F-test. Constant systematic error is measured by the y-intercept, and proportional systematic error is measured by the slope. The paired t-test measures total systematic error.

Diagnostic Validity

Diagnostic or predictive validity compares the ability of a new assay method (test method) to accurately diagnose or predict the presence or absence of disease with that of an established method (reference method). Diagnostic value results include diagnostic sensitivity and specificity, diagnostic efficiency, and positive and negative predictive values. For the calculation of diagnostic values, one compares the test results with the "true" results as defined by an external method considered to be the reference method. For example, one could compare the results of a tumor antigen assay (test results) with those obtained by the physician using histologic analysis of biopsy material (true results). Alternatively, one could compare the results of a new tumor antigen assay (test results) with those obtained by a reference or in-house tumor antigen assay (true results). Individual patient assay results from the new method are then assigned to one of four categories (true positives [TP], true negatives [TN], false positives [FP], or false negatives [FN]) from which the diagnostic values are derived/calculated.

TP = a positive result for a patient who has the disease

TN = a negative result for a patient who does not have the disease

FP = a positive result for a patient who does not have the disease

FN = a negative result for a patient who does have the disease

Diagnostic sensitivity is the percent of patients with the disease who test positive by the new assay. Diagnostic specificity is the percent of patients without the disease who test negative by the assay. Diagnostic efficiency is the percent of all test results that are either true positives or true negatives. Positive predictive value is the percent of all positive test results that are true positives. Negative predictive value is the percent of all negative test results that are true negatives.

$$\text{Diagnostic \% sensitivity} = \frac{TP}{TP + FN}(100\%)$$

$$\text{Diagnostic \% specificity} = \frac{TN}{TN + FP}(100\%)$$

$$\text{Diagnostic \% efficiency} = \frac{TP + TN}{TP + TN + FP + FN}(100\%)$$

$$\text{Predictive value } (+) = \frac{TP}{TP + FP}(100\%)$$

$$\text{Predictive value } (-) = \frac{TN}{TN + FN}(100\%)$$

Diagnostic sensitivity tests the probability that a test result will be positive when the disease is present. Diagnostic specificity tests the probability that a test result will be negative when the disease is not present. Diagnostic efficiency is a combination of these and reflects the probability that one will obtain a correct positive or negative result. The positive predictive value tests the ability of a positive test to correctly predict disease, and negative predictive value tests the ability of a negative test to correctly predict a lack of disease. Diagnostic studies should involve a large number of patient samples, and the prevalence of the disease tested for in the patient sampling does affect the positive and negative predictive values.

Normal (Healthy) Reference Intervals

Normal or healthy reference intervals should be established for the test method using a patient population seen in the specific hospital or area. Often it is necessary to establish different reference intervals for different age brackets (neonatal, pediatric, adult, geriatric), different genders (male, female), and the presence or absence of pregnancy. In addition, some differences have been attributable to genetic/ethnic origin (African American, Native American, Asiatic, Hispanic, European, etc.), diet, and geographic location. The normal reference intervals serve as the standard against which one interprets individual patient results. In order to establish a normal (healthy) reference interval for an analyte using a new assay method (test method), one calculates a ninety-five-percent confidence interval (mean plus or minus 2 SD) on assay results from a population set known to be in good health. Subsequently, any patient result that falls within this interval is considered to be normal (healthy), whereas patient results that fall outside (above or below) the limits of this interval are considered to be abnormally increased or decreased respectively. Typically one establishes the cutoff between normal (presumed negative for disease) and abnormal (presumed positive for disease) results by using the mean plus or minus two SDs. Occasionally one will establish a tighter set of cutoff values in an effort to correctly identify all patients with a particular pathology, although one will increase the number of false positive cases (e.g., cutoff points for phenylketonuria [PKU] babies). The reference interval should be established using a minimum of 100 different subjects.

$$\text{Reference interval} = \bar{x} +/- 2SD$$

where: $\bar{x}$ = the mean of the results obtained on healthy individuals
SD = standard deviation

Once all of the data has been collected and analyzed, a letter should be sent to all physicians and other health-care workers (i.e., nursing services) who have direct patient contact within your institution alerting each of the change in methodologies. Include in the letter

- the effective date of change
- if applicable, reference and control ranges for the new test method
- any other changes, such as sensitivities of the reagent to certain drugs, interference sources, new collection methods or any other pertinent information that may be of vital importance to the physician and other health-care workers

The process of evaluating a new test method is different from performing routine quality control (QC). Daily QC is a process that is established to detect any systematic errors that may interfere with reporting patient samples. It should serve as a baseline to verify that all parameters on an automated instrument are correct and in working order.

Criteria have been presented within this chapter as to whether a method validation should be performed to justify the addition of a new test method. The manager of the laboratory should weigh each one of these criteria very carefully before the decision is reached. Technical staff within the laboratory, physicians, and other members of the health-care team should also be consulted regarding the need to add the new test. Once the decision to add a new test method has been made, statistical analysis must be performed comparing the old and new methods. But throughout this decision process, the main focus should not detour from the major goal, which is improving patient care.

BIBLIOGRAPHY

Cembrowski, Anne M. Sullivan. 2000. Quality control and statistics. In *Clinical chemistry principles, procedures, correlations*, ed. Michael L. Bishop, Janet L. Duben-Engelkirk, and Edward D. Fody. 4th ed. Philadelphia: Lippincott, Williams & Wilkins.

Coleman, Mary. 2003. Method evaluation and preanalytical variables. In *Clinical chemistry concepts and applications*, ed. Shauna C. Anderson and Susan Cockayne. 2d ed. New York: McGraw-Hill Medical.

Coulter Corporation and Instrumentation Laboratory: Partners for Excellence. Coulter II/ACL™ Coagulation Instruments. February 1997. *Implementation guide and documentation records*. Section 8, Comparison Study. Miami, Fla.: Coulter.

Forrest General Hospital Hematology Procedure Manual. May 2002. Hattiesburg, Miss: Forrest General Hospital.

Garber, Carl C., and R. Neill Carey. 2003. Evaluation of methods. In *Clinical chemistry theory, analysis, correlation*, ed. Lawrence A. Kaplan, Amadeo J. Pesce, and Steven C. Kazmierczak. 4th ed. St Louis, Mo.: Mosby.

Kaplan, Lawrence A., and Amadeo J. Pesce. 1996. *Clinical chemistry: Theory, analysis, correlation.* 3d ed. St. Louis, Mo.: Mosby.

Koch, David A., and Theodore Peters. 1996. Selection and evaluation of methods: With an introduction to statistical techniques. In *Tietz Fundamentals of Clinical Chemistry*, ed. Carl A. Burtis and Edward R. Ashwood. 4th ed. Philadelphia: W. B. Saunders.

Solberg, Helge Erik. 1996. Establishment and use of reference values. In *Tietz Fundamentals of Clinical Chemistry*, ed. Carl A. Burtis and Edward R. Ashwood. 4th ed. Philadelphia: W. B. Saunders.

Shultz, Edward K. 1996. Clinical interpretation of laboratory procedures. In *Tietz Fundamentals of Clinical Chemistry*, ed. Carl A. Burtis and Edward R. Ashwood. 4th ed. Philadelphia: W. B. Saunders.

INTERNET RESOURCES

David G. Rhodes Associates, Inc. <www.dgrhoads.com/>

University of Pittsburgh School of Medicine, Department of Pathology. <http://path.upmc.edu/showcase/posters/li.html>

Westgard QC. <www.westgard.com/basicmvbook.htm>

QUESTIONS

1. In the current literature, comparison studies are referred to as _____. *(Objective 1, Level I)*

2. What is a comparison study? *(Objective 1, Level I)*

3. Discuss the purpose of a comparison study. *(Objective 2, Level I)*

4. What criteria must be met in order to justify switching to a different methodology? *(Objective 3, Level I)*
   a. _____
   b. _____
   c. _____
   d. _____

5. What questions must be asked to determine if it is feasible to switch methodologies? *(Objective 4, Level I)*
   a. _____
   b. _____
   c. _____
   d. _____

6. Why are new analytical methods developed? *(Objective 5, Level II)*

7. Who grants approval for a new test method? *(Objective 6, Level I)*

8. In order for a new test method to be granted approval, the company developing the new method must *(Objective 7, Level I)*
   a. submit application and fees
   b. test the general population
   c. have the clinical laboratory association approval
   d. submit experimental data

9. State the function for each of the following statistical tests: *(Objective 8, Level I)*
   a. Precision

   b. Accuracy

   c. Analytical sensitivity

   d. Analytical specificity

   e. Diagnostic validity

10. Once the "new" method is adopted, the letter to the physicians and other health-care workers (i.e., nursing services) who have direct patient contact of your institution stating that there is a change in reagents should include *(Objective 9, Level I)*
    a. new reference levels
    b. estimated date of change
    c. any other changes
    d. all of the above

EXERCISES

Completion of the exercises will enhance your knowledge of evaluation of new test methods.
(Objective 10, Level III and Objective 11, Level III)

1. Obtain data on a previous comparison study and analyze whether the new test method can be used.

2. Develop a proposal to justify a comparison study for a new method.

3. Interview a department supervisor and a chief technologist to determine when a comparison study should be done and what should be included. If possible, study a comparison study that has been completed to determine the elements of the process.

CASES

Analyze and propose solutions for the following case studies. *(Objective 12, Level III)*

1. Several of the internal medicine physicians went to a workshop recently and learned about a new test method. They returned to the hospital and came to the laboratory requesting that you implement the method. Compose a recommendation and give your reasons for your recommendation. The following are the facts you determine after researching the new method:

Old Method	New Method
Cost per specimen = $5.00/test	Cost per specimen = $20.00/test
Diagnostic Specificity = 90%	Diagnostic Specificity = 98%
Diagnostic Sensitivity = 95%	Diagnostic Sensitivity = 98%
Already have instrumentation	Would require purchase of a new instrument
Tech time = 2 hrs.	Tech time = 1.5 hrs
Technically simple to perform	Technically difficult to perform

2. You have just accepted the position as administrative chief technologist at Tishomingo Lake Medical Center in Corinth, Mississippi. This facility is a sixty-eight-bed acute-care facility that includes general medical, surgical, cardiac, and emergency services. The nearest two medical facilities are approximately 100 miles in proximity (one is located to the west in Southaven, Mississippi, with a bed size of 160, and one is located to the south in Tupelo, Mississippi, with a bed size of 450). Your facility is staffed with fifteen full-time physicians, forty-five nurses, three phlebotomists (one for each laboratory shift), and twelve clinical laboratory scientists: six on day shift, three on evening shift, and three on night shift. There are no section supervisors, and all changes in laboratory policy and procedure, whether it is purchasing or leasing new equipment, changing testing methods, or requesting time off must meet with your approval. This facility may not be compared to the 650-bed acute-care facility in Memphis, Tennessee, where you previously worked as transfusion services supervisor. At that facility, you were a specialist in blood bank and rarely performed any type of testing in other departments in the laboratory and only made decisions in regard to updating or changing blood bank policy and procedure.

   A sales representative from JADA Corporation is currently soliciting your laboratory to purchase a new D-Dimer test for the detection of deep vein thrombosis and/or pulmonary embolism.

   a. What is the first thing you should do before implementing this particular assay?

   b. What questions should you ask the sales representative concerning this new test?

   c. What other type of research may be necessary before deciding to add this particular assay to your laboratory test menu?

   d. Formulate a "generic" procedure for the test.

Chapter 28

Quality Control

Margot Hall, Ph.D., F.A.I.C., CChem MRSC

OBJECTIVES

Upon completion of this chapter the learner will be able to

1. Define *quality control*. *(Level I)*
2. Differentiate between internal and external quality control. *(Level II)*
3. Define the following terms: *(Level I)*
   a. accuracy
   b. central tendency
   c. coefficient of variation
   d. confidence intervals
   e. imprecision
   f. mean
   g. median
   h. mode
   i. normal or Gaussian distribution
   j. precision
   k. random error
   l. range
   m. reliability
   n. shift
   o. skewed distribution
   p. standard deviation
   q. systemic error
   r. trend
   s. variance
   t. Westgard rules
4. Assess the use of quality control and its impact on quality assurance. *(Level III)*
5. Calculate the following values associated with quality control when given laboratory data: *(Level II)*
   a. coefficient of variation
   b. mean
   c. median
   d. standard deviation
   e. variance
6. Relate the Westgard rules to specific situations. *(Level II)*
7. Choose the appropriate action based on the quality control data and analysis for the case studies. *(Level III)*

TOPIC SUMMARY

Background

Quality assurance involves all processes that a laboratory uses to ensure quality test results. This includes planning, assessment, and monitoring to ensure the quality of the preanalytical, analytical, and postanalytical processes. The quality planning should involve the creation, selection, and validation of the laboratory processes and methods. Examples of laboratory processes and methods might include personnel policies, procedures to be followed by the personnel, methods of specimen collection and handling, selection of instruments and analytical methods, and so on. Quality assessment involves a formal systematic measurement and monitoring of the performance of laboratory processes. It emphasizes the assessment of pre- and postanalytical processes such as patient and specimen identification, sample collection and processing, and reporting and interpretation of results. By contrast, quality control involves the monitoring of the analytical phase or process (i.e., the actual measurement of the analyte) and is usually accomplished using statistical techniques. Clearly, when quality assessment and quality control approaches suggest that there is a problem, then quality improvement measures must be used to determine the cause of the problem and quality planning used to eliminate the problem. Quality control (QC) is the process by which one monitors analytical procedures in order to ensure the accuracy and precision of test results and thus the validity of patient results prior to their reporting. Typically this is accomplished by monitoring QC materials such as serum, urine, and cerebrospinal fluid (CSF) concomitantly with patient samples. QC can be subdivided into internal and external QC.

Internal QC involves

1. establishing the mean ($\bar{x}$) and standard deviation (SD) for the QC material, verifying the accuracy and precision of the control material, and establishing acceptable statistical limits for each analytical method using that control material.
2. assaying the QC material concomitantly with patient samples and verifying that the control material results fall within the acceptable limits prior to accepting or rejecting a given assay run (test analysis).
3. monitoring control results over time for changes in precision (random error) or accuracy (systematic error) using prescribed methods and then addressing the problem, when one exists, by finding and correcting the source of error and reanalyzing the patient and control samples.

External QC involves

1. the comparison of a lab's assay results from unknown test samples with the mean results of those obtained on the same samples by other labs.
2. the comparison of a lab's assay results from unknown test samples with those obtained by an external agency using a reference method. This is often part of a proficiency testing program.

QC Materials

QC material is prepared by pooling either human or animal source body fluids. Typical controls are serum and urine. Other controls include whole blood, plasma, and CSF. Liquid, frozen, and lyophilized QC materials exist and should be stored at the appropriate temperatures. Commercially available QC material exists for most assays. Typically the control material comes in either two or three concentrations (levels) of analyte. The normal control will have analyte concentration(s) in the "normal" or healthy reference interval, and the analyte concentration(s) of the abnormal control will be in the expected range of common pathologies.

Controls should be stable over a period of time (more than six months), should be free of diseases such as human immunodeficiency virus (HIV) and hepatitis, and should not be turbid, hemolyzed, or discolored.

Both assayed (measured) and unassayed (unmeasured) commercially available controls exist. Assayed control material will have been randomly tested by the manufacturer and the means and standard deviations determined for each of a variety of common instruments and test methods. It is recommended that one check these values when first introducing a new batch (lot number) of control material into the lab. Naturally, the lab must determine the means, SDs, and reference intervals for unassayed control materials. It is good practice to assay an old lot number of control alongside a new lot number of control when first using it. Likewise, controls should be assayed with every manual test and at regular intervals on automated instruments to ensure the reliability (accuracy and precision) of the test results and therefore the validity of patient test results.

Definitions and Statistics

Accuracy

A measure of how closely a test result agrees with the "true" value for that sample. This is determined by comparing the mean of repeated testing values with the true value determined by a reference method such as gravimetric analysis.

Precision

A measure of how closely repeated measurements of a sample (replicates) agree with each other. This is determined by calculating the SD for the replicates.

Imprecision

Measurements do not closely replicate, and the SD will be larger.

Reliability

A measure of both the accuracy and precision of a method.

Central Tendency

Represents a large group of data points that are equal to or very nearly the same as one data point (cluster of data points) and are represented by a peak on a frequency diagram.

Normal or Gaussian Distribution

Implies that there are approximately the same number and distribution of data points to either side of the peak (symmetrical spread of data points around the peak). This is represented by a bell-shaped curve and approximately equal values for the mean, median, and mode. (See Figure 28–1.)

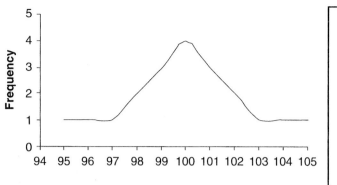

FIGURE 28–1. Normal or Gaussian Distribution

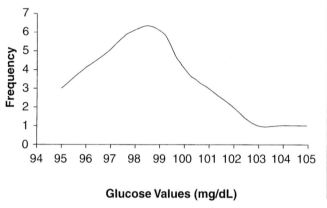

FIGURE 28–2. Skewed Distribution

The following is a data set for a blood urea nitrogen control:

Day	Value (mg/dL)
01	16
02	15
03	18
04	17
05	16
06	16
07	17
08	14
09	15
10	16

$$\bar{x} = \frac{\sum x_i}{n}$$

where: $\bar{x}$ = mean

$\sum$ = sum of

x_i = individual value

n = number of values or data points

Sum of the data points = 160
Mean = 160/10 = 16 mg/dL

FIGURE 28–3. Calculation of a Mean

Skewed Distribution

Refers to the asymmetrical spread of data points around the peak. The mean, median, and mode are not equal. (See Figure 28–2.)

Mean

The average of all data points in a data set calculated by the following:

$$\bar{x} = \frac{\sum x_i}{n}$$

where: $\bar{x}$ = mean

$\sum$ = sum of

x_i = individual value

n = number of values or data points

(See Figure 28–3.)

Median

The middle data point of all the data points arranged in numerical order. (See Figure 28–4.)

The following is a data set for a serum chloride control:

Day	Value (MEq/L)	Order	
01	98	97	
02	102	98	
03	101	98	
04	99	99	
05	104	99	middle
06	99	99	middle
07	97	101	
08	103	102	
09	99	103	
10	98	104	

The median is the middle data point and therefore equals 99 Meq/L.

FIGURE 28–4. Determination of the Median Value

Mode

The most frequent number or value found in a data set. (See Figure 28–5.)

Range

The difference between the high and low values of data points in a data set. (See Figure 28–6.)

The following is a data set for a serum potassium control:

Date	Value (Meq/L)	Order	
01	3.5	3.5	
02	3.7	3.6	
03	3.8	3.7	
04	4.2	3.8	most frequent
05	3.9	3.8	most frequent
06	4.0	3.8	most frequent
07	3.6	3.9	
08	3.8	4.0	
09	4.1	4.1	
10	3.8	4.2	

The value 3.8 Meq/L is found the most frequently in the data set and therefore represents the mode.

FIGURE 28–5. Determination of the Mode

The following is a data set for a serum creatinine control:

Day	Value (mg/dL)	Order	
01	0.7	0.7	lowest value
02	0.8	0.8	
03	1.0	0.8	
04	0.9	0.9	
05	1.2	0.9	
06	1.1	1.0	
07	1.0	1.0	
08	0.9	1.0	
09	0.8	1.1	
10	1.0	1.2	highest value

Range = the difference between the highest and the lowest value of the data points in a set

Range = 1.2 − 0.7 = 0.5 mg/dL

FIGURE 28–6. Determination of the Range

Variance

A mathematic representation of the dispersion or degree of tightness of data points around the mean or peak in a data set. It is the square of the SD and is calculated by the following:

$$s^2 = \frac{\sum(x_i - \bar{x})^2}{n - 1}$$

where: s^2 = variance
$\sum$ = sum of
x_i = individual value
$\bar{x}$ = mean
n = number of values or data points

(See Figure 28–7.)

The following is a data set for a serum PSA control:

Day	Value (ng/mL)	Value − Mean	Square of the (Value − Mean)
01	4.0	4 − 4 = 0	0
02	3.0	3 − 4 = −1	1
03	4.0	4 − 4 = 0	0
04	5.0	5 − 4 = +1	1
05	4.0	4 − 4 = 0	0

Mean ($\bar{x}$) = 20/5 = 4

Number of Values Minus One = 4
Sum of the Squares = 2

$$s^2 = \frac{\sum(x_i - \bar{x})^2}{n - 1}$$

where: s^2 = variance
$\sum$ = sum of
x_i = individual value
$\bar{x}$ = mean
n = number of values or data points

Variance = 2/4 = 0.5

FIGURE 28–7. Calculation of the Variance

Standard Deviation

A mathematic representation of the dispersion or degree of tightness of data points around the mean or peak in a data set. It is the square root of the variance and is calculated by the following:

$$s \text{ or } SD = \sqrt{\frac{\sum(x_i - \bar{x})^2}{n - 1}}$$

where: s or SD = standard deviation
$\sqrt{}$ = square root of
$\sum$ = sum of
x_i = individual value
$\bar{x}$ = mean
n = number of values or data points
(See Figure 28–8.)

Confidence Interval

Refers to the limits (high and low values) between which a specified proportion of the data points in a data set will fall. In a data set with normal distribution 68%, 95%, and 99%, confidence intervals (CI) will have the following ranges:

68% CI = mean ± 1 SD
95% CI = mean ± 2 SD
99% CI = mean ± 3 SD

In the chemistry lab one often uses a 95% CI as a reference interval, and this implies that for replicate measurements on the same control one would expect one of every twenty measurements to fall outside the limits. (See Figure 28–9.)

Coefficient of Variation

The SD divided by the mean and multiplied by 100 to obtain a percentage. It is calculated by the following:

$$\%CV = \frac{(SD)}{\bar{x}}(100)$$

where: %CV = coefficient of variation
SD = standard deviation
$\bar{x}$ = mean

It allows one to compare methods of analysis with very different means. Typically it should be less than 5%. (See Figure 28–10.)

Levey-Jennings Charts

An approach to monitoring method performance for precision and long-term accuracy involves plotting control values on a Levey-Jennings chart. The chart consists of a solid line representing the target mean value and dashed lines (on either side of the solid line) that represent plus and minus 1, 2, and 3 SD from the

---

The following is a data set for a serum sodium control:

Day	Value (MEq/L)	Value – Mean	Square of the (Value – Mean)
01	142	142 – 140 = +2	4
02	138	138 – 140 = –2	4
03	140	140 – 140 = 0	0
04	138	138 – 140 = –2	4
05	142	142 – 140 = +2	4

Mean ($\bar{x}$) = 700/5 = 140

Number of Values Minus One = 4

Sum of the Squares = 16

Variance is

$$s^2 = \frac{\sum(x_i - \bar{x})^2}{n - 1}$$

where: s^2 = variance
$\sum$ = sum of
x_i = individual value
$\bar{x}$ = mean
n = number of values or data points

Variance = 16/4 = 4

And the SD is the square root of the variance or

$$s \text{ or } SD = \sqrt{\frac{\sum(x_i - \bar{x})^2}{n - 1}}$$

where: s or SD = standard deviation
$\sqrt{}$ = square root of
$\sum$ = sum of
x_i = individual value
$\bar{x}$ = mean
n = number of values or data points

Thus the square root of 4 is 2, and the SD equals 2.

FIGURE 28–8. Calculation of the Standard Deviation

mean. Values are plotted against time. That is to say that the Y-axis goes from –3 SD to +3 SD, whereas on

A serum control for alanine transaminase has a mean of 16 U/L and an SD of 2 U/L at 30 degrees centigrade. The CI equal the following:

68% CI = mean ± 1 SD
95% CI = mean ± 2 SD
99% CI = mean ± 3 SD

Thus a 68% CI is
16 U/L − 2 U/L = 14 U/L
16 U/L + 2 U/L = 18 U/L
and the 68% CI = 14 to 18 U/L

Similarly the 95% CI is
16 U/L − 4 U/L = 12 U/L
16 U/L + 4 U/L = 20 U/L
and the 95% CI = 12 − 20 U/L

And the 99% CI is
16 U/L − 6 U/L = 10 U/L
16 U/L + 6 U/L = 22 U/L
and the 99% CI = 10 − 22 U/L

FIGURE 28–9. Determination of a Confidence Interval

A serum control for glucose has a mean of 100 mg/dL and an SD of 6 mg/dL. The coefficient of variation (%CV) is calculated as

$$\%CV = \frac{(SD)}{\bar{x}}(100)$$

where: %CV = coefficient of variation
SD = standard deviation
$\bar{x}$ = mean

Thus the %CV = (6 mg/dL/100 mg/dL) (100)
= 6%

FIGURE 28–10. Calculation of the Coefficient of Variation

the X-axis one plots days of the month or some other convenient time frame such as the hospital shifts. Values are added to the plot to signify the target values for a particular assay. For example, if the mean was 10 mg/dl and the SD was 0.1 mg/dl, then the chart

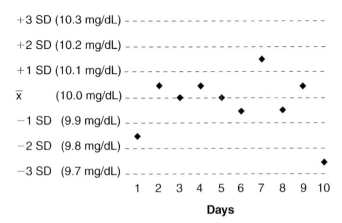

FIGURE 28–11. Example of a Levy-Jennings Chart
(Adapted with permission from Levey, S., and E. R. Jennings. 1950. The use of control charts in the clinical laboratories. *American Journal of Clinical Pathology* 20: 1059–65.)

would go from 9.7 mg/dl to 10.3 mg/dl. The clinical scientists would then plot the actual values for control materials assayed alongside the patient samples in each run. (See Figure 28–11.)

Precision and long-term accuracy exist when the values of data points for the control material are close to the target mean and approximately equally distributed on either side of it. Mathematically, precision is represented by a low SD. Imprecision exists when the values of data points for the control material exhibit more scattering, and their SD is therefore greater. This usually involves less than optimal technique on the part of the technologist. Generally, precision is lower for manual assays as compared with those performed using automated instrumentation. Inaccuracy occurs when the mean for the control material is changing and is reflected by either a trend or shift in control values.

Trend

A small but steady and continuous change of the control values in one direction. If left unchecked, the control values will go off the chart over time. Trends often indicate reagent or calibrator deterioration or gradual instrumental failure. (See Figure 28–12.)

Shift

A change of the mean for the control material. The new mean is continuous but different from the original mean. This can reflect the resetting of an instrument, a small but consistent flaw in the instrument, or a change of lot number of control material. (See Figure 28–13.)

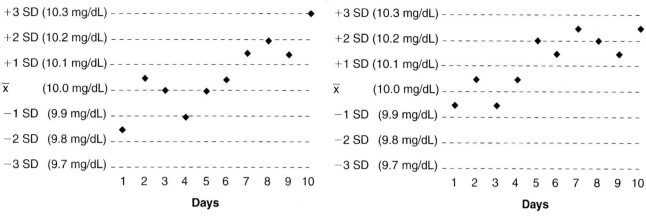

FIGURE 28–12. Example of a Trend

FIGURE 28–13. Example of a Shift

The 95% CI Rule

A commonly accepted rule of thumb is that the control value should fall within $\bar{x}$ 2SD for the analysis to be accepted and the patients' results to be reported out. (See Figure 28–14.)

A Level I carcinoembryonic antigen (CEA) control serum had a mean of 4.0 ng/mL and an SD of 0.25 ng/mL. Thus assays in which the Level I CEA control value was between 3.50ng/mL (mean minus 2SD) and 4.50 ng/mL (mean + 2SD) would be acceptable, whereas assays in which the Level I CEA control lay outside this range would be unacceptable.

FIGURE 28–14. Example of the 95% CI Rule

Westgard Rules

A set of criteria by which one can monitor test performance and accept or reject the run (i.e., release or not release the patient data). It is also useful in determining if the problem is random error (addressed by rules R4S and 13S) or systematic error (addressed by rules 2_{2S}, 4_{1S}, and $10_{\bar{x}}$). (Westgard applied these rules using two controls with each analysis/run.) The Westgard rules include the following: (See Table 28–1 and Figure 28–15.)

Random Error

Error occurring on a unique sample or without any defined pattern. It is represented on a Levey-Jennings chart by a data point that is significantly different from the values of other data points, and by a violation of the 13S and R4S Westgard rules. Repeating the assay (calibrators, controls, and patient samples) often serves

---

1_{2S}	One control value lies outside the mean ±2SD. Warning flag tells the technologist to check the other rules. If they are not violated repeat the controls.
1_{3S}	One control value lies outside the mean ±3SD. Reject the analysis/run.
2_{2S}	Two consecutive control values lie outside the mean +2SD or the mean −2SD (must be in the same direction). Reject the analysis/run.
R_{4S}	One control value exceeds the mean +2SD and another control value exceeds the mean −2SD (i.e., they are more than 4SD apart from one another) and they were assayed consecutively. Reject the analysis/run.
4_{1S}	Four consecutive control values lie outside the mean +1SD or the mean −1SD. Reject the analysis/run.
$10_{\bar{x}}$	Ten consecutive control values lie on the same side of the mean. Reject the analysis/run.

(Westgard, J. O., P. L. Barry, M. R. Hunt, and T. A. Groth. 1981. Multi-rule shewhart chart for quality control in clinical chemistry. *Clinical Chemistry* 27: 493–501.)

TABLE 28–1 Westgard Rules

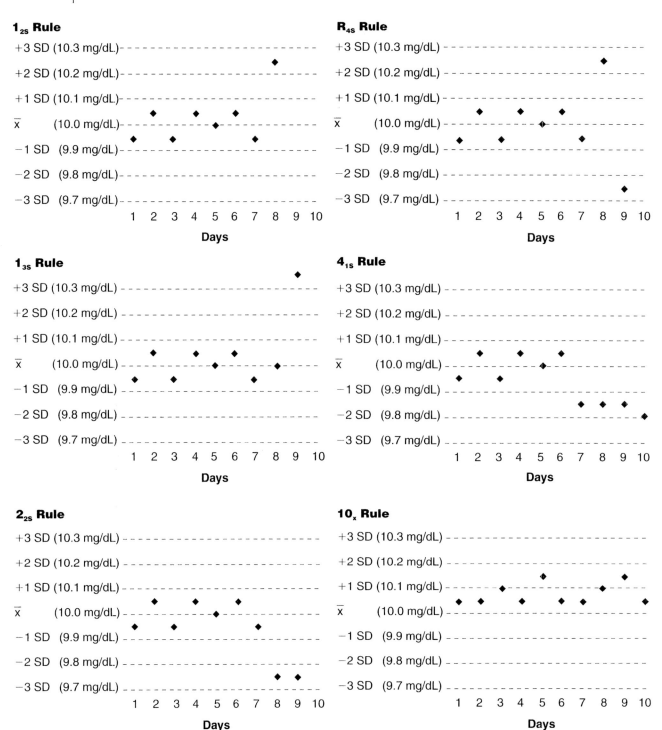

FIGURE 28-15. Examples of the Westgard Rules

to correct the problem (i.e., one obtains an acceptable control value). (See Figure 28-16.)

Systematic Error

Error that is present in all samples and affects those samples approximately equally. It is represented by a trend or shift pattern on Levey-Jennings charts and by a violation of the 22S, 41S, or $10_{\bar{x}}$ Westgard rules. Repeating the assay does not correct the problem.

One needs to investigate the source of error. (See Figure 28-17.)

BIBLIOGRAPHY

Bakes-Martin, R. C. 1993. Quality assurance. In *Clinical chemistry concepts and applications*, ed. [S. C. Anderson and S. Cockayne] (38–71). Philadelphia: W. B. Saunders.

Cembrowski, G. S., A. M. Sullivan, and T. L. Hoffer. (2000) Quality control and statistics. In *Clinical chemistry*

The following is a data set for a serum calcium control that has a mean of 9.2 mg/dL and an SD of 0.2 mg/dL.

Target value is 9.2 mg/dL

mean ± 1 SD = 9.0 – 9.4 mg/dL

mean ± 2 SD = 8.8 – 9.6 mg/dL

mean ± 3 SD = 8.6 – 9.8 mg/dL

Order of Control	Value (mg/dL)
1	9.2
2	9.3
3	9.1
4	9.2
5	9.3
6	9.9

FIGURE 28–16. Example of Random Error

The following is a data set for a serum bilirubin control that has a mean of 1.00 mg/dL and an SD of 0.10 mg/dL.

Target value is 1.00 mg/dL

mean ± 1 SD = 0.90 – 1.10 mg/dL

mean ± 2 SD = 0.80 – 1.20 mg/dL

mean ± 3 SD = 0.70 – 1.30 mg/dL

Order of Control	Value (mg/dL)
1	1.00
2	1.05
3	0.95
4	1.10
6	1.28
7	1.27

FIGURE 28–17. Example of Systematic Error

principles, procedures, correlations, ed. [M. L. Bishop, J. L. Duben-Engelkirk, and E. P. Fody]. 4th ed. (40–76). Philadelphia: Lippincott, Williams and Wilkins.

Levey, S., and E. R. Jennings. 1950. The use of control charts in the clinical laboratories. *American Journal of Clinical Pathology* 20: 1059–65.

Westgard, J. O., P. L. Barry, M. R. Hunt, and T. A. Groth. 1981. Multi-rule shewhart chart for quality control in clinical chemistry. *Clinical Chemistry* 27: 493–501.

Westgard, J. O., and G. G. Klee. 1996. Quality management. In *Tietz fundamentals of clinical chemistry*, ed. C. A. Burtis and E. R. Ashwood. 4th ed. (211–23). Philadelphia: W. B. Saunders.

INTERNET RESOURCES

Westgard Quality Control. <www.westgard.com>

Virtual Hospital. <www.vh.org/Providers/CME/CLIA/CLIAHP.html>

QUESTIONS

1. Quality control is defined as _____

   (Objective 1, Level I)

2. Differentiate between internal and external quality control. *(Objective 2, Level II)*

3. Define *(Objective 3, Level I)*

   a. accuracy: _____

   b. precision: _____

   c. reliability: _____

d. mean: _____

e. median: _____

f. mode: _____

g. range: _____

h. variance: _____

i. standard deviation: _____

j. confidence intervals: _____

k. coefficient of variation: _____

l. trend: _____

m. shift: _____

n. central tendency: _____

o. normal distribution: _____

p. skewed distribution: _____

q. imprecision: _____

r. Westgard rules: _____

s. random error: _____

t. systematic error: _____

EXERCISES

Completion of the exercises will enhance your knowledge of quality control. *(Objective 4, Level III)*

1. Review QC documents in the clinical chemistry department noting the application of the calculations and definitions that you have learned in this chapter.

2. Interview the individual or individuals in each department of the lab responsible for maintaining the QC information, and assess how the information is used in that department. The departments may be divided among the class participants. Discuss this as a class to determine the similarities and differences of use of QC information among departments.

3. Interview the individual responsible for maintaining and reviewing the QC information for the entire laboratory. What is the role of this person? How does this person use this information? What impact does the quality control data have on quality assurance or total quality management?

CASES

For each of the following cases, perform the calculations and answer the questions, as appropriate. *(Objective 5, Level II, Objective 6, Level II, and Objective 7, Level III)*

1. You are the chief technologist for a clinical chemistry lab. You have a new batch (lot number) of control, and you wish to know whether you should use it. You assay it and obtain the following QC data for the sodium analyses on Wonder Control Level I:

Sodium mmol/L

145	135	143	146
151	136	137	133
148	142	134	140
138	146	141	138
140	138	139	142

Determine the mean, median, and mode and decide whether they represent a normal (Gaussian) distribution or not. Should you introduce this into the lab as the new control?

2. You are the chief technologist of a clinical chemistry laboratory. You must chose between two different glucose test methods for use in the lab. You assay a specific normal glucose control by both methods and obtain the following results:

Glucose mg/dL Method A

100	105	101	99
102	98	104	96
101	97	99	103
100	98	102	101
99	95	100	100

Glucose mg/dL Method B

107	100	93	99
110	105	91	94
89	108	111	92
102	98	96	104
95	97	105	103

For each method, determine the mean, median, mode, and SD. Are both methods exhibiting a normal distribution? Which method is more precise? The manufacturer has listed a mean of 100 mg/dL and an SD of ± 3 mg/dL. Which method is more accurate? Which method would you choose for your laboratory?

3. You are charged with selecting between two methods for prostatic acid phosphatase analysis. One is an immunologic test measuring mass, and the other is a kinetic test measuring enzyme activity. The results obtained on control samples (levels 1 and 2) supplied by the manufacturers are

Prostatic Acid Phosphatase ug/L

Mean	SD
2.84	0.40
21.56	0.89

Prostatic Acid Phosphatase U/L

Mean	SD
1.61	0.06
8.20	0.05

Calculate the %CV for each control and determine which is the better test method.

4. As the QC officer for your clinical chemistry laboratory, you have reviewed the Levey-Jennings charts for potassium and noticed that the technologists have obtained the following data for the normal control (days 1–20).

Day	Potassium mmol/L	Day	Potassium mmol/L
1	3.5	11	3.7
2	3.4	12	3.9
3	3.8	13	3.8
4	3.6	14	4.0
5	3.7	15	4.2
6	3.4	16	4.5
7	3.3	17	4.6
8	3.9	18	4.6
9	3.6	19	4.8
10	3.5	20	4.9

The target value has a mean of 3.6 mmol/L with an SD of 0.2 mmol/L. What is the 95% CI for this batch of control? Plot the data and determine whether this represents a shift, a trend, or an acceptable QC record. What should you do next?

5. Your laboratory uses the Westgard Multirule System for its QC. A new technologist asks you to look at the QC results for blood urea nitrogen (BUN) and decide whether one should release the patient data to the physician or not. The BUN results for the Level I QC material ($\bar{x}$ = 16 mg/dL, SD = 1 mg/dL) were the following:

Day	Urea mg/dL	Day	Urea mg/dL
1	14	4	16
2	15	5	20
3	17	6	19

Should you release the patient data? Why or why not?

6. Your lab has been participating for some time in a national proficiency testing program. Results on proficiency testing samples have been generally good until this month. Your lab's results on each of the proficiency testing samples analyzed this month have been considerably lower than was expected. What source(s) of error could explain this? What should you do and in what order?

Chapter 29

Quality Management

Gayle Curtis, M.S., MT(ASCP), CPHQ

OBJECTIVES

Upon completion of this chapter the learner will be able to

1. Define *quality*. *(Level I)*
2. According to Gerteis, list items important for patient satisfaction. *(Level I)*
3. Identify the ultimate agent who evaluates the quality of health care provided by the professional. *(Level I)*
4. List and describe components of the care-delivery process. *(Level II)*
5. Name four types of complexity that a process or system may experience. *(Level I)*
6. Discuss how one might reduce variation. *(Level II)*
7. Discuss the components of Westgard's quality management. *(Level II)*
8. List Langley and associates' three questions regarding continuous quality improvement. *(Level I)*
9. List characteristics needed by the laboratory professional to contribute to quality. *(Level I)*
10. Create an approach to improve a process in the clinical laboratory or the hospital. *(Level III)*
11. Analyze the case studies and propose solutions. *(Level III)*

TOPIC SUMMARY

Quality is a value. Quality management is a learned body of knowledge, skills, and practices aimed at achieving excellence in products, service, and environment based on the requirements, perceptions, and future needs of customers. Quality principles and practices impact how each clinical laboratory team member understands and implements his or her role. In this regard, quality is how we do our work. Quality is doing the right things right and making continuous improvements.

Managing quality in a service business such as health-care delivery is inherently challenging. First, service businesses do not produce a "thing" whose quality can be measured, weighed, and tested. Quality is determined by the transaction between "servers" and customers. Service quality is subjective and personal. It depends on how happy the "server" is and on whether he or she perceives the job as satisfying. It depends on how the customer's expectations are being met. These expectations might not be clear nor mutually appreciated by both the customer and the server. Second, because service quality is intangible, it is difficult to measure. The tangible measures such as numbers of customers served, cost of providing the service, and revenue generated lead to "looking good without being good" in the eyes of the customer—the patient.

Quality begins with the customer. Although the laboratory professional's customers include coworkers and physicians, the ultimate customers in health care are the patients. They are who we serve. They are why we are here. *Quality* happens when we meet or exceed customer requirements through the entire episode of care. In the book *Through the Patient's Eyes*, Gerteis et al. (1993) reports what they learned from patients about what matters to them. She found that information, choice, participation, coordination of transitions, and knowing that preferences would be respected and honored were the critical measures of satisfaction for patients.

Ultimately, it is the patient who will evaluate the quality of health care provided by the professional. Each clinical laboratory professional must understand that it is the experience of care that the patient values. The interaction with the patient when blood is being collected, when a glucose tolerance test is being explained, or when instructions are being given for collecting a clean urine specimen is what the patient perceives as care. It is this interaction as perceived by the patient that defines quality for the patient. Equally important to the laboratorian's understanding is that the quality of the patient's experience does not replace the need for optimal clinical quality. For the patient, clinical quality and analytical quality is an expected foundation of his or her care.

To create quality in health care most organizations use a combination of quality management initiatives. Measurement, assessment, and improvement may be at the discipline (departmental) level, hospitalwide (involving multiple departments or functions), and/or the communitywide level (dealing with entire patient populations). The clinical laboratory professional must accept the challenge of becoming a health-care team member who can help create and manage quality health care.

It is important for the clinical laboratory professional to understand that he or she must build and sustain a solid foundation of quality control, quality assessment, and quality management within the clinical laboratory improving the technical management of analytical processes. In addition, the laboratory professional must collaborate with other health-care professionals in the improvement of patient outcomes. The collaborative work of the clinical laboratory professional is to provide an essential component to a comprehensive, quality care delivery system. In this framework, the care-delivery process is what we do. It is why health-care delivery exists. Care delivery and its improvement are team efforts. Excellence in healthcare delivery results from an atmosphere of respect, interdisciplinary interaction, and cooperation.

The care-delivery process includes accessing; assessing and diagnosing; planning; treating; reentering a hospital, home, or another care facility; and evaluating.

- **Accessing** is the process of acquiring the information, communicating with a knowledgeable provider, getting an appointment, or entering a care site.
- **Assessing and diagnosing** include clinical (hands-on), laboratory, radiologic, and other diagnostic processes. Clinical data and information created by the laboratory are essential to effective decision making about the care of individual patients and populations of patients.
- **Planning** includes strategic/quality plans and the patient/family plan of care. Laboratorians contribute to planning by consulting on appropriate lab tests for specific patients or populations. Another example of planning would be participating in screening of populations in community outreach efforts.
- **Treating** includes drugs, procedures, counseling, teaching, and care in support of patient oxygenation, circulation, behavior, perception, mobility, nutrition, elimination, and immunity.
- **Reentering** is the process of an informed patient moving to another level of care, site of care, agency, or provider relationship.
- **Evaluating** is the process used to determine whether interventions were effective and helpful to the patient and family served.

Deming's (1986) view of an organization is a group of systems designed to serve customers. The systems are made up of processes and tasks that are linked together and affect one another. To excel at meeting customer needs, an organization must constantly improve these processes and systems. Quality management in health care begins with patient needs and expectations. These needs are then balanced with the professional standards and requirements that are used in designing, implementing, and improving important patient care processes and systems.

Deming (1986) advises us to study and understand the processes of production or service that we are delivering. His 85/15 rule declares that eighty-five percent of a worker's effectiveness is determined by the system he works within. Only fifteen percent of his contribution is due to his own skill. To break down systems into meaningful blocks for analysis, we should consider the "internal customers" of processes. Quantitative analysis of processes using statistical process control and repetitions of a Plan/Do/Check (Study)/Act cycle provide the improvement method (Langley and associates 1996) of quality management. (See Figure 29-1.)

When implementing the improvement model, three questions drive the process.

- **What are we trying to accomplish?** Improvement begins with setting aims. The aim should be stated in simple terms (e.g., fifty percent reduction in rejected specimens). Agreement on the aim and allocation of people and resources are crucial to aim accomplishment.

Quality Management 179

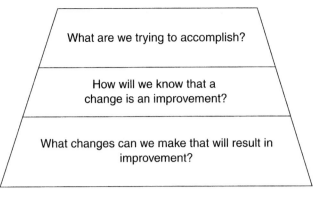

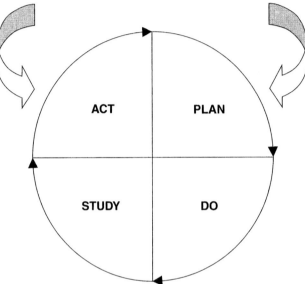

FIGURE 29–1. Improvement Model
(Adapted with permission from Langley, G. J., T. W. Nolan, C. Norman, and L. P. Provost. 1996. *The improvement guide: A practical approach to enhancing organizational performance.* San Francisco: Jossey-Bass.)

- **How will we know that a change is an improvement?** Measurement is an important part of testing and implementing changes. Measures need to be identified to tell whether a change that is made actually leads to an improvement. Measures are used for learning which improvement steps worked and which improvement steps did not make a difference. For example, we may simplify the steps in the specimen collection process to improve the number of specimens that have to be rejected and re-collected. By measuring or counting the number of specimens rejected we can tell whether or not there was actual improvement in the specimen collection process. If the number of specimens that have to be rejected was reduced, we would likely say that there had been a successful change with improvement noted. If the number of specimens that have to be rejected was increased, we would likely say there had been no improvement and continue to work on improving the specimen collection process.

- **What changes can we make that will result in improvement?** All improvement requires making a change, but not all change results in improvement. Achieving new goals requires changing the system. It is important to be able to identify the most promising changes.

A series of progressive cycles of experimentation based on the Plan/Do/Study/Act cycle of process improvement help answer the questions. Hunches, theories, and good ideas become changes that result in real improvement in the processes of care. Data and measurement form the foundation for cycles. Ongoing collection and reflection on information drives the action elements of the cycles.

When we repeatedly try to improve a process without any systematic plan, complexity arises. We may solve one piece by adding or rearranging a step, not realizing that we are distorting other parts of the process. Almost all processes include work that would not be necessary if systems worked flawlessly. An understanding of complexity is then applicable to us when trying to manage or improve quality.

There are four types of complexity: (1) mistakes and defects, (2) breakdowns and delays, (3) inefficiencies, and (4) variation. The odds are that a process or system will have at least one or more of these problems. Deming (1986) suggests that we examine processes to identify areas, tasks, and jobs that fall into one of these categories, then work to track down the root causes.

The Pareto principle is valuable in process improvement. It teaches that 80% of the trouble comes from 20% of the problems. Sometimes called the 80/20 rule, Joseph Juran (1989) advises us to apply this rule and concentrate on the "vital few" sources of problems and not be distracted by those of lesser importance.

When defects occur or someone makes an error, work has to be repeated and extra steps added to correct the error or dispose of the damage. The solution lies in finding ways to error-proof the process, preventing them in the first place.

Even when products or services are not harmed but supply or production systems break down, real work is put on hold and displaced with repair or waiting—and eventually rework. When products or services are not defective and the workflow is not interrupted, it may be that more material, time, and movement is used than absolutely essential.

One of the main culprits working to make processes unreliable or erratic is variation. Every process has some variation. There are a number of potential causes of variation in every process. Although we can't hope to eliminate all the variation in a process, we do have tools that allow us to get rid of much of it. The goal is to reduce variation as much as possible.

One way to reduce variation is standardization: getting everyone to use the same procedures, materials, equipment, and so forth. Another way is to study the process as it now operates, look for potential sources of variation, and gather data to see if these factors do affect the output. Statistical process control is a useful tool for reducing or eliminating variation. Statistically designed experiments are often helpful.

James O. Westgard (2000) has applied concepts and techniques of quality management to the medical laboratory. He delineates a quality management framework that involves quality laboratory processes, quality control, quality assessment, quality improvement, quality planning, and quality goals. Westgard points out that quality assurance is the outcome of this whole quality management process rather than being a component in the process.

Westgard (2000) suggests that these components work together like a feedback loop. **Quality planning** is concerned with establishing and validating processes that meet customer needs. Selection and evaluation of new methods and instruments are examples of quality planning. **Quality laboratory processes** are the policies, procedures, personnel standards, and physical resources that determine how work gets done in the laboratory. **Quality control and quality assessment** measure how well the work is getting done. When problems are detected, **quality improvement** determines the root causes, which can then be eliminated by implementing effective changes in **quality laboratory processes.**

Accreditation and regulatory agencies have specific quality assessment requirements with which medical laboratories must comply to be certified to perform testing on human specimens. These quality rules for laboratory services are designed to enhance patient safety and promote higher-quality care. The requirements pertain to laboratory testing in all settings including commercial labs, hospitals, and physician offices.

Conditions that must be met for laboratories to be certified under the Clinical Laboratory Improvement Amendments of 1988 (CLIA) are delineated in the CLIA Regulations published in the *Federal Register* and the *Code of Federal Regulations* (2003). Generally, the regulations call for laboratories to do the following quality assessment activities:

1. Monitor and evaluate the overall quality of the laboratory systems and correct identified problems.
2. Ensure confidentiality of patient information.
3. Ensure positive specimen identification and maintain optimum specimen integrity.
4. Investigate complaints and problems reported to the laboratory.
5. Identify problems that occur as a result of a breakdown in communication between the laboratory and the ordering individual.
6. Assess employee and consultant competency.
7. Meet specific applicable preanalytic, analytic, and postanalytic system requirements.

The quality management principles described in this chapter provide tangible approaches to compliance with CLIA requirements for quality assessment. Quality assessment when used in concert with the statistical techniques of quality control and the tools of quality improvement provides a powerful way to improve the quality and safety of patient care.

What is expected of the clinical laboratory professional in the pursuit of quality? There are implications for practitioners and leaders of clinical laboratory services. All clinical laboratory professionals need

- personal mastery of the clinical competencies required to practice clinical laboratory science
- a mental "big picture" of the health-care delivery system and a close-up view of the processes that make it happen
- a working definition of quality from the perspective of what matters to the patient
- team skills that allow for team learning and contribution to improvement initiatives
- tools and techniques for active participation in process improvements to eliminate error and waste

In addition, clinical laboratory leaders need

- skills to build shared vision and commitment to align clinical laboratory professional goals with that of the organization
- skills to build and participate in teams
- skills to recognize and reward quality performers

Understanding and practicing quality management principles, tools, and techniques is an essential competency for the clinical laboratory professional. We impact quality by paying attention to each patient's needs and expectations during care interactions. Excellence in laboratory services depends on how we apply quality management tools and techniques on a daily basis. The challenge is great. The resulting value added for the patient and the intrinsic reward of a job well done for the laboratorians make the effort worthwhile.

BIBLIOGRAPHY

Deming, W. E. 1986. *Out of the crisis.* Cambridge: Massachusetts Institute of Technology, Center for Advanced Engineering Study.

Federal Register. 2003. 68, 16, pp. 3704–14. Retrieved March 19, 2003, from <www.phppo.cdc.gov/clia/regs/toc.asp>

Gerteis, Margaret, Susan Edgman-Levitan, Jennifer Daley, and Thomas L. Delbanco. 1993. *Through the patient's eyes.* San Francisco: Jossey-Bass Health Series.

Juran, J. M. 1989. *Juran on leadership for quality: An executive handbook.* New York: Free Press.

Langley, G. J., T. W. Nolan, C. Norman, and L. P. Provost. 1996. *The improvement guide: A practical approach to enhancing organizational performance.* San Francisco: Jossey-Bass.

Westgard, James O. 2000. *The Westgard web lessons: Assuring quality through total quality management.* Retrieved July 25, 2002, from <www.Westgard.com>

INTERNET RESOURCES

CDC. Division of Laboratory Systems. <www.phppo.cdc.gov/dls/default.asp> (enter "quality" in the search box of this last resource) and <www.phppo.cdc.gov/clia/regs/toc.asp>

Institute for Healthcare Improvement. <www.ihi.org>

International Organization for Standardization. <www.iso.ch/iso/en/ISOOnline.frontpage>

Louis B. Caruana. Clinical Laboratory Science Internet Resources. <http://members.tripod.com/~LouCaru/index-5.html>

Westgard QC. <www.westgard.com>

QUESTIONS

1. Define *quality*. *(Objective 1, Level I)*

2. According to Gerteis, items important to patient satisfaction include *(Objective 2, Level I)*
   a. doctor's personality, information, hospital's reputation, price of care
   b. information, choice, participation, coordination of transition, knowing preferences
   c. health-care provider's accessibility, price of care, location of provider, outpatient facilities
   d. volume of procedures done yearly, doctor's reputation, ability to coordinate with insurance company.

3. _____ is the ultimate agent who evaluates the quality of health care provided by the professional. *(Objective 3, Level I)*

4. List and describe components of the health-care delivery process. *(Objective 4, Level II)*

5. The four types of complexity that a process may possess include all of the following EXCEPT *(Objective 5, Level I)*
   a. mistakes and defects
   b. breakdowns and delays
   c. cost controls
   d. inefficiencies
   e. variation

6. Discuss how one might reduce variation. *(Objective 6, Level II)*

7. List and discuss the components of Westgard's quality management framework. *(Objective 7, Level II)*

8. Langley and associates' three questions that drive continuous quality improvement are *(Objective 8, Level I)*

    a. _____

    b. _____

    c. _____

9. List five characteristics that the laboratory personnel need in order to contribute to quality. *(Objective 9, Level I)*

    a. _____

    b. _____

    c. _____

    d. _____

    e. _____

EXERCISES

Completion of the exercises will enhance your knowledge of quality management. *(Objective 1, Level I and Objective 10, Level III)*

1. Interview technologists about their views of the definition of quality and what quality means to the patient. Summarize your findings.

2. Interview a hospital's performance improvement coordinator or director of quality management about the model used for performance improvement. Prepare a report summarizing your findings.

3. Observe processes of health care within the clinical laboratory or the hospital and identify an example of an opportunity for improvement. Determine the focus for this improvement and determine the approach that might be used to improve.

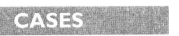

Analyze the following case studies and propose solutions. *(Objective 11, Level III)*

1. As the laboratory manager, you review the inpatient survey results. From the inpatient survey results for the last three months, you note that patients are very unhappy regarding the service they receive from the laboratory. The complaints all seem to stem from the morning phlebotomy rounds. Patients complain of having to delay their breakfast because the laboratory is late in collecting blood. Some patients indicate this is especially disturbing because they cannot even have their first morning cup of coffee. As the laboratory manager, how would you address this situation?

2. As laboratory manager, upon reviewing your monthly incident reports in the laboratory, you note that physicians are requesting that prothrombin time tests be rerun approximately five times per week. Repeated testing results indicate an error in the original data. In investigating this situation, you determine that the nursing staff has drawn the blood for these samples, processing of the specimen is being done in the laboratory processing section by the on-job-trained laboratory assistants, and the plasma is being delivered to the coagulation technologists/scientists promptly. Sometimes the value in error is above the true value and sometimes the value is below the true value, thus there is no consistency to the error. Is this situation a problem? Does it address quality? What would you do to solve this situation?

Chapter 30

Problem Solving

Sabrina H. Bryant, M.S., MT(ASCP), CLS(NCA)

OBJECTIVES

Upon completion of this chapter the learner will be able to

1. List the steps in problem solving. (*Level I*)
2. Discuss each problem-solving step. (*Level II*)
3. Evaluate problem-solving skills used in a clinical laboratory. (*Level III*)
4. Choose a problem and plan its solution using the problem-solving steps presented in this chapter. (*Level III*)
5. Analyze the problem and design a solution for the case studies. (*Level III*)

TOPIC SUMMARY

Problem solving, critical thinking, troubleshooting, decision making, analytical thinking, and strategic planning are all terms used to describe the same premise. But what precisely is meant by these terms? A problem may be defined as a question, a challenge, a conflict, or an improvement. The term "problem" is generally associated with a negative event, which is rapidly resolved or completely avoided. According to Dirkes (1993), **problem solving** is a general approach for making things happen whether the objective is satisfying school requirements or finding ways to improve life situations. The scientific method is an example of problem solving used in the laboratory.

As laboratorians, problem solving is a major portion of our professional responsibility. As individuals, dealing with problems is just part of everyday life. Situations often occur, in personal and professional settings, that must be handled quickly, thus resolution is generally performed in short order with little or no difficulty. Individuals perceive events differently, so the seriousness of a problem may vary from person to person. As with problems, solutions may be simple or complex. A solution may be a simple reaction to a roadblock hindering task completion, or maybe a more complex reaction resulting in a cascade of problems due to a hasty unformed plan of action in response to the original conflict.

Although only one specific outcome is desired, problem solving is considered open-ended and may be approached from many angles. A valid train of thought is to resolve the problem as quickly as possible with as little discussion as possible. Although this train of thought may be effective for some situations, it is not always the best approach when one or more problems exist or when more than one variable is present. Taking a little time to secure the most effective solution for all parties involved with respect to the variables may provide greater benefits. A few key steps to aid in developing problem-solving skills follow:

Steps in Problem Solving

1. Define the problem.
2. Create scenarios.
3. Implement solution.
4. Examine solution.
5. Reflect (on problem/solution).

Define Problem

The first order of business is to determine if a problem exists and to decide what is the precise problem. Restate any predefined situations to clarify variables.

Write down the facts to verify if one or more problems exist. Research the problem to determine the specifics of the initial incidence as well as any other occurrences. Choose pertinent information from the data gathered to use as a basis for brainstorming and discussion.

Create Scenarios

As an individual, brainstorm the potential approaches that might be considered. Then identify the desired outcomes of others affected by the problem. Refine the ideas to create a variety of potential solutions. Create written and illustrated scenarios to depict the problem and the solutions. Analyze the scenarios for resultant problems generated by the solution.

Solution Implementation

Choosing the most appropriate answer to the problem is not always easy. If at all possible, test the solution on an individual or small group before allowing full-scale implementation. This small-scale test will indicate how the solution works and identify threats to complete problem resolution. If the test does not seem to rectify the problem, test another of the scenarios using any new data collected during the trial. Keep a record of the solutions that may resolve the conflict as a backup and as a reference.

Examine the Solution

Consider the following questions when examining the solution. Is the solution effective? Are there any new conflicts that have developed since the solution was implemented? What might be the most effective part of the solution? Is the fix permanent or temporary? Does more work need to be done to completely resolve the problem?

Reflection

After a period of time, reconsider the original conflict. Look at the possible resolution scenarios developed. Set specific times to evaluate the situation and monitor the effectiveness of the solution (e.g., one day, one month, three months, etc.). If the solution worked, was it the best choice? Can the solution be generalized to other situations?

An example of problem solving in the clinical laboratory follows: A new PRN (pro re nata which means "as needed") tech is assigned to work in chemistry. The only experience prior to this job was her clinical education, which was three years ago. In the two months since she was hired, she has worked 12 four to six hour shifts. Every time she works on the evening or night shift, approximately one hour of downtime is required the next morning for repairs on the main chemistry analyzer. No problems occur with the main analyzer when she works on the day shift and another person processes all the chemistry specimens. There is a backup analyzer, but it is not operated because it takes twice as long to run the same tests as on the main analyzer.

Define the Problem

The problem is actually multifaceted. First, the tech was inadequately trained to prepare the specimens and run the analyzer, resulting in lost tech time to repair the instrument. But the main problem is that the downtime is delaying patient care and treatment.

Create Scenarios

- Scenario #1—Schedule the PRN tech to work with the chemistry supervisor to be properly trained on all of the instruments in that department.
- Scenario #2—Have the PRN tech use only the backup instrument for the small number of tests run on her night shift.
- Scenario #3—Have the PRN tech do a rotation in specimen processing to refresh her skills in this area.

Solution Implementation and Examination

After solution implementation (Scenario #1), the tech still had a few instrument problems. But after more hands-on experience during the day shift, she realized that she had not been allowing the specimens to clot and/or to be centrifuged for the required length of time. She read the specimen handling and processing manual and worked a few extra shifts in specimen processing. The combination of scenarios #1 and #3 made the best possible solution. Remember, not every problem or question can be solved with the first approach, but with careful examination the major conflict can usually be resolved.

Reflect

- Would any other scenarios resolve the problem?
- Could any permanent solution be used for other new employees?
- Are other problems obvious?

Now take a moment to reflect on the problem-solving steps presented in this chapter by working through the example situations, mentally checking off the steps from the problem-solving list. Clearly define the primary problem. Develop potential written or illustrated scenarios that might be used to solve the problem. Choose and implement the best solution or combination of solutions. After a designated period of time, examine the solution for completeness. Finally, spend some time in reflection with reference to the problem and the effectiveness of the solution.

BIBLIOGRAPHY

Baron, J., and R. Brown. 1991. *Teaching decision making to adolescents.* Mahwah, N.J.: Lawrence Erlbaum Associates.

Dirkes, M. Ann. 1993. *Self-directed problem solving.* Lanham, Md.: University Press of America.

Fogarty, Robin. 1997. *Problem-based learning and other curriculum models for the multiple intelligences classroom.* Arlington Heights, Ill.: Skylight Training and Publishing.

Sternberg, Robert J. 1992. *Teaching for thinking: The thinking cycle.* Reston, Va.: National Association for Secondary School Principals.

INTERNET RESOURCES

Ball State University Teaching Strategies. <www.bsu.edu/teachers/burris/iwonder/strategies/strategies.html>

Deepthunder. <www.deepthunder.com/frsttrng/prbslve.htm>

Pearson Education. <www.pearsoned.com>

San Francisco State University, Response Sets in Learning and Problem Solving. <http://online.sfsu.edu/~psych200/unit4/46.htm>

Skylight Professional Development (check What's New or Site Search). <www.skylightedu.com>

QUESTIONS

1. The steps in problem solving include all EXCEPT *(Objective 1, Level I)*
   a. define the problem
   b. create scenarios
   c. implement solution
   d. examine resolution
   e. publish employee's problem

2. Discuss each step in problem solving. *(Objective 2, Level II)*

EXERCISES

Completion of the exercises will enhance your knowledge of problem solving. *(Objective 3, Level III and Objective 4, Level III)*

1. Using the problem-solving steps outlined in this chapter, evaluate the specimen processing for your laboratory. Points to consider include collection and delivery to the lab as well as delivery to the department. Could this system be more efficient? What steps would you employ to make the system most time and cost effective?

2. Over the past ten years the number of students interested in a career in the clinical laboratory has decreased. Brainstorm and develop two scenarios (one written and one illustrated) depicting recruitment tools that might attract and interest young people.

3. Discuss with a department supervisor or laboratory manager the approach to problem solving used. Compare this approach with the list outlined in this chapter. Are the lists similar? Describe any differences with regard to the positive or negative effect on the solution.

4. Choose a personal or professional problem and work through using the problem-solving steps.

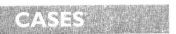

Following are three clinical laboratory cases. Using the given information, each learner should determine the problem and design a resolution for each case. Work groups of three to four individuals may be formed for the resolution design portion. Both written and illustrated depictions of the resolution should be attempted. Groups should develop at least three solution scenarios for the cases. (Remember, the first solution may not solve the problem. Also keep in mind that a combination of scenarios may be needed to fix the problem.)

You may use role play for cases to evaluate your understanding of the problem and the effects of the solution. Individuals may want to approach the situation from different perspectives. *(Objective 5, Level III)*

1. The chemistry department supervisor noticed that the daily and weekly quality control reports were not completed when she was on vacation. She has also received calls from nurses looking for test results. Patients had tests ordered in the hospital computer, but no results had been received, and the laboratory computer has no results for the tests that were ordered. The techs were questioned and reported that they had done a great deal of work in her absence and that they remembered some of the patient names. The barcode work list shows that the workload had been very heavy for the time the supervisor was out. Upon further investigation, the supervisor found that the main chemistry instrument was no longer accessible by the hospital information system due to the implementation of a new management software system.

    What is the main problem?
    What is the desired outcome?
    What are three possible solution options?
    What solution is the best of those devised, and why?
    Should any other factors be considered? (What? And why?)

2. A small hospital laboratory has one permanent full-time day shift hematology position available, and two techs are interested in the position. One tech is on night shift and the other tech is on evening shift. The techs are equally qualified for the position. Their hire dates are the same. The evening shift person is married and has a small child not yet in school. She plans to quit if she is not given the position. The night shift tech is newly married and is interested in starting a family in the near future. The hospital policy is to hire from within if at all possible.

    What is the main problem and the desired outcome?
    What are three possible solution options?
    What solution is the best of those devised, and why?
    Should any other factors be considered? (What? And why?)

3. A very large and active medical center has within the last six months doubled the amount work they are sending to the main laboratory. Turnaround time has increased to about one and one half hours from time of collection to results. The main lab has hired two new techs that will start within two weeks. The emergency room (ER) physicians are interested in having a STAT lab in the ER because they feel that the workload will continue to increase, and they are displeased with the increased turnaround time. They would like to have limited services such as CBC, UA, ABGs, wet preps, pregnancy tests, and Chem 7 performed in the ER. The lab manager has suggested that increasing lab staff and upgrading instrumentation in the main lab will not only effectively combat this problem but will work toward a long-term solution for future expansion.

What is the main problem?
What is the desired outcome?
What are three possible solution options?
What solution is the best of those devised, and why?
Should any other factors be considered? (What? And why?)

Chapter 31

Preanalytical, Analytical, and Postanalytical Phases

Jane Hudson, Ph.D., MT(ASCP)SM, CLS(NCA)

OBJECTIVES

Upon completion of this chapter the learner will be able to

1. Define preanalytical, analytical, and postanalytical in regards to laboratory testing. *(Level I)*
2. Discuss the role of the laboratory in preanalytical, analytical, and postanalytical phases. *(Level II)*
3. Critique a laboratory's preanalytical, analytical, and postanalytical activities by describing areas in which the laboratory might improve activities. *(Level III)*
4. Differentiate the three phases (preanalytical, analytical, and postanalytical) and the laboratory actions in each phase, then formulate solutions to address the issues raised in the case studies. *(Level III)*

TOPIC SUMMARY

The medical technologist/clinical laboratory scientist has always satisfied and excelled in the analytical testing component of patient care. The laboratory has always been the place where the specimen was sent and where data was generated regarding that specimen. That data was usually very reliable and contributed to the patient's care. As medical technologists/clinical laboratory scientists, we prided ourselves on our specimen preparation, analysis of the specimen, and quality control used to verify the results. This is the analytical component of our jobs, and we are experts.

As the health-care system has changed, medical technologists/clinical laboratory scientists have realized that they must also be involved in the preanalytical and postanalytical components of patient care. Therefore, we now recognize three components of patient care: **preanalytical (input), analytical (process),** and **postanalytical (output).** Figure 31–1 shows a diagram of the three phases.

The preanalytical component is critical because at this stage the clinical question is formulated. The medical technologist/clinical laboratory scientist can provide information regarding the types of tests available to address the question, the efficiency and cost of the different types of tests, the specimen required, and the procedure for specimen collection. This information must be considered in the present health-care environment to avoid unnecessary costs and unnecessary delay in answering the clinical question. Medical technologists/clinical laboratory scientists are valuable members of the preanalytical team, and many are now serving on teams developing clinical pathways.

The postanalytical component is somewhat addressed in our reporting of data with information regarding normal/abnormal ranges and panic values, and we even notify the physician regarding result

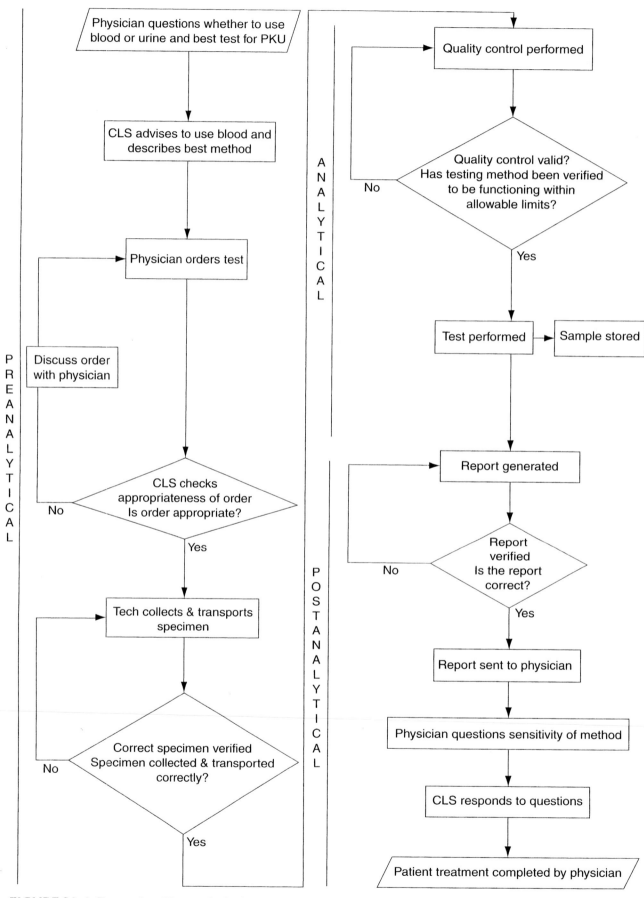

FIGURE 31-1. Example of Preanalytical, Analytical, and Postanalytical Phases

probabilities. However, we often fail to consult with the physician regarding the action taken and the effect on the patient as a result of the testing data we provided. Patient outcomes are critical in the health-care environment today, and this is an essential step in the postanalytical component.

Patient outcomes are used to justify the need for laboratory testing. Elevitch (1998) indicates that most inpatients receive clinical laboratory tests, and as many as one of five outpatients also are impacted by the clinical laboratory tests. According to Mass (1999), laboratory testing information is involved in approximately seventy percent of the medical decisions. Therefore, assessment of patient outcomes is critical in critiquing and modifying laboratory services. The medical technologist/clinical laboratory scientist must be involved with the medical team that reviews data regarding patient outcomes in order to provide quality medical care and accountability.

In order to provide competent practice in all three components of the job, the medical technologist/clinical laboratory scientist must know more than just the mechanics of the laboratory tests. Knowledge of body systems, including anatomy and physiology of each, must be mastered. In addition, the cutting-edge technology such as that found in genetic testing and molecular testing also must be mastered. Health-care cost is a major factor that must also be considered. The ability to problem solve, interpret, and think "outside of the box" is an essential ingredient to providing quality service to the patient. Medical technologists/clinical laboratory scientists who possess these skills should seek out ways to be involved with other health-care practitioners such as accompanying physicians on rounds and serving on critical pathway teams, safety committees, quality assurance committees, cost analysis committees, performance improvement committees, and so on. As the medical technologist/clinical laboratory scientist performs all the components of the job—preanalytical, analytical, and postanalytical—the patient and the institution are served more effectively.

BIBLIOGRAPHY

Barr, Judith T. 1999. Clinical laboratory utilization: Rationale. In *Principles of clinical laboratory utilization and consultation*, ed. B. Davis, D. Mass, and M. Bishop. Philadelphia: W. B. Saunders.

Elevitch, Franklin. 1998. Impact of managed care on laboratory economics. *Laboratory Medicine* 29, no. 12: 747–52.

Luckey, I., and B. G. Davis., (1999) Clinical laboratory utilization: Implementation. In *Principles of Clinical Laboratory Utilization and Consultation*, ed. B. Davis, D. Mass, and M. Bishop. Philadelphia: W. B. Saunders.

Mass, Diana. 1999. MT/MLT programs decreasing as laboratory needs change. *Vantage Point* 3, no. 17: 1, 3–6.

INTERNET RESOURCES

American Association for Clinical Chemistry, Clinical Laboratory News.
<www.aacc.org/cln/features/97features/aug97feat.html>

American Society for Clinical Laboratory Science.
<www.ascls.org/labtesting/labintro.asp>

Biomedical Clinical Pathology.
<www.biomedcentral.com/1472-6890/1/5>

The Journal of the International Federation of Clinical Chemistry and Laboratory Medicine.
<www.ifcc.org/ejifcc/vol13no1/1301200107n.htm>

Virtual Hospital, The University of Iowa. <www.vh.org>

Westgard Quality Control.
<www.westgard.com/qcapp6.htm>

QUESTIONS

1. The preanalytical component is *(Objective 1, Level I)*
   a. formulation of the clinical question
   b. choices are made regarding clinical testing
   c. quality control is performed
   d. a and b
   e. all of the above

2. The analytical component is *(Objective 1, Level I)*
   a. specimen preparation
   b. analysis of specimen
   c. quality control performed
   d. a and b
   e. all of the above

3. The postanalytical component is *(Objective 1, Level I)*
   a. *analysis of effect of testing data on patient outcomes*
   b. performing quality control
   c. performing tests
   d. selecting the clinical question

4. Give examples of the role of the laboratory in preanalytical, analytical, and postanalytical phases. *(Objective 2, Level II)*

EXERCISES

Completion of the exercises will enhance your knowledge of preanalytical, analytical, and postanalytical phases. *(Objective 3, Level III)*

1. Develop a detailed flowchart starting with the patient's first visit to the physician through completion of treatment and return to health. Use your own experiences or use a patient case history—a diabetic case history is an excellent one. After the detailed flowchart is developed, insert a red arrow at each step that laboratory services should be involved. Describe the involvement needed at each step.

2. Visit a meeting of the clinical pathways committee or review the minutes of a meeting, and write a report on your observations. Share your report with the class.

3. Visit a meeting of the patient outcomes committee or review the minutes of a meeting, and write a report on your observations. Share your report with the class.

4. List the laboratory's present involvement in preanalytical, analytical, and postanalytical tasks and recommend additional involvement that may be needed. Describe areas where your laboratory might improve. Defend your position.

CASES

In the following case situations, differentiate the three phases (preanalytical, analytical, and postanalytical) and the laboratory's action in each phase, then formulate solutions to address the issues raised. *(Objective 4, Level III)*

1. A survey was conducted of physicians ordering outpatient urinalysis tests in the month of June. The physician survey revealed that several times with healthy young females, a colony count of less than 100,000 cfu/ml was reported when the physician believed an infection was present. The patients received antibiotic therapy based on clinical symptoms, even though the culture did not support the diagnosis. The physicians in the survey are questioning the culture technique. Should these findings be investigated? How would you investigate this finding to resolve this dilemma? Is this a preanalytical, analytical, or postanalytical situation?

2. Many of the pediatric physicians recently attended a conference regarding reducing substances found in the urine. Now you are receiving five to ten orders daily for paper chromography analysis for galactosemia on children younger than one year. You use Clinitest tablets, which indicate if any reducing substance is present, as a screening test on the urine of all children under two years of age. How would you go about working with the physicians? Is this a preanalytical, analytical, or postanalytical situation?

3. You do CK Isosenzymes in-house by batch testing every morning or every other morning depending on volume and tech time. Tryoponin I testing, considered the "gold standard" test, is sent out to a reference laboratory and requires eight hours turnaround time. After several months of study regarding the ordering pattern, you note that the physicians are ordering both CK Isosenzymes and tryoponin I testing STAT on their cardiac patients. Would you have recommendations for the chief technologist regarding these tests? Would you have suggestions for the physicians based on your knowledge? Is this a preanalytical, analytical, or postanalytical situation?

4. When hematocrits are ordered, you do them on an instrument that gives you the total CBC results. You note on a patient that there are critical platelet and WBC results; however, the hematocrit is normal. Do you report the critical values even though they are not requested? How would you handle this situation? Is this a preanalytical, analytical, or postanalytical situation?

5. In plotting your quality control information, you note a trend developing. What would you do? Is this a preanalytical, analytical, or postanalytical situation?

Chapter 32

Instrument Selection

Carolyn Beck, Ed.D., MT(ASCP)SBB

OBJECTIVES

Upon completion of this chapter the learner will be able to

1. List several factors that must be taken into consideration when purchasing an instrument for a specific type of laboratory. *(Level I)*
2. Discuss the various types of individuals who should be invited by the lab manager to participate in a teamwork approach to developing a needs assessment and conducting research on instruments available in the marketplace. *(Level II)*
3. Discuss several of the major cost considerations related to instrument acquisition. *(Level II)*
4. Explain how networking with fellow laboratorians and managers can be helpful during the process of selecting an instrument. *(Level II)*
5. Given cases, develop a needs assessment for the purchase of a specific type of instrument for a specific laboratory facility. *(Level III)*
6. Investigate methods of financing the acquisition of a given instrument. *(Level II)*
7. Analyze case studies and propose solutions. *(Level III)*

TOPIC SUMMARY

There are three main steps in the selection of a laboratory instrument for purchase: performing an inclusive needs assessment, researching the availability of instruments in the marketplace, and evaluating all the data gathered to determine which instrument will be the acquired.

Performing a **needs assessment** is the process of determining exactly which features and characteristics of an instrument are necessary to satisfy the needs requirements for a specific laboratory. The assessment should attempt to define both present and future needs to be met by a new instrument. Since numerous factors contribute to the list of desired qualities, a team approach will provide a greater diversity of opinions and concerns. Therefore, the assessment team should include representatives of personnel on all shifts using and supervising the use of the instrument in addition to individuals on the management team. Other team members may be the lab information specialist, quality assurance officer, safety officer, and others with special expertise. The participation of organizational management individuals knowledgeable about expansion plans for the facility within the next five years is critical to the assessment stage. When considering future expansion, the team should allow for expansion of the lab test offerings and new tests that may be added over the next few years, including tests that do not exist now. The desires of physicians for additional tests, increased speed, or increased stat capacity should also be considered.

Key factors to be considered when determining your needs are the **characteristics of the individual laboratory.** Bowie (1993) and Quale (1993) provide detailed discussions on such factors as the lab test menu needed in the future, the current and future lab workload, the test mix of the lab, the work-flow situation (e.g., what STAT capabilities are needed). In addition, *labor considerations* such as minimal sample loading times, walk-away features, automatic sample dilution, instrument quality control features and data generation features, ease of troubleshooting, and maintenance downtime are always critical. The impact of an instrument on **the laboratory environment** should also be considered: its size, special electrical or plumbing needs, and the amount of heat generated during operation must be studied. As part of the assessment, **quality of performance** issues should be addressed. Quality of performance factors include such issues as setting minimum standards for acceptable instrument performance regarding linearity, sensitivity, specificity, accuracy, precision, stability of electronics, and stability of reagents used.

Additional instrument features of importance include the instrument throughput, the sample processing method of the instrument (such as sequential vs. simultaneous, random vs. fixed ordering of samples, and batching capabilities), bar coding, and sample identification features. Safety features such as primary tube sampling should be evaluated. Based on past experiences, personnel may have preferences for photometric versus electrochemical methodologies. A major consideration today is the compatibility of the instrument with the Laboratory Information System (LIS), and its ability to communicate by both uploading and downloading. Data storage capabilities may be critical to some facilities. Current textbooks are available with comprehensive information on numerous additional factors to be examined, including the details of how various instruments process and analyze samples (Bowie 1993; Quale 1993: Haven et al. 1995; Fink and Narayanan 1994). After gathering all of the input from the needs assessment, a detailed list of desired characteristics of the instrument can be generated. This list serves as a guide for the activities in the remaining steps.

The second step in the selection process is **research.** This process should be more than simply meeting with sales personnel, although such contacts can be used as an initial step in determining what is available in the marketplace. From literature supplied by the manufacturer of an instrument, many of the quality of performance details can be found and discussed. In addition, many manufacturers have Web sites for research on their products. There are also Web sites that research the manufacturing company. An example would be the Healthcare Product Comparison System found at www.ecri.org. Some professional organizations also maintain information related to locating sources for instruments, reagents, and other products (e.g., the American Association of Blood Banks Buyer's Guide at www.aabb.org). Other Web sites hope to develop information for comparing numerous instruments within one site (e.g., www.labboss.com). An alternative approach to this research procedure is the process of developing a request for proposal (RFP). This approach should also use a team to develop the RFP, which is essentially a list of questions to which each vendor replies. Vendors may assist the team by providing sample RFP questions and formats, especially from other labs purchasing similar instruments. All team members should have input on the types of questions asked so that no details or specifications are omitted. An RFP document can easily be ten to twenty pages in length. Because each vendor answers the same questions, comparisons of the instruments can be made easily. Barglowski (2001) discusses this procedure in detail and provides sample instrument evaluation forms and side-by-side comparison forms.

Next, the instrument features should be compared using the information collected. A chart could be helpful to compare each of the features on the needs list. After comparing the many features of models on the market obtained by research, the list of acceptable instruments should be narrowed. Before the final selection is made another type of information should be collected.

This second type of research should focus on networking with technologists and managers in facilities of similar size and function as the lab seeking the new instrument. This approach helps one lab learn from the mistakes or successes of others. If your sales representative does not encourage you to pursue this avenue of research, use caution in following his or her recommendations. Discussing instruments with others is also an avenue in determining the satisfaction of other consumers with manufacturer support services, timeliness of repairs, reagent problems, and actual instrument downtime. A comparison of actual user findings to company claims may then be made. Networking with others at instrument exhibits and at meetings can be a powerful research tool. Some meetings schedule instrument user groups for specific instruments to foster informal discussions that can be enlightening to those considering purchasing the instrument.

A manager must also be concerned with costs, not only of the instrument itself but also of the reagents, service contracts, labor, and many other factors in the cost equation. The purchase cost of an instrument may just be the tip of a very large iceberg (Bowie 1993). Cost is often the most limiting factor in determining how many of the desired features of the instrument are realistic for the setting. Cost may determine what is really "needed" versus what is "wanted." Thorough research into all the details of cost will avoid surprises in the future. It might be appropriate to evaluate costs of outsourcing various low-frequency tests at this time, using projected costs with the new instrument (Bowie 1993; Quale 1993; O'Brien 2000).

With the rapid changes in technology today, the old concept of using an instrument until it becomes inoperable or maintenance becomes too expensive may not be viable. Instrument changes may occur more frequently in the future. It may not be feasible to purchase instruments for a variety of reasons. Most manufacturers have a variety of programs available for financing, including several types of leases (O'Brien 2000). Reconditioned instruments may also be considered. Numerous companies now offer used instruments. The manager must consider all these options in determining costs of the instrument and a realistic useful lifetime (O'Brien 2000).

When the needs assessment and research stages have been completed, only the **evaluation and decision-making steps** remain. Based on the developed needs list and the comparison data on various instruments developed through the research process, a number of unacceptable instruments should have been eliminated from consideration. Again, a consensus decision with those using the instrument and with managers may be a wise strategy, especially if the final decision between two or three instruments will be based on minor considerations. Worker input makes it "our" instrument rather than the manager's new instrument. When the final decision is made, a discussion of which factors influenced the final decision made by management answers many questions for the staff and enhances feelings of staff inclusion in the process. Because instrument purchases are some of the largest laboratory expenditures, the selection process should allow time for extensive research and evaluation.

BIBLIOGRAPHY

Barglowski, Mark. 2001. The instrument selection process: Beyond the sales pitch. *Medical Laboratory Observer* 33, no. 2: 45–51.

Bowie, Lenuel J. 1993. *Selection of laboratory instruments.* In: *Principles of laboratory instruments*, ed. Larry E. Schoeff and Robert H. Williams. St. Louis, Mo.: Mosby.

Fink, Joseph G., and Sheshadri Narayanan. 1994. Preventive maintenance and troubleshooting. In *Clinical laboratory instrumentation and automation: Principles, applications, and selection*, ed. Kory M. Ward, Craig A. Lehmann, and Alan M. Leiken. Philadelphia: W. B. Saunders.

Haven, Mary C., Gregory A. Tetrault, and Jerald R. Schenken. 1995. *Laboratory instrumentation.* 4th ed. New York: Van Nostrand Reinhold.

O'Brien, Judith A. 2000. *Common problems in clinical laboratory management.* New York: McGraw-Hill.

Quale, Marguerite. 1993. *Definitions, concepts and approaches.* In *Principles of laboratory Instrument*, ed. Larry E. Schoeff and Robert H. Williams. St. Louis, Mo.: Mosby.

Ward, Kory M., Craig A. Lehmann, and Alan M. Leiken, eds. 1994. *Clinical laboratory instrumentation and automation: Principles, applications, and selection.* Philadelphia: W. B. Saunders.

INTERNET RESOURCES

Selected Manufacturers

Abbott Laboratories. <www.Abbott.com>
Advanced Instruments, Inc. <www.Aitests.com>
Beckman Coulter. <www.beckmancoulter.com>
Olympus. <www.olympus.com>

Refurbished/Used Laboratory Instruments

Lab Boss. <www.labboss.com>
ACT Diagnostics. <www.actdiagnostics.com>
Spectron Corporation. <www.spectroncorp.com>
See a more comprehensive guide to internet resources in O'Brien 2000. Also, additional links are found on some of the previously listed sites.

QUESTIONS

1. List the various factors that must be taken into consideration when purchasing an instrument for a specific type of laboratory. *(Objective 1, Level I)*

    a. _____

    b. _____

    c. _____

2. Discuss the various individuals who should become involved in a teamwork approach to developing a needs assessment and conducting research on instruments available in the marketplace. *(Objective 2, Level II)*

3. Discuss several of the major cost considerations related to instrument purchase. *(Objective 3, Level II)*

4. Explain how networking with fellow laboratorians and managers can be helpful during the process of selecting an instrument. *(Objective 4, Level II)*

EXERCISES

Completion of the exercises will enhance your knowledge of the instrument selection process. *(Objective 5, Level III and Objective 6, Level II)*

1. Develop a needs assessment for the purchase of a specific type of instrument for a specific facility. Be sure to consider characteristics of the laboratory, lab environment, quality of performance, and safety features. This may be done individually or as a group. After you have developed a specific needs assessment, interview a vendor that sells an instrument that will address your needs. This can be done at a professional meeting or by inviting a sales representative to address the group. If this is not possible, gather information by researching the vendor's Web site and/or literature. Then interview a medical technologist operating that particular instrument. Compare vendor information with the user information that you gather.

2. Evaluate and choose (or not choose) an instrument based on a needs assessment and research information.

3. Investigate methods of financing the acquisition of a given instrument by interviewing laboratory managers at several institutions.

CASES

Analyze the following case studies and propose solutions. *(Objective 7, Level III)*

1. You are the supervisor of a laboratory in a thirty-bed hospital that is located fifty miles from a major medical center. Your facility has no emergency room and airlifts critical patients to the medical center. There is no obstetrics service, but there are two operating rooms, and approximately fifteen surgeries are performed per week. There is no outpatient clinic, so all samples tested are from patients in your facility. The bulk of the work is

routine testing (general chemistries) presurgery and testing of routine medical patients (diabetics, alcoholics, the elderly, physical exams, etc.) The average number of chemistry tests per week is around 3,500. Approximately eighty-five percent of testing is done on the 7 A.M. to 3 P.M. shift. Less than ten percent of the testing is done on a STAT basis.

Your old instrument for chemistry testing is on its last legs. You need to determine what type of new instrument to buy. In a meeting with the pathologist, he states that no expansion is planned for the next five to seven years, that cost containment is a primary consideration (especially labor costs), and that the patient load should remain about the same. The physicians at the facility feel more profits could be generated if a greater variety of tests were available instead of sending so many tests to the reference lab. They especially wish to monitor the drug levels (for prescribed medications) in their elderly patients. They also would like more exotic tests done besides electrolytes and general chemistries. Which instrument would you recommend for purchase?

2. You are a medical technologist in a large reference lab in a major metropolitan area. You collect samples in your facility, but the majority are collected from physicians offices in fifteen surrounding counties. Most of the samples enter your facility after 3 P.M. Because of the distances traveled from office to you, few of the samples are emergencies. One of your advertised policies is that all routine hematology and chemistry panels (such as a twenty-four-test panel) will be performed and the data transmitted to the physician's office before 8 A.M. the next day. Special and unusual tests are guaranteed within two days. Your supervisor has asked you as a technologist working in the chemistry laboratory to serve on an advisory committee to determine which new chemistry analyzer the laboratory needs. Currently you perform chemistry panels on approximately 1,600 patients a night, and most are twenty-four tests per panel. Your goal is to complete all testing between 3 P.M. and 6 A.M. At the first committee meeting the pathologist outlines his concerns, which include improved safety, increasing the workload ten percent a year for the next five years, and keeping personnel costs minimal. No new technologists will be hired in the next two years although workload will increase. Routine test panels are the main emphasis and job of this lab, and other instruments will handle the special and unusual testing. Which instrument would you recommend for purchase?

3. You are a technologist in a very large medical center and have been working in clinical chemistry for ten years. The medical center has in excess of 1,500 beds in three buildings and also has very large day surgery and ambulatory care centers. The center has a class I trauma center and treats more than 600 cases per month of life-threatening trauma and 6,000 less serious emergency room cases per month. The five-year management plan for the center includes expansion of emergency services. During the planning stage of the expanded trauma facility, the committee has discovered that the doctors at the emergency facilities are dissatisfied with the lab services provided. They are pleased with the large array of specialty and unusual tests the large lab can provide but do not feel that the tests needed in an emergency (usually Na, K, CO_2, Cl, glucose, BUN, and enzymes for heart

attacks) are done quickly enough. It has been proposed that a new lab facility for emergency testing only be opened in the new trauma center. You have been asked to become the chemistry supervisor of this new lab and are to present a proposal detailing the kind of instrumentation you will need. Cost is not an important factor, but complete computerization is. Which instrument would you recommend for purchase?

4. You are a technologist working in a medical center clinical lab. For many years there were really three laboratories under one management that provided services for patient testing. The first lab handled emergency testing only. The larger main lab performed the majority of the routine tests and also did all the rare and exotic tests. Finally, a third lab existed to perform tests on the patients in the outpatient clinic. The clinic contains multiple disciplines and the practices of 200 physicians. Three years ago the medical center decided to consolidate all areas of the hospital, and all of the labs were combined into one very large facility. Now the physicians in the medical center are very unhappy with lab services. They complain that emergency tests are not done promptly enough and that clinic patient tests are often lost in the system, and results are not completed by the time the patient is ready to see the clinic doctor. You have been asked to help design a new lab for the clinic to do routine chemistry tests and panels and ensure that results will be ready with a two-hour-or-less turnaround time. The doctors have asked for at least thirty-two different tests to be available. To speed communications, the physicians want the instrument to be able to interface with the hospital computer. They state that less than ten percent of tests will be STAT. Most tests will be screening panels of twenty to twenty-four tests or routine general chemistry tests as follow-up testing (such as glucoses for diabetes or a BUN for a patient with kidney disease). With 200 doctors each seeing thirty patients a day and seventy percent needing lab tests, a large number and a large variety of tests will be needed. The pathologist also suggested barcoding of patient tubes due to the large volume of patients seen each day for chemistry panels. Safety is a major concern because of the large hepatitis and AIDS sections of the clinic. The doctors are satisfied with the turnaround time for the rare and exotic tests, which will not be a part of the new lab for the clinic. Which instrument would you recommend for purchase?

5. You are the med tech supervisor in a lab in a large kidney dialysis center. You see sixty to eighty patients a day for dialysis. For those that are dialyzed, the doctors prefer to have blood tests done before and after the treatment. The tests that need to be done on each patient are Na, K, Cl, CO_2, BUN, Creatinine, Glucose, and Calcium. Speed of testing is critical because the patient must wait to get on the dialysis machine until the tests are completed. After treatment, the patient cannot be dismissed until the lab values are known. Other tests, which are not STAT, are sent to another lab. This is a very specialized lab that does only a very few tests, but the lab must have great speed and accuracy. You have an Dupont Automated Clinical Analyzer IV (ACA IV) now, and the doctors want it replaced to make life easier for everyone at the center. Biohazardous samples are a big concern because dialysis patients have higher rates of hepatitis than most patients. Computer

interfacing is not possible now, but it would help speed results to the nurses. The center has minimal numbers of lab personnel and is always behind on plotting quality assurance charts. Another problem has been a lack of electronic data storage of patient results from the previous week. The lab supervisor has also been told to try to reduce reagent costs, which have been high with the ACA. Which instrument would you recommend for purchase?

Chapter 33

Establishing Preventive and Corrective Maintenance Programs

Carolyn Beck, Ed.D., MT(ASCP)SBB

OBJECTIVES

Upon completion of this chapter the learner will be able to

1. Define the term *preventive maintenance*, combining the concepts of maintenance as a process and a program. *(Level II)*
2. Discuss several reasons why preventive maintenance programs for instruments are important and beneficial to the clinical laboratory. *(Level II)*
3. Discuss the purpose of buying service contracts for major instruments. *(Level II)*
4. Describe some of the key steps in implementing a preventive maintenance program. *(Level II)*
5. Define the term *corrective maintenance*. *(Level I)*
6. Define the term *troubleshooting* and describe its relationship to instrument repair. *(Level II)*
7. Name several voluntary accreditation agencies and national government regulatory agencies that have standards related to instrument maintenance and repair. *(Level I)*
8. Define the term *good manufacturing practices* and give an example of how such practices impact laboratory instrumentation. *(Level II)*
9. Review and summarize the components of an instrument manual. *(Level II)*
10. Analyze the case studies and propose solutions. *(Level III)*

TOPIC SUMMARY

One of the challenges of modern laboratory management is the diversity of components that are managed. Individual components include management of personnel, materials, finances, facilities, inventories, and equipment. Each component has several subcategories. Equipment management includes three major subcategories: selection and acquisition, maintenance, and repair of instruments (Fink and Narayanan 1994).

Surprisingly, maintenance of instruments was not normally discussed in the literature until 1968 when Baer suggested that laboratory directors should protect themselves from prolonged breakdown and repair periods by establishing programs of preventive maintenance. Since the 1970s, instrument preventive maintenance (PM) programs have become more and more intermingled with the quality control issues in total quality management programs. In reality, PM is a separate issue and should not be confused with performance verification and function verification, which are quality control issues. Both verification and instrument maintenance are necessary (Fink and Narayanan 1994).

Beginning in the 1980s, dramatic changes occurred in two areas: in the instruments themselves and in regulatory oversight. Both large and small laboratory instruments are marvels of high technology. Certainly more of the instruments of today perform part of their own maintenance, especially checking electronic components through self-testing procedures. Instruments do some self-cleaning and notify operators of numerous types of problems. Modern instruments should require less maintenance downtime than the instruments of previous decades. However, due to their complexity, instruments of today usually cannot be completely taken apart and repaired by the technologist like the simpler spectrophotometers, continuous-flow instruments, and cell counters of the past. This increased complexity requires the purchase of a service contract that contributes substantially to the cost of equipment management. The service contract usually covers the costs of major repairs, replacement parts, and some PM activities performed by the technicians of the manufacturer. Such contracts focus on repairs beyond the ability of most technologists to diagnosis and correct. Various types of service contracts are available, and timeliness of repairs is a critical component of the agreement.

Although the time required for actual hands-on maintenance may have decreased for some instruments, the time required for documentation necessary to meet regulatory requirements has grown. Even the simplest of instruments such as centrifuges, autoclaves, ovens, and heating baths require thoroughly documented PM activities to meet the regulations in the modern lab environment (O'Brien 2000).

PM has numerous definitions. An extensive and thoughtful discussion of both the terminology and history of maintenance in the laboratory is presented by Fink and Narayanan (1994). PM as a term can be used in two ways. First, PM can be defined as a **program**. Program definitions stress the planned nature of scheduled activities. Examples of activities include cleaning, adjusting parts, checking mechanical operations, and so on. PM is also defined as a **process.** The process definitions of PM focus on a specific series of activities (such as step-by-step guides of tasks) to be performed at specific intervals to obtain the goals of instrument maintenance. Maintenance implies keeping the instrument in good condition, in an operating and functional state, and avoiding failures. When combining these ideas, PM becomes a planned program of scheduled activities (cleaning and minor repairs) to prevent instrument dysfunction and failure (Fink and Narayanan 1994; Karselis 1994; O'Brien 2000).

PM is a commitment of both time and money. What justifications are there for PM programs? First, as in any business, time is money. Downtime means financial loss, as no product is being produced when the instrument is not operating. Labor costs are wasted if employees have idle time and production schedules are disrupted. In this business, disruptions can be detrimental to patient care. Other considerations include lower repair costs when maintenance prevents breakdowns and perhaps longer instrument life with routine care. Breakdowns can place employees at risk of injury, so safety is also a concern. Above all, product quality depends on a functional, stable, and reliable instrument. A major goal of PM is to prevent malfunctions before the quality of testing is compromised (Fink and Narayanan 1994; Karselis 1994; O'Brien 2000).

Many voluntary accreditation organizations, government agencies, textbook authors, and laboratory managers have developed sample PM programs consisting of numerous steps and flowcharts. A new manager does not need to reinvent the wheel. There are many sources to help establish and implement PM programs (Fink and Narayanan 1994; Karselis 1994; O'Brien 2000). The manager should delegate the responsibilities of the PM activities and scheduling to supervisors and instrument operators while retaining the responsibility for oversight and evaluation.

Instrument manuals provided by manufacturers detail which maintenance tasks should be performed and at what intervals. In addition, the schedule of PM frequency must meet regulatory criteria that may differ from some manufacturers' recommendations. To implement the PM program, the supervisor should first identify every piece of equipment to be maintained. A documentation form should be developed that details daily, weekly, monthly, and other PM activities for each of the identified pieces of equipment. Often such forms are supplied by the manufacturer. Samples of such forms are readily available (O'Brien 2000). One such example is shown in Figure 33–1.

Next, the PM tasks should be assigned to personnel who are then trained to perform the tasks and complete appropriate documentation. Management should seek to include all workers in the PM program so that all learn the importance of these activities (Fink and Narayanan 1994). Less experienced individuals can be assigned to simpler instruments (centrifuges, heating baths, thermometers, etc.). Instruments of greater complexity should be maintained by technologists knowledgeable in instrument theory and familiar with operational details. More than one individual should be able to perform PM on any given instrument, and training of new employees should be an ongoing activity. Most labs are fortunate enough to have one or more individuals who have an almost innate ability to understand mechanical workings. The key to successful PM

Month: January   Year: 2003   Instrument: Chemistry   Serial No.: 2222

Daily

Shift 1	1	2	3	4	5	6	7	8	9	10	11	12	13	14	15	16	17	18	19	20	21	22	23	24	25	26	27	28	29	30	31
Clean probes	x		x	x	x	x	x	x	x	x		x	x	x	x	x	x	x	x	x		x	x	x	x	x	x	x	x	x	
Empty waste containers	x	x	x	x	x	x	x	x	x	x	x	x	x	x	x	x	x	x	x	x	x	x	x	x	x	x	x	x	x	x	x
Update inventory	x	x	x	x	x	x	x	x	x	x	x	x	x	x	x	x	x	x	x	x	x	x	x	x	x	x	x	x	x	x	x
Initials	jh	jh	jh	jh	jh	jh	jh	ph	ph	ph	ph	ph	dt	dt	dt	dt	dt	bw	bw	bw	bw	bw	cb	cb	cb	cb	cb	cb	cb	cb	cb

Weekly

	Date/Initials	Date/Initials	Date/Initials	Date/Initials
Clean sample segments	1/6/03 jh	1/13/03 ph	1/20/03 dt	1/27/03 bw
Clean sample cup adaptors	1/6/03 jh	1/13/03 ph	1/20/03 dt	1/27/03 bw
Clean air filters	1/6/03 dt	1/13/03 bw	1/20/03 cb	1/27/03 jh
Clean outside of probe	1/6/03 ph	1/13/03 dt	1/20/03 jh	1/27/03 cb

Monthly

	Date Completed/Initials
Tubing decontamination	1/20/03 cb

FIGURE 33–1. Partial PM Log Sheet

programs for complex instruments may well depend on a knowledgeable operator who not only knows the theory of the instrument but can also quickly recognize departures from normal functioning (Karselis 1994).

The final stage of PM is oversight of the program by the supervisor and the manager. Not only should records be reviewed to ensure the performance of PM tasks, but trends in instrument performance and failures should also be identified and investigated. Surveillance is also necessary to confirm regulatory compliance. Laboratory accreditation agencies require documented PM programs. The agency accreditation manuals (e.g., Manual of CAP or JCAHO) discuss PM requirements and necessary documentation. Maintenance records for instruments are so important that they should be kept for the entire lifespan of the instrument (O'Brien 2000).

Notice that this topic so far has dealt only with PM. The other half of this picture is instrument troubleshooting and repair. Repair is also referred to as corrective maintenance. In contrast to PM, repair is not a planned series of activities and does not occur according to a schedule. Corrective maintenance occurs when the instrument malfunctions or fails. Such incidents are inevitable despite the best PM programs. The most difficult part of repair is determining where in the instrument the fault resides. That is, the diagnosis of the problem is the key to rapid repair and return of the instrument to operation. The process of locating the malfunction is known as troubleshooting. There are numerous sources that outline steps in beginning the troubleshooting process. The process should follow logical steps and assumptions rather than random repair attempts. Before the problem can be located, it must be defined clearly. In addition, the most obvious and common solutions should be attempted before more exotic faults are considered. Most manufacturers supply a troubleshooting guide within the instrument manual, often with suggestions for finding the fault using a step-by-step elimination procedure. In addition to troubleshooting guides in manuals or online, many companies have technical assistance phone lines available twenty-four hours a day to assist with repair procedures and to confirm that the repair should be attempted in-house. For safety reasons, technologists should never attempt repairs beyond their abilities. As with PM, repairs and troubleshooting activities must be carefully documented and records stored with the history of that instrument (Schoeff 1993; Fink and Narayanan 1994; Karselis 1994; O'Brien 2000). An example of a repair documentation form is shown in Figure 31–2. Voluntary accreditation and governmental inspection agencies require documentation of PM and repair activities. During inspections by these agencies, PM and repair records will be scrutinized, especially if the laboratory produces a product (such as blood components). In the case of product preparation, the laboratory must also meet the standards required of all other medical products. These standards are called good manufacturing practices (GMP).

With the large amount of automation in the laboratories of today, both PM and corrective maintenance are critical to providing uninterrupted, quality health care to the clients of laboratory services.

Bibliography

Baer, D. M. 1968. Repair and maintenance of instruments. *Bull Pathology* 9, no. 10: 196–197.

Fink, Joseph G., and Sheshadri Narayanan. 1994. Preventive maintenance and troubleshooting. In *Clinical laboratory instrumentation and automation: Principles, applications, and selection*, ed. Kory M. Ward, Craig A. Lehmann, and Alan M. Leiken. Philadelphia: W. B. Saunders.

Karselis, Terence C. 1994. *Pocket guide to clinical laboratory instrumentation.* Philadelphia: F. A. Davis.

O'Brien, Judith A. 2000. *Common problems in clinical laboratory management.* New York: McGraw-Hill.

Schoeff, Larry E. 1993. Maintenance and repair. In *Principles of laboratory instruments.*, ed. Larry E. Schoeff and Robert H. Williams. St. Louis, Mo: Mosby.

Date/Initials	Problem Description	Resolution
1/8/03 cb	Improper lamp intensity	Replaced lamp and checked
1/25/03 cb	Transfer arm broken	Replaced with new transfer arm
1/28/03 cb	Cell jam	Cleared and restarted
1/31/03 cb	Crashed sampling probe	Changed probe

FIGURE 33–2. Partial Repair Log

INTERNET RESOURCES

Example Vendor Sites with Troubleshooting Guides

Beckman Coulter. <www.beckmancoulter.com>
Abbott Laboratories. <www.abbott.com>

Example Sites for Instrument Repair and/or Calibration (some also sell refurbished instruments)

Fisher Hamilton. <www.fisherhamilton.com>
Allometrics, Inc. <www.allometrics.com/services>
Medical Equipment Repair Associates.
   <www.meraserv.com>
MedStore. <www.medstore.com>

QUESTIONS

1. Define the terms *preventive* and *corrective maintenance*, including the major differences between these two types of instrument maintenance. *(Objective 1, Level II)*

2. List some of the benefits to the laboratory of a successful preventive maintenance program. *(Objective 2, Level II)*

3. Explain why it is necessary to purchase service contracts on major pieces of laboratory equipment. *(Objective 3, Level II)*

4. List steps the laboratory supervisor should include in setting up a preventive maintenance program. *(Objective 4, Level II)*

5. Corrective maintenance is *(Objective 5, Level I)*
    a. scheduled program of activities
    b. steps to be performed at specific intervals
    c. repair/replacement of parts when a failure occurs
    d. ongoing activity

6. Define *troubleshooting* and relate it to instrument repair. *(Objective 6, Level II)*

EXERCISES

Completion of the exercises will enhance your knowledge of establishing preventive and corrective maintenance programs. *(Objective 7, Level I; Objective 8, Level II; and Objective 9, Level II)*

1. Interview several laboratory supervisors to determine which government regulations have impacted the maintenance and repair of laboratory instruments and which government agencies (both federal and state) are involved in regulation of their laboratory. During the interview, ask to see typical documentation of PM and repair for one lab instrument in which you are interested. Determine from your interview what types of deficiencies inspectors cite most often related to PM and repair programs.

2. Perform a survey of clinical laboratories and blood banks/blood drawing centers in your area to determine which voluntary accrediting agencies perform inspections of various types of labs. Ask area lab managers why they participate in these voluntary inspections and why they choose one organization over another.

3. Discuss GMPs with the manager of a blood donation center. Determine how these standards and their documentation differ from routine instrument PM and repair programs. Determine how these regulations have increased the workload in blood centers.

4. Obtain an instrument manual for a complex chemistry or hematology instrument and examine the manufacturer's schedule for PM. Determine if that particular manufacturer supplies log books/documentation forms to record the results of PM procedures. Examine the troubleshooting guide to determine its organizational structure and ease of use.

5. Compare the instrument manual of a complex instrument with that of a smaller piece of equipment such as a centrifuge or a microscope. Determine if the PM schedule and the troubleshooting guide are supplied in detail by the manufacturers of both pieces of equipment.

CASES

Analyze the following case studies and propose solutions. *(Objective 10, Level III)*

1. The supervisor of the chemistry division of a clinical laboratory in a 500-bed hospital was doing her monthly review of the PM charts for the chemistry instruments. She noticed that again this month the AGX9000 instrument had been taken out of service for a brief period due to the failure of the instrument to produce acceptable results with all three control samples (normal, abnormal high, and abnormal low) at 5 A.M. on Sunday morning. This was the third month in a row that the instrument had failed to produce acceptable quality control results suddenly and without warning. All of the failures had occurred between 2 A.M. and 5 A.M. on Sundays. The records documented that the instrument had performed satisfactorily all day on Saturday and on Sunday after instrument self-checks were performed as outlined in the troubleshooting manual. Levy-Jennings charts showed no trends or shifts in the control data in the days and hours before the failure. The failures seemed to occur when the lab was not busy and the instrument had been idle. The PM charts documented that all PM activities had been completed on schedule and no unusual or exotic maintenance had been documented. On the most recent form documenting the

failure, the technologist had noted that during the instrument self-check the instrument reported an electrical anomaly had occurred since the last self-check. What should the supervisor do now?

2. As the supervisor in charge of the cerebrospinal fluid examinations, you note that the cellular elements are beginning to appear fragmented and distorted. The laboratory purchased the cytocentrifuge about six months ago. When you check the PM and corrective maintenance records, there are no records found for the cytocentrifuge. What steps would you take to solve the immediate problem, and how could you prevent this situation from occurring in the future?

Chapter 34

Organization and Time Management

Hermolee Thomas Barnes, M.Ed., MT(ASCP)

OBJECTIVES

Upon completion of this chapter the learner will be able to

1. Define the first step in organization. *(Level I)*
2. Describe the use of the main list and secondary list. *(Level II)*
3. Identify areas that may be cluttered. *(Level I)*
4. Discuss time savers. *(Level II)*
5. Discuss how one might avoid time wasters. *(Level II)*
6. Analyze his or her organization and time management skills. *(Level III)*
7. Formulate a list of organization and time management skills essential for the effective manager. *(Level III)*
8. Analyze the situations in the case studies. *(Level III)*

TOPIC SUMMARY

The Tortoise and the Hare is an Aesop fable, featuring a race between a slow but steady tortoise and a fast and boastful hare. The Hare was the anticipated winner who, surprisingly, lost. Did the Tortoise have a secret weapon? Some would say that the Tortoise's experience in evaluating situations gave him an edge. He had mastered the art of planning ahead and taking one step at a time. He therefore was able to endure the hardships of the journey and realize his goal. The impudent Hare took off in a burst of speed and was soon exhausted. The Hare had relied solely on his agility and speed to outrun the "slowpoke Tortoise." Although the Hare desired to win the race, he had not taken the steps needed to realize that goal. The Hare had not even considered that the Tortoise might reach the finish line first. If only the Hare had known that the key to getting things done is to "work smarter—not harder."

This chapter will focus on organization and time management skills for the workplace. Techniques discussed in this chapter are also applicable to non-job-related responsibilities. Good organizational skills and time management go hand in hand. The first step in organizing is to set goals and define the tasks necessary to reach those goals. All tasks should be assigned a priority status, with "essential" or "greatest need" tasks being completed first. It is important to maintain realistic expectations when developing and ranking tasks.

Many successful planners use a two-list system, consisting of a **main list** (master list) and a **secondary list** (work list or daily planner). The main list is comprehensive. It contains *all* tasks to be done in a given time (e.g., daily, weekly, monthly, semiannually, or yearly). Tasks on the main list may be listed in no particular order, as long as *everything* to be done is included. At the beginning of each workday/shift, or at the end of the previous workday/shift, the main list should be referenced to make the secondary list.

Tasks on the secondary list are ranked according to importance; for example, instrument start-up and quality control (QC) procedures are processed ahead of test runs, and STATS and timed procedures are processed prior to routine runs. Emergency procedures are examples of tasks that are not usually listed on main or secondary lists. Emergency procedures are given priority as they occur. Because emergencies are not predictable, workers should be careful about setting inflexible time limits.

A group of *like* procedures should be considered as a single task, for example, the plating of microbiology cultures is one task on the secondary list. Each task on the secondary list should be accorded a time line or a time in which it must be completed. It is not "good" work practice to wait until its time limit is near to begin a task. A beginning worker should practice working step by step, performing one task at a time, until proficiency has been attained. A proficient worker can usually accomplish several small tasks simultaneously, running shorter procedures while longer ones are processing. However, no matter how good one becomes at organizing and managing time, every task will not get done all of the time.

Tasks on the secondary list should be crossed off as they are completed. Tasks on the secondary list that were not accomplished should be reevaluated and ranked on another secondary list or (if no longer needed) eliminated altogether. As proficiency with maintaining the main and secondary lists increases, personal and workplace task lists may be combined for greater overall efficiency. Keep in mind that the fastest worker does not always complete the job *first*—and the slowest worker does not always do the job *best*. The goal is to be thorough, accurate, *and* timely. Accomplished tasks should be diligently removed from the main list to avoid clutter (be careful not to remove ongoing or repeating tasks from the Main List).

Clutter can cause havoc in an otherwise organized world. Although clutter is most visible when it occurs in the work areas, it is just as damaging in the less visible spaces. One of the less visible spaces for clutter is the computer hard drive. The computer has become a necessity in the workplace, and like other equipment, it must be cleaned, updated, and maintained constantly to operate properly. This means removing and replacing unused/outdated software, expanding memory and purging outdated files according to established protocols.

The least visible of cluttered spaces is the *mind*. In the workplace, focus should be on job responsibilities. Each task should have the worker's undivided attention. It is both undesirable and unsafe for a worker to tackle procedures that yield life-altering results if the worker's mind and emotions are permeated by personal problems. Good health, a clear mind, a rested body, and proper nutrition are important factors for peak performance. Foregoing meals and breaks to utilize a few extra minutes is neither healthy nor responsible. Nourishment fuels the body just as gasoline fuels a car. Neither car nor body will travel far on empty.

The key to doing the best job in the least amount of time is good organization. Following are some helpful hints for developing good organizational skills:

1. Setting goals—State what is to be accomplished.
2. Identifying tasks—Identify steps needed to reach the goals.
3. Setting priorities—Assign urgency status (most important to least).
4. Using time wisely—Work to be efficient, not just busy.

Time savers are measures that help a worker prepare to be more accomplished in less time. An average workday consists of eight to ten hours, so if "time is money," it should be spent wisely. Common time-saving measures include the following:

1. Set goals—Make goals specific and measurable.
2. Set priorities—Do the most important (highest priority) tasks *first*.
3. Organize—Arrange workload to accomplish what is expected.
4. Delegate—"Free up" time for handling more important tasks.
5. Get started—Do it now. The sooner it is started, the sooner it will be finished.

Time wasters are nonproductive interferences in the work routine. They leave less time to accomplish important tasks. Common time wasters include the following:

1. Procrastination—Putting off until later what should be done *now*.
2. Interruptions—Results may be delayed due to frequent interruption by telephone and people.
3. Clutter—Mental or work-space clutter may hinder processing.
4. Disorganization—Not knowing where to begin.
5. Lack of goals—Not knowing what is important to do, or when it should be done.

Bibliography

Covey, Stephen R. 1994. *First things first*. New York: Simon & Schuster.

Gilbert, Sara. 1990. *Go for it: Get organized*. New York: Morrow Junior Books.

Mayer, Jeffrey J. 1999. *Time management for dummies*. Foster City, Calif.: IDG Books Worldwide.

Olson, Jeff. 1997. *Getting organized.* Bristol, Vt.: Velocity Business Publishing.

Winston, Stephanie. 1995. *Stephanie Winston's best organizing tips.* New York: Simon & Schuster.

Internet Resources

About, Inc. <http://telecommuting.about.com/library/tips/aa010103.htm>

Paauwerfully Organized. <www.orgcoach.net/improve_organize.html>

Virginia Polytechnic Institute and State University, Division of Student Affairs. <www.ucc.vt.edu/stdysk/htimesug.html>

QUESTIONS

1. The first step in organization is _____. *(Objective 1, Level I)*
2. Describe the use of the main list and the secondary list. *(Objective 2, Level II)*
3. Clutter areas may include _____ and _____ in addition to workplaces. *(Objective 3, Level I)*
4. Discuss time savers. *(Objective 4, Level II)*
5. Discuss how one might avoid time wasters. *(Objective 5, Level II)*

EXERCISES

Completion of the exercises will enhance your knowledge of organization and time management. *(Objective 6, Level III and Objective 7, Level III)*

1. Analyze your organization and time-management skills. Are your organization and time-management skills more like the Tortoise's or more like the Hare's? Explain.
2. Select an effective manager and interview the individual to determine what organization and time-management skills he or she uses. Make a list and share with other class members.
3. If you were this effective manager, what organization and time-management skills would be important to you, and how would you improve upon those skills already being used?

CASES

For the following cases, analyze each situation for organization and time management skills and problems. *(Objective 8, Level III)*

1. The administrative technologist who is responsible for hiring and evaluating techs working in the laboratory is always very busy and difficult to approach. Your evaluation sessions seem to be rushed and mechanical, and the phone is constantly ringing. You receive good evaluations, but you leave each evaluation session feeling that the session is a waste of time and just something that must be done. There are always many papers on the administrative technologist's desk. Papers even have to be moved from a chair for you to sit down. When you ask for a copy of your evaluation, it sometimes takes weeks to receive it. Given this situation, analyze the organization and time-management problems.

2. The administrative technologist in charge of the laboratory often walks through the laboratory and expresses an interest in your tasks. This individual always lets you know when you do a good job and encourages you when you need to improve. An administrative technologist is required to attend many meetings, including budget planning sessions and consultative sessions with the section supervisors and other hospital staff. Therefore, you know that the individual is really busy, but still takes time to notice your work. Given this situation, analyze the organization and time-management skills being utilized by the administrative technologist.

Chapter 35

The Laboratory Information System: Choosing the Right One

Beth Parham White, B.S., MT(ASCP), CLS(NCA)

OBJECTIVES

Upon completion of this chapter the learner will be able to

1. Name five benefits of using a laboratory information system (LIS). *(Level I)*
2. Identify the first step in choosing an LIS. *(Level I)*
3. Discuss the components of a request for proposal (RFP). *(Level II)*
4. Name two groups external to the clinical laboratory who would provide valuable input into the selection process. *(Level I)*
5. Describe the necessity of the input of these other groups. *(Level I)*
6. Create a list of items to be used in evaluating an LIS. *(Level III)*
7. Propose solutions for the case studies. *(Level III)*

TOPIC SUMMARY

The laboratory information system (LIS) has become an essential tool in most modern clinical laboratories. Laboratories rely on the LIS to perform numerous tasks, from technical to clerical to accounting. A good LIS can aid the laboratory in many ways. For example, it can allow the laboratory to "do more with less" by reducing time-consuming paperwork required by manual reporting methods, and it may possibly allow the laboratory to add new procedures without increasing personnel. It can store patient data for easy reference by lab personnel, and some systems can store quality control (QC) data to help the technologists with their QC programs. By providing immediate access to results, it can greatly reduce the turnaround time of STAT testing. It also standardizes the format of test results, which can reduce confusion for those reading the reports. And when used in conjunction with the bar code capability of many of today's laboratory analyzers, it can reduce the chances of an assay being run on the wrong patient.

For the laboratory manager, the task of choosing the right LIS for the laboratory is extremely important and complex. According to McClatchey (1994), the first step the manager must take is the selection of an LIS team to work together to find the right system. This team should include members from every section of the laboratory, including the pathologists. Also, because the LIS will need to interface with the hospital information system (HIS), the team should include someone from that area of the hospital who has extensive knowledge of that system. As the leader of this team, the laboratory manager can guide the members through all the steps necessary for making a good choice for the laboratory. Initially, the team members must decide what services the laboratory needs from its LIS. Not every laboratory will require the same services. For example, the needs of a lab in a small community hospital will differ greatly from those of a lab in a large medical center with many satellite labs. The selection team members must assess all laboratory operations, from the ordering of tests to specimen collection to actual analysis to reporting of results to patient billing. It is important for the LIS team to seek input from as many laboratory staff members as possible to help those who will eventually be users of the new system to feel that they have had a say in the choice of which system will be chosen. This approach may aid in overall acceptance of the new LIS and may provide an easier transitional stage when it is put into use. At a minimum, the LIS should accomplish the following:

- Require two different access codes or passwords per user for access to the system. Two codes may include a unique user identification (ID) (e.g., first initial plus last name, plus last four digits of a social security number) and a password created by the user. Using two codes or passwords allows for increased security of the system and confidentiality of the patient records contained within as mandated by the Health Insurance Portability and Accountability Act (HIPAA) of the federal government.
- Assign a unique accession number to each patient sample received and/or each test ordered.
- Provide a clear result screen/page for each lab result that includes normal/therapeutic ranges and flagging of critical values.
- Provide a unique file for each assay that provides information about the assay, such as sample type, sample volume required, normal/therapeutic ranges, where to send sample if sent to a reference lab, and any other special instructions needed.
- Record for each test time collected and initials of phlebotomist, time received in lab and initials of person who received it, time results were released and technologist's initials.
- Allow techs to create worksheets for testing.
- Create lists of pending and overdue tests.
- Print bar-coded labels for specimens.
- Interface with major instruments so that demographics and tests ordered may be downloaded.
- Allow for reports to be pulled, such as number of tests ordered per month, workload units, and so on.
- Allow for additional tests to be added to an existing order.
- Allow access to past laboratory results.
- Allow for comments to be entered in test result field, such as documentation of critical value notification.
- Back up all files daily.

Once the selection team has a general idea of how it wants the LIS to function in the laboratory, they must begin the task of finding the right system. Professional publications can provide information about LISs through articles and advertisements. Frequently, LIS vendors will display their systems at national and regional meetings. Also, members of the team can talk to lab professionals at other institutions for recommendations of which systems to consider. From this research, the selection team members should choose a few vendors who have systems that seem feasible for their particular laboratory. The next step then is to contact those vendors and send them a request for proposal (RFP). In the RFP, it is necessary to provide the vendors with detailed information about what the laboratory will require from the system, what kind of service will be expected during and after installation, and what financial limitations exist. The laboratory requirements should take future laboratory growth and expansion of services into consideration. Any special services needed such as faxing of reports, instant printing of reports at remote printers, interfacing of laboratory analyzers and the HIS, and ability to handle specialized departments that need complex reporting such as blood bank, microbiology, cytology, and histology should also be considered. It is also important to include the input of members of the hospital medical staff concerning the configuration of lab reports. The vendors will use the information in the RFP to form their own proposal for the laboratory with details of what services their system and company can offer and at what cost.

Once all proposals have been received, the LIS team must make the final choice of which LIS to purchase. The team must closely examine each vendor's proposal to see which one offers the most services while remaining within the constraints of the laboratory budget. In addition to technical specifications, the vendor should offer a plan for the future service of their system. Initial training of laboratory personnel, repair service, and providing future upgrades should be included. The vendor should also provide a plan for bringing the system into the laboratory and helping the lab as it prepares to "go live." If possible, team members should visit other laboratories using each system under consideration to see it in action and to talk with some of the professionals who use it on a daily basis and who have had experience in dealing with each company over a period of time. After all proposals have been carefully reviewed and all possible information has been gathered, the selection team can then make a final decision.

The process of choosing an LIS for a laboratory is a very long and difficult one for everyone involved. The manager, as LIS team leader, must make sure that the team is very thorough and considers every aspect in detail. Selection of an LIS system is critical because, once the LIS is in place, it will impact virtually every employee and procedure in the laboratory and will play a large role in how the lab functions and progresses for many years to come.

Bibliography

Burtis, Carl A., and Edward R. Ashwood. 1996. *Tietz fundamentals of clinical chemistry*. 4th ed. Philadelphia: W. B. Saunders.

McClatchey, Kenneth D. 1994. *Clinical laboratory medicine*. Baltimore: Williams & Wilkins.

Ware, John. 2001. *A comparative review of Per Se Ultra System, Star Laboratory, and Meditech LIS*. Unpublished manuscript.

Internet Resources

Braley Consulting Services, Inc.
    <www.braley.com/braley/pub/index.htm>
On-Line Consultant Software, Laboratory Information Systems (LIS) Directory.
    <www.health-infosys-dir.com/yphclis.asp>

QUESTIONS

1. What are five benefits a laboratory can gain by acquiring an LIS? *(Objective 1, Level I)*
    a. _____
    b. _____
    c. _____
    d. _____
    e. _____

2. The first step in the process of choosing a new LIS for the laboratory is *(Objective 2, Level I)*
    a. contacting all the vendors
    b. selecting an LIS team to evaluate the systems
    c. deciding the budget for the project
    d. defining the needs of the laboratory

3. What is an RFP? What should it include? *(Objective 3, Level II)*

4. Name two groups from outside the laboratory whose input is needed in choosing the specifications of the LIS? Why is their input important? *(Objective 4, Level I)*

5. Why are visits to other laboratories so important in the process of making the final choice of an LIS? *(Objective 5, Level I)*

EXERCISES

Completion of the exercises will enhance your knowledge of the laboratory information system. *(Objective 6, Level III)*

1. As a research exercise, the class should divide into groups. Each group should interview (in person or by telephone) the manager of a local or affiliated hospital laboratory to find out what steps were taken in choosing that laboratory's LIS, and what factors were most important in making the final decision as to which LIS to purchase. The groups should then report back to class and discuss how and why each laboratory made the choice they did. A list should be created of items to consider when selecting an LIS.

2. Visit a vendor at a professional meeting and gather data individually and in groups and report back to the entire class regarding the items the vendor stresses as important in LIS selection.

3. Research the literature individually or in groups and report to the class regarding the items found that should be considered in selecting an LIS.

CASES

Examine the following case study and propose solutions for the various situations. *(Objective 7, Level III)*

The laboratory of a 300-bed hospital has just had a new LIS installed. The LIS was chosen, despite objections of the laboratory manager, by the HIS department, with the choice being made based on cost and how well the new system will interface with the hospital system. As soon as the new LIS goes on-line, problems begin to occur. For each of the following problems, tell which part of the **correct** process for choosing an LIS could have prevented the problem, and how the problem could be solved by a better system.

1. The trauma emergency department is unhappy because all emergency reports print on a printer that is two hallways away in the chest pain emergency department.

2. Four different physicians have called stating that they cannot figure out how to read the urinalysis reports.

3. The chemistry supervisor has threatened to quit because the system takes six minutes to accept data from her main instrument, delaying every report coming from that department.

4. The newly appointed supervisor of the LIS team has reported that it takes two days for the LIS company to respond to phone calls and questions.

5. The laboratory manager has noticed a sudden increase in complaints from nursing about tests that have been missed or greatly delayed.

Chapter 36

Epidemiology in the Clinical Laboratory

Margaret McDonald, Ph.D., MT(ASCP)

OBJECTIVES

Upon completion of this chapter the learner will be able to

1. Define *epidemiology*. *(Level I)*
2. State the overall purpose of epidemiology. *(Level I)*
3. Identify how epidemiology is used. *(Level I)*
4. Discuss the role of the clinical laboratory in epidemiology. *(Level II)*
5. Define *(Level I)*
    a. validity
    b. "gold standard"
    c. sensitivity of a test
    d. specificity of a test
    e. reliability
    f. interrater reliability
    g. kappa statistic
    h. surveillance
6. Describe how predictive value positive and predictive value negative are used. *(Level II)*
7. Describe the purpose of the Notifiable Infectious Disease Surveillance program. *(Level II)*
8. Discuss the role of the laboratory in surveillance. *(Level II)*
9. Calculate sensitivity, specificity, predictive value positive and negative of a screening test. *(Level II)*.
10. Calculate kappa test statistic for a laboratory test. *(Level II)*
11. Analyze notifiable disease reporting trends in the laboratory. *(Level III)*
12. Analyze the case studies and propose solutions. *(Level III)*

TOPIC SUMMARY

Illness and disease outcomes are not chance occurrences in people, but are assumed to be due to a wide variety of factors or determinants, including behavioral and biological characteristics (Gordis 2000). Because the presence or absence of these factors and the levels to which they are present may differ in population subgroups, patterns of disease frequency and distribution may vary within a population. The science that investigates this variability in disease occurrence is epidemiology and, as defined by Last (1995), it is the study of determinants and distribution of disease in population groups. Epidemiology, in essence then, investigates the who, what, where, and when of disease outcomes. Disease outcomes may be considered as any altered health state, such as injury, illness, or death.

Epidemiology provides information useful for disease prevention and control efforts and for establishing the causes of disease. For example, epidemiology is routinely used by public health scientists and healthcare providers for planning strategies, for program evaluation, as well as for disease surveillance. Other researchers use epidemiology methods to establish the etiologic agents of disease. Clinical laboratories integrate these activities because they provide essential screening and diagnostic test services used to assess the health status of the public. Further, epidemiology methods are routinely applied in the clinical laboratory to assess the quality and accuracy of these tests as well as to monitor mandatory disease reporting to state agencies.

The purpose of this chapter is to illustrate the following epidemiology principles and methods used in the clinical laboratory:

1. Evaluation of screening test validity
   a. Sensitivity
   b. Specificity
   c. Predictive value positive
   d. Predictive value negative
2. Evaluation of interrater reliability-kappa
3. Surveillance compliance

Evaluation of Screening Test Validity

Test **validity** measures how closely the test value is to the true measure—in other words, accuracy (Last 1995). In the laboratory, a screening test is valid when the result correctly identifies a patient with the disease as positive and a patient without the condition as negative. The screening test must then be validated using a highly accurate diagnostic test or procedure, generally known as a "**gold standard**" (the most accurate measure currently available, Last 1995). Examples of gold standards include the process of collecting bone marrow aspirations, clinically diagnosed cases of myocardial infarction, and a positive streptococcal B result from culture.

Table 36–1 illustrates the relationship between a screening test and a gold standard. As shown, test validity is measured by **sensitivity** and **specificity** (Hennekens, Buring, and Mayrent 1987). The sensitivity of a screening test, its ability to detect positives among the truly diseased, is calculated $a/(a + c)$, and is measured as a proportion (0.0–1.0). A high sensitivity (values closer to 1.0) indicates that a greater proportion of those truly diseased are correctly screened positive. Here, the small proportion of those with the disease who are erroneously screened negative are considered "false negatives." As sensitivity decreases, the screening test will detect fewer truly diseased persons as positive, resulting in a high proportion of "false negatives." The specificity of a screening test, its ability to detect negatives among the truly nondiseased, is calculated $d/(b + d)$, and it, too, is a proportion (0.0–1.0). Screening tests with high specificity correctly identify a large proportion of truly disease-free individuals as negative. The remaining disease-free individuals classified incorrectly by the screen as positive are "false positives." A screening test with low specificity will produce a high proportion of "false positive results." The example in Table 36–2 illustrates a screening test for disease with high sensitivity (0.90)—ninety percent of those with the disease are correctly screened positive—and there are ten percent "false negatives," 10/100. Specificity is high too (0.85)—eighty-five percent of those without the disease are correctly screened negative, with fifteen percent "false positive" results (15/100).

Should all laboratory screening tests demonstrate both high specificity and sensitivity? Although this might be considered desirable initially, in reality it is often not possible or necessary. It depends on the disease in question and the consequences of missing a true positive result (i.e., low sensitivity) or misclassifying truly negative results as positive (i.e., low specificity). For example, to minimize the spread of sexually transmitted diseases, it is advantageous to use screening tests with high sensitivity at the expense of lowered specificity. This trade-off increases the number of persons who screen positive but also includes some who are truly negative. The latter group—the false positives—

TABLE 36–1. Characteristics of Screening Test Results		
	GOLD STANDARD	
SCREENING TEST	**DISEASE PRESENT (+)**	**DISEASE ABSENT (−)**
Test Positive	a	b
Test Negative	c	d

a = those with the disease who screen positive (true positive)
b = those without the disease who screen positive (false positive)
c = those with the disease who screen negative (false negative)
d = those without the disease who screen negative (true negative)

Sensitivity = $a/(a + c)$ *Specificity* = $d/(b + d)$

Predictive Value Positive = $a/(a + b)$ *Predictive Value Negative* = $d/(c + d)$

(Adapted from Henneken, C. H., J. E. Buring, and E. S. Mayrent. 1987. *Epidemiology in medicine*. Philadelphia: Lippincott, Williams and Wilkins.)

TABLE 36–2. Example—Characteristics of Screening Test Results

	GOLD STANDARD	
SCREENING TEST	DISEASE PRESENT (+)	DISEASE ABSENT (−)
Test Positive	90 (a)	15 (b)
Test Negative	10 (c)	85 (d)

Sensitivity of screening test for disease = 90/100 = 0.90
Specificity of screening test for disease = 85/100 = 0.85
Predictive Value Positive = a/(a + b) = 90/105 = 0.86
Predictive Value Negative = d/(c + d) = 85/95 = 0.89

would be correctly classified as negative upon subsequent testing by a diagnostic gold standard. Choosing a screen with high sensitivity provides a conservative approach and is warranted to reduce the potential of further spreading disease. Similarly, it is essential that a PAP smear screening for cervical cancer have high sensitivity to ascertain all positives even though a small portion of true negatives (false positive) will be erroneously included in the group. However, the magnitude of this error is far less serious than the consequences of missing a true positive screening result for cancer. In general, for serious or life-threatening diseases such as cancer, it is essential to have screening tests with high sensitivity at the expense of specificity.

Two additional measures, **predictive value positive** and **predictive value negative** are better indicators of the *yield* of the screening test. That is, among those who screened positive, what proportion actually had the condition, and among those screened negative, what proportion were truly disease free. Predictive value positive is calculated a/(a + b) and predictive value negative is calculated d/(c + d). Both of these measures are proportions (0.0–0.1) and depend on disease specificity and prevalence (i.e., number of existing cases of disease at a specified time) in the study population. If, for example, the prevalence of a condition is very low in the study population, say one in a million, the screening test will not pick up many positive results (the yield will be low, predictive value positive will be low) simply because there are so few with the targeted condition in the study population. So, these predictive value measures are more appropriately used to decide whether or not a screening test is useful for the population at hand. The example in Table 36–2 shows a predictive value of 0.86, indicating that eighty-six percent of those screened positive actually had the condition, and 0.89 of those who screened negative were truly free from disease.

Evaluation of Interrater Reliability-Kappa

Test **reliability** is the repeatability or reproducibility of tests results, and **interrater reliability** measures the degree to which two or more assessors agree on test results (Last 1995; Sackett et al. 1991). Both measures are routinely applied in laboratories as part of quality control and quality assurance programs indicating how closely two raters (e.g., medical technologists/clinical laboratory scientists, pathologists) agree when interpreting test results from the same patients. This test does not measure accuracy, as two raters might report the same but incorrect result, but increased reliability may produce more confidence in reporting results. For example, if two medical technologists/clinical laboratory scientists perform a serology slide test with categorical outcomes (positive, negative) on the same 100 patients, result agreement should be high. The overall percent agreement for these outcomes can easily be calculated as shown in Table 36–3. Cell A represents positive agreement for observer 1 and observer 2 and cell D indicates negative result concurrence for both assessors. The total percent agreement, then, is the sum of the positive and negative agreement divided by the total number of observations, or A + D/N. Although this information is helpful, the percent overall agreement does not show how the results differed between raters: did observer 1, for example, find more positives than observer 2? Moreover, how much agreement should one expect simply by chance alone, and how can one measure this agreement (presumably high among well-trained laboratory personnel) once chance has been considered?

To answer these questions, a **kappa statistic** can be calculated for categorical test results, which provides the agreement level between two raters once chance

TABLE 36–3. Characteristics of Agreement Levels between Two Observers

		OBSERVER 1		
		Positive	Negative	Total
OBSERVER 2	Positive	A	B	A + B
	Negative	C	D	C + D
	Total (N)	A + C	B + D	A + B + C + D = N

Identification of cells and calculations:

A = positive/positive rater *agreement*
B = negative/positive rater disagreement
C = positive/negative rater disagreement
D = negative/negative rater *agreement*

A + D = rater agreement (**A_o**)

A + B + C + D = maximum possible agreement (**N**)

A_o/N = overall percent agreement

[(A + B)(A + C)]/(A + B + C + D) = cell A agreement expected by chance

[(C + D)(B + D)]/(A + B + C + D) = cell D agreement expected by chance

Cell A agreement expected by chance + cell D agreement expected by chance = Total agreement expected by chance (**A_e**)

Kappa = $(A_o - A_e)/(N - A_e)$

(Adapted from Cohen, J. 1960. A coefficient of agreement for nominal scales. *Educational and Psychological Measurement* 20: 37–46.)

agreement has been taken into account (Sackett et al. 1991; Cohen 1960). The kappa statistic ranges from −1 (perfect disagreement between raters) to +1 (perfect agreement between raters) with 0 indicating agreement no better than chance. The numerator in the kappa statistic is the level of rater agreement once chance is accounted for, shown in Table 36–3 as the observed agreement (A_o) minus the total agreement due to chance alone (A_e), and the denominator consists of the maximum level of agreement possible after chance is considered ($N - A_e$). Kappa levels above 0.60 are generally considered to indicate moderate or higher agreement (Sackett et al. 1991).

The serology slide test example mentioned earlier is used to demonstrate the kappa test statistic in Table 36–4. As shown in the table, both technologists agree on eighty-five test results (A_o), the expected agreement based on chance alone is seventy-eight (A_e), and the *observed* improvement after taking chance into account is not substantial (85 − 78 = 7). The maximum improvement possible over chance (100 − 78 = 22) serves as the denominator for kappa, and the kappa result of (7/22 = 0.32) indicates the modest agreement level between technologists/scientists after taking chance agreement into account.

As part of a laboratory quality assurance program, the kappa test could be used as a supplemental indicator to determine a technologist's/scientist's success level when learning new test procedures. Many serology, hematology, and immunology test results can be categorized (e.g., positive and negative; 1+, 2+, 3+; titer endpoints) and interpreted for agreement levels by technically experienced and lesser-trained technologists/scientists.

Surveillance Compliance

Public health surveillance is an ongoing process where data are systematically collected, analyzed, and interpreted for health improvement purposes (Thacker and Berkelmen 1988). Typically the data include information on disease cases and risk factors or determinants related to disease. Results are maintained by local and state health departments. Some surveillance activities are also conducted on a national level to monitor trends in disease incidence (i.e., new cases of disease

TABLE 36–4. Example—Agreement between Two Medical Technologists/Clinical Laboratory Scientists Regarding a Serology Test Result Performed on 100 Patients.

		MEDICAL TECHNOLOGIST 1				
		Positive		Negative		Total
MEDICAL TECHNOLOGIST 2	Positive	80	(a)	5	(b)	85
	Negative	10	(c)	5	(d)	15
	Total	90		10		100

$80 + 5 = 85$ = rater agreement (A_o)

$80 + 5 + 10 + 5 = 100$ = maximum possible agreement (**N**)

$85/100 = 0.85$ = overall percent agreement

$[(80 + 5)(80 + 10)]/(80 + 5 + 10 + 5) = 76.5$ = cell A agreement expected by chance

$[(10 + 5)(5 + 5)]/(80 + 5 + 10 + 5) = 1.5$ = cell D agreement expected by chance

$76.5 + 1.5 = 78$ = Total agreement expected by chance (A_e)

Kappa = $(85 - 78)/(100 - 78) = 7/22 = 0.32$

---

within a specified time period) and reduce morbidity and mortality. One such program is the **Notifiable Infectious Disease Surveillance program,** established through the Centers for Disease Control and Prevention (CDC) to monitor the incidence of specific infectious conditions throughout the United States (CDC 2002, 1997). These conditions are chosen based on illness severity, infectivity, and other factors. Table 36–5 lists the specific conditions that comprise this program and require mandatory reporting to the CDC.

The clinical laboratory plays a basic and crucial role in this important CDC surveillance program, serving as the link between the physician's test request and result reporting to the local and state health department, where, at the latter, counts for each condition are tabulated and forwarded to the CDC for national reporting. In addition, the laboratory must also ensure that the information accompanying each report is complete, accurate, and sent within the imposed time limit.

The laboratory can establish its own quality assurance program to measure surveillance compliance for notifiable diseases. On a monthly basis, for example, a tally of all notifiable disease results reported through the laboratory could be totaled and the percent forwarded (to the state health department) within the mandated time frame. If reports were not sent within a timely basis, reasons for noncompliance should be sought and corrected for the next reporting review period. In a similar manner, the forms used for such reporting can be reviewed to assess completeness in required information fields (e.g., full names, address, date of test, date sampled obtained).

When laboratories are required to report specific disease conditions to the state health department, they must strive for 100% reporting compliance within the required time and should monitor the reporting compliance level through some quality assurance system.

In conclusion, methods to evaluate the accuracy and reliability of screening tests and methods for disease surveillance illustrate the critical role laboratories have in public health practice. As such, the laboratorian must ensure quality performance in these areas.

BIBLIOGRAPHY

Centers for Disease Control and Prevention. 1997. Case definitions for infectious conditions under public health surveillance. *MMWR* 46, no. RR-10.

Centers for Disease Control and Prevention. Epidemiology Program Office. 2002. *Nationally notifiable infectious diseases: United States.* Retrieved July 26, 2002, from <www.cdc.gov/epo/dphsi/PHS/infdis2002.htm>

Cohen, J. 1960. A coefficient of agreement for nominal scales. *Educational and Psychological Measurement* 20: 37–46.

Gordis, L. 2000. *Epidemiology.* 2d ed. Philadelphia: W. B. Saunders.

TABLE 36–5. Nationally Notifiable Infectious Diseases—United States 2002

- Acquired Immunodeficiency Syndrome (AIDS)
- Anthrax
- Botulism
  - Botulism, foodborne
  - Botulism, infant
  - Botulism, other (wound & unspecified)
- Brucellosis
- Chancroid
- *Chlamydia trachomatis*, genital infections
- Cholera
- Coccidioidomycosis
- Cryptosporidiosis
- Cyclosporiasis
- Diphtheria
- Ehrlichiosis
  - Ehrlichiosis, human granulocytic
  - Ehrlichiosis, human monocytic
  - Ehrlichiosis, human, other or unspecified agent
- Encephalitis, Arboviral
  - Encephalitis, California serogroup viral
  - Encephalitis, Eastern equine
  - Encephalitis, Powassan
  - Encephalitis, St. Louis
  - Encephalitis, Western equine
  - Encephalitis, West Nile
- Enterohemorrhagic *Escherichia coli*
  - Enterohemorrhagic *Escherichia coli*, O157:H7
  - Enterohemorrhagic *Escherichia coli*, shiga toxin positive, serogroup non-O157
- Giardiasis
- Gonorrhea
- *Haemophilus influenzae*, invasive disease
- Hansen disease (leprosy)
- Hantavirus pulmonary syndrome
- Hemolytic uremic syndrome, post-diarrheal
- Hepatitis, viral, acute
  - Hepatitis A, acute
  - Hepatitis B, acute
  - Hepatitis B virus, perinatal infection
  - Hepatitis, C; non A, non B, acute
- HIV infection
  - HIV infection, adult (> = 13 years)
  - HIV infection, pediatric (< 13 years)
- Legionellosis
- Listeriosis
- Lyme disease
- Malaria
- Measles
- Meningococcal disease
- Mumps
- Pertussis
- Plague
- Poliomyelitis, paralytic
- Psittacosis
- Q Fever
- Rabies
  - Rabies, animal
  - Rabies, human
- Rocky Mountain spotted fever
- Rubella
- Rubella, congenital syndrome
- Salmonellosis
- Shigellosis
- Streptococcal disease, invasive, Group A
- Streptococcal toxic-shock syndrome
- *Streptococcus pneumoniae*, drug resistant, invasive disease
- *Streptococcus pneumoniae*, invasive in children < 5 years
- Syphilis
  - Syphilis, primary
  - Syphilis, secondary
  - Syphilis, latent
  - Syphilis, early latent
  - Syphilis, late latent
  - Syphilis, latent unknown duration
  - Neurosyphilis
  - Syphilis, late, non-neurological
- Syphilis, congenital
  - Syphilitic Stillbirth
- Tetanus
- Toxic-shock syndrome
- Trichinosis
- Tuberculosis
- Tularemia
- Typhoid fever
- Varicella (deaths only)
- Yellow fever

Hennekens, C. H., J. E. Buring, and E. S. Mayrent. 1987. *Epidemiology in medicine.* Philadelphia: Lippincott, Williams and Wilkins.

Last, J. M., ed. 1995. *A dictionary of epidemiology.* 3d ed. New York: Oxford University Press.

Sackett, D. L., R. B. Haynes, G. H. Guyatt, and P. Tugwell. 1991. *Clinical epidemiology: A basic science for clinical medicine.* 2d ed. Philadelphia: Lippincott, Williams and Wilkins.

Thacker, S., and R. Berkelman. 1988. Public health surveillance in the United States. *Epidemiology Reviews* 10: 164–190.

Internet Resources

General

CDC Wonder. <wonder.cdc.gov/>
Department of Epidemiology and Biostatistics, University of California, San Francisco. <www.epibiostat.ucsf.edu/epidem/epidem.html>
Gideon Informatics, Inc. <www.gideononline.com>
Journal of The Society for Healthcare Epidemiology of America, Slack, Incorporated. <www.slackinc.com/general/iche/ichehome.htm> (enter "laboratory and role and epidemiology" in search box)

Surveillance and tools to monitor surveillance

CDC Epidemiology Program Office. <www.cdc.gov/epo/dphsi/index.htm>
<www.cdc.gov/epo/dphsi/phs/infdis2002.htm>
<www.cdc.gov/epo/dphsi/netss.htm>
<www.cdc.gov/epiinfo/index.htm>
CDC Morbidity and Mortality Weekly Report. <http://www.cdc.gov/mmwr/mmwr_wk.html>
CDC National Center for Infectious Disease. <http://www.cdc.gov/ncidod/osr/index.htm>

Sensitivity, specificity, predictive value

CDC. <www.cdc.gov/hiv/pubs/rt/sensitivity.htm>
Medical University of South Carolina. <www.musc.edu/dc/icrebm/sensitivity.html>

QUESTIONS

1. Epidemiology is _____ .

   (Objective 1, Level I)

2. The overall purpose of epidemiology is to *(Objective 2, Level I)*
   a. provide basis for public health disease prevention
   b. provide basis for control measures for groups at risk of disease
   c. provide information to pathologists
   d. provide information for cost analysis
   e. a and b
   f. all of the above

3. Epidemiology is used *(Objective 3, Level I)*
   a. in public health planning
   b. for disease surveillance
   c. to evaluate health programs and medical technologies
   d. to perform etiological research
   e. all of the above

4. Discuss the role of the clinical laboratory in epidemiology. *(Objective 4, Level II)*

5. Define the following terms: *(Objective 5, Level I)*
   a. validity: _____
   b. "gold standard": _____

c. sensitivity of a test: _____

d. specificity of a test: _____

e. reliability: _____

f. interrater reliability: _____

g. kappa statistic: _____

h. surveillance: _____

6. Describe how predictive value positive and predictive value negative are used in the clinical laboratory. *(Objective 6, Level II)*

7. Describe the purpose of the Notifiable Infectious Disease Surveillance program. *(Objective 7, Level II)*

8. Discuss the role of the laboratory in surveillance. *(Objective 8, Level II)*

EXERCISES

Completion of the exercises will enhance your knowledge of epidemiology in the clinical laboratory. *(Objective 9, Level II; Objective 10, Level II; and Objective 11, Level III)*

1. Regarding measures of validity for current laboratory screening tests and those under consideration, determine the sensitivity, specificity, predictive value positive and negative of a screening test currently used in your laboratory. Note that test results from a gold standard must be available to compare with the screening test. Examples of screening tests that you might study are:

Example: Select thirty microbiology specimens cultured for B streptococcus and perform the serological screening test for B strep. Construct a table similar to that shown in Table 36-1 and calculate measures of validity.

Example: Compare the results from hemoglobin electrophoresis on thirty specimens, with a corresponding sickle cell screening test. Construct a table similar to that shown in Table 36-1 and calculate measures of validity.

Example: These measures may be used to compare one screening test with another. If considering a new screen for a diagnostic test, apply the gold standard test results to the current screening test and ones under consideration. Differences in sensitivity and specificity aid in the decision-making process. Construct a table similar to that shown in Table 36-1 and calculate measures of validity.

2. Regarding kappa test statistic in the laboratory:
   a. Select a slide test with a positive and negative outcome. Consider using two experienced technologists for this test. Have each technologist perform this test on the same twenty patients, recording results for each test by each technologist. Calculate the kappa test statistic.
   b. As part of a program to train technologists unfamiliar with the test, use the same slide test and patient samples from #1.; maintain the twenty test results from one of the trained technologists. Compare these results with those of a technologist being trained in this test procedure. Calculate kappa for these two raters.

3. Regarding monitoring trends in reporting notifiable diseases—setting up a monitoring system in the lab:
   a. On a monthly basis, tally all results reportable to the state health department. Of these, calculate the overall percent that were reported within twenty-four, forty-eight, seventy-two, or more than seventy-two hours. Were there particular results reported seventy-two hours or later upon completion? Consider the reasons for these delays: Were these results reported from a specific department? Was there a shift or day of the week where compliance was lacking? Implement measures to correct the situation.
   b. The reporting forms used to forward notifiable disease results to the state have required fields of information, including demographic and clinical data. Analyze these forms in a laboratory for reporting completeness, identify problems, and recommend how the reporting process might be improved.

CASES

Analyze the following case studies and propose solutions. *(Objective 12, Level III)*

1. The microbiology supervisor reports to you, the laboratory manager, that large, white pigmented, slightly beta hemolytic colonies have been isolated from blood cultures on four newborns. The colonies appear to be staphylococcus, but are catalase negative. Upon further investigation, the microbiologist reports that the microorganism is sodium hippurate positive. Are there any steps you need to take regarding this situation? Is this considered a notifiable infectious disease?

2. You, as laboratory manager, must decide whether to add in-house performance of the Western Blot to the antibody screening test you presently do in the laboratory for human immunodeficiency virus (HIV). Some of your physicians are complaining because their patients had false positive results on the screening test you perform and they are requesting that the Western Blot be done in-house. In order to serve your physician clients, you decide to address them as a group this afternoon. What kind of information would you present, and what questions would you ask?

Chapter 37

Accreditation

John Curry, M.Ed., MT(ASCP)DLM

OBJECTIVES

Upon completion of this chapter the learner will be able to

1. Define *accreditation*. *(Level I)*
2. Describe the purpose of accreditation. *(Level I)*
3. Discuss the role of each of the following organizations related to laboratory accreditation: *(Level II)*
   a. Joint Commission on Accreditation of Healthcare Organizations (JCAHO)
   b. College of American Pathologists (CAP)
   c. American Association of Blood Banks (AABB)
   d. National Accrediting Agency for Clinical Laboratory Sciences (NAACLS)
4. Discuss the Clinical Laboratory Improvement Amendments of 1988 (CLIA '88) and its impact on the clinical laboratory. *(Level II)*
5. Analyze one section of the laboratory using either JCAHO or CAP guidelines. *(Level III)*
6. Evaluate the educational program using the *Guidelines to Accreditation* and *NAACLS Standards*. *(Level III)*
7. Analyze the situations and recommend solutions for the case studies. *(Level III)*

TOPIC SUMMARY

Accreditation for medical technology/clinical laboratory science specifically addresses the approval of a health-care facility or an institution of higher learning. Accrediting agencies cover all aspects of the clinical laboratory, hospital, and programs/schools for allied health. These agencies are important in ensuring that laboratories, hospitals, physician offices, and programs/schools of allied health provide not only quality personnel, but also improve the quality of care. Some of the accrediting agencies specific to the laboratory include Joint Commission on Accreditation of Healthcare Organizations (JCAHO), College of American Pathologists (CAP), and American Association of Blood Banks (AABB). The JCAHO and CAP review all aspects of the laboratory operation. This includes quality control, performance improvement, proficiency testing, safety, personnel requirements, policies and procedures, the facility, specimen collection and handling, quality of water used for testing, computer services (if applicable), storage of patient information, reporting of patient information, and ordering of tests on the patient. In addition to requirements that must be met for the general laboratory, each section of the laboratory (i.e., hematology, chemistry, microbiology, etc.) must meet specific requirements. The AABB accredits blood bank services only and includes both transfusion services and donor/processing of blood and blood products. Areas specifically addressed are transfusion procedures, therapeutic phlebotomies, blood storage, blood component modification, blood donors, parentage testing, and personnel. The National Accrediting Agency for Clinical Laboratory Sciences (NAACLS) is responsible for accrediting clinical laboratory science education programs. Educational programs that hold NAACLS accreditation must meet minimum criteria called standards.

A brief review of each of these accrediting agencies is included with a discussion of Clinical Laboratory Improvement Amendments (CLIA) requirements.

Joint Commission on Accreditation of Health Care Organizations (JCAHO)

The JCAHO evaluates and accredits more than 19,500 health-care organizations in the United States, including hospitals, health-care networks, managed care organizations, and health-care organizations that provide home care, long-term care, behavioral health, laboratory, and ambulatory care services. It is a nonprofit organization and is the world's leading health-care standard-setting and accrediting organization.

The JCAH, now JCAHO, was formed in 1951 by the American College of Physicians, The American Medical Association, and the American College of Surgeons. Its primary purpose was to provide voluntary accreditation. In 1953 the first "Standards for Hospital Accreditation" were published. The Joint Commission began charging for the surveys in 1964. The charges were based on the size and type of service provided by the hospitals or health networks. The surveys are conducted by hospital administrators, nurses, and laboratory professionals. These are voluntary surveyors that have their expenses reimbursed only.

The Social Security Amendments of 1965 included an amendment that all hospitals accredited by the JCAHO were deemed to be in compliance with most of the Medicare Conditions of Participation for hospitals and were able to participate in Medicare and Medicaid programs.

The accreditation cycle initially was every two years; however, in 1983, the cycle changed to every three years for hospitals and every two years for labs. In 1993, the standards were changed again to emphasize performance improvement concepts and to require a policy to prohibit smoking in all hospitals.

If the laboratory is accredited by the CAP and the hospital is accredited by the JCAHO, the laboratory will not have to undergo the full JCAHO inspection. The JCAHO will however check the laboratory for the transfusion service, quality assurance, employee competency and education, and pathology services.

In 1995, the federal government recognized the JCAHO laboratory accreditation survey as meeting the requirements for the CLIA '88 certification.

Citations under JCAHO are identified as type I. For a type I recommendation, the laboratory must provide evidence in six months to JCAHO that the laboratory is in compliance with the standard. JCAHO allows six months because of the requirement to document four months of compliance in the response. For example, if a type I deficiency was obtained because no proficiency testing was done for a particular analyte, a copy of the proficiency test purchase order and documentation of proficiency testing performance during the six months would be required.

College of American Pathologists (CAP)

The CAP is a medical society that serves more than 15,000 physician members and the laboratory community throughout the world. It is the largest association composed exclusively of pathologists and is considered the leader in providing laboratory quality improvement programs.

The CAP was established in December 1946 by a committee of the American Society of Clinical Pathologists. The first chemistry survey was conducted in 1949 with subsequent surveys covering all aspects of the clinical laboratory. In 1967 the JCAHO adopted the CAP lab accreditation standards. The CAP inspection and accreditation program was declared equivalent to the CLIA-67 standards in 1969.

The accreditation survey for the CAP is on a two-year cycle. The cycle is developed with a self-evaluation every other year and an on-site inspection done in the second year. The charges for the survey are based on the number of checklists needed for the inspection. The inspection is performed by laboratory professionals on a voluntary basis. These volunteers are from other CAP accredited laboratories. Their expenses are reimbursed.

CAP identifies deficiencies as phase I or phase II. Any phase I deficiencies noted in the survey do not have to be corrected within the two years prior to the next site visit; however, written documentation must be provided indicating what actions will be taken and a time table for the correction. Phase II deficiencies must be corrected within thirty days in order for the laboratory accreditation to continue and the laboratory must demonstrate compliance on the next site visit. A limited space situation might be considered a phase I deficiency if the limited space did not compromise the patient care. However, it would be considered a phase II deficiency if laboratory employees do not have enough space for the equipment or to safely perform the work.

A phase II deficiency might be cited if a laboratory did not have proof of proficiency testing for the last two years for an analyte. To correct this problem, the laboratory would order the correct test from the proficiency test provider and show proof by sending a copy of the purchase order to CAP. Lack of proper safety checks on equipment is also considered a phase II deficiency, and correction would require proof that the biomed or engineering department had completed these checks within the thirty-day period.

In 1994 CAP was given deemed authority for laboratory accreditation under the CLIA '88.

American Association of Blood Banks (AABB)

The AABB was established in 1947 as an international association of blood banks, including hospitals and community blood centers, transfusion and transplantation services, and the individuals involved in activities dealing with transfusion and transplantation. It was established to promote the highest standard of care for patients and donors in all aspects of blood banking.

In 1986 the CAP and the AABB began conducting joint accreditation inspections. The fees for the AABB inspection are based on the size of the hospital and the number of units transfused. The inspector is usually a blood banker from another accredited blood service. The inspection is done every two years. The deficiencies are handled the same as with CAP.

The AABB also publishes several books used in most blood banks. These include the *Technical Manual* and *Standards of Blood Banks and Transfusion Services*.

National Accrediting Agency for Clinical Laboratory Sciences (NAACLS)

The purpose of NAACLS is the accreditation of educational programs for clinical laboratory science. This accreditation includes university/colleges and hospital programs for medical technologist/clinical laboratory scientist, medical laboratory technician/clinical laboratory technician, histotechnologist, histologic technician, pathologists' assistant, phlebotomists, and diagnostic molecular science.

The NAACLS self-study readers and site visitors are professionals from peer programs and institutions who volunteer their services. Their expenses are reimbursed.

Accreditation can be awarded for up to seven years. A self-study report and a site visit is completed prior to the end of the assigned accreditation period. A *Guide to Accreditation* is available that explains the process and states the standards. The fees are based on the type of program being accredited and the number of affiliated institutions.

If a program is not in compliance with a standard, the program must submit a progress report within a specified period of time documenting compliance. Continued accreditation is contingent upon a satisfactory progress report.

Clinical Laboratory Improvement Amendments of 1988 (CLIA '88)

CLIA '88 was established in 1988 to amend the Clinical Laboratory Improvement Act of 1967, which was established originally to govern laboratories involved in interstate commerce. CLIA '88 covers all laboratories performing laboratory testing regardless of where these labs are based. This includes private labs, hospital-based labs, and physician office labs.

CLIA '88 also established minimum requirements that must be met in order to perform laboratory testing. The requirements cover quality assurance, quality control, proficiency testing, record retention, complexity of tests (high, moderate, and waived), job categories, and personnel requirements to perform testing, supervise, and direct laboratory services. These requirements can be found in the *Federal Register*.

All of the CLIA '88 requirements did not go into effect until the early part of the 1990s. CLIA is directed by the Centers for Medicare and Medicaid Services (CMS), which was previously HCFA (Health Care Financing Administration). The surveys are done by the state health departments. The inspectors are medical technologists/clinical laboratory scientists employed by the state board of health. The fees are based on the number of tests performed by the lab and the type of testing done.

There are several types of CLIA certificates:

1. CLIA Certificate—issued to a laboratory that is in compliance with CLIA requirements.
2. Certificate of Physician Performed Microscopy—used for labs where the physician only performs microscopic exams.
3. Certificate of Accreditation—issued on the basis of the laboratory being accredited by an organization approved by CMS such as CAP and JCAHO.
4. Certificate of Registration—issued to a laboratory pending accreditation by CLIA.
5. Certificate of Waiver—issued to laboratories performing only waived tests such as capillary blood glucose, urine dipstick, and other waived testing.

In almost all aspects of health care some type of accreditation is required. It is most important that as health-care professionals we educate ourselves on accreditation requirements and procedures if we are to be effective in our jobs.

BIBLIOGRAPHY

Accreditation Manual for Pathology and Clinical Laboratory Services. 1993. Oak Brook Terrace, Ill. Joint Commission on Accreditation of Healthcare Organizations.

Guide to Accreditation. 2001. Chicago: National Accrediting Agency for Clinical Laboratory Sciences.

Laboratory Inspection Manual. 1993. Gaithersburg, Md.: Aspen Publishers.

Survey Procedures and Interpretive Guidelines for Laboratories and Laboratory Science—Appendix C. 1990. Baltimore: Health Care Financing Administration.

U.S. Department of Health and Human Services. February 1992. *Federal Register* 57, 40. Washington, D.C: Government Printing Office.

INTERNET RESOURCES

American Association of Blood Banks. <www.aabb.org>
California Department of Health Services. <www.dhs.cahwnet.gov>
Centers of Medicare & Medicaid Services. <www.cms.hhs.gov>
College of American Pathologists. <www.cap.org>
Joint Commission on Accreditation of Healthcare Organizations. <www.jcaho.org>
National Accrediting Agency for Clinical Laboratory Sciences. <www.naacls.org>

QUESTIONS

1. Accreditation is *(Objective 1, Level I)*
   a. approval of an institution
   b. acceptance of a person into the profession
   c. qualification of an individual
   d. institutional membership in a professional organization

2. The purpose of accreditation is *(Objective 2, Level I)*
   a. to recognize quality
   b. to inform the public that an institution has met minimum standards
   c. to improve quality care
   d. all of the above

3. Discuss the role of each of these organizations in relations to laboratory accreditation. *(Objective 3, Level II)*

   JCAHO:

   CAP:

   AABB:

   NAACLS:

4. Discuss CLIA '88 and its impact on the clinical laboratory. *(Objective 4, Level II)*

EXERCISES

Completion of the exercises will enhance your knowledge of accreditation. *(Objective 5, Level III and Objective 6, Level III)*

1. Using either the JCAHO or CAP guidelines, analyze one section of the laboratory and report your findings to the class. This may be performed individually or in groups.

2. The class assumes the role of inspectors for a JCAHO or CAP inspection for the entire laboratory. A team captain is selected who divides the responsibilities for the inspection. The class conducts a mini-inspection of each laboratory and writes a report.

3. Using the *Guide to Accreditation* and the NAACLS *Standards* obtained from the Web site, individually or as a group evaluate an educational program's compliance with the standards. If performed as a group, the standards can be distributed among the members of the group. If performed as an individual, only a few standards for evaluation should be addressed.

CASES

Analyze the following case studies and recommend solutions. *(Objective 7, Level III)*

1. You have just been surveyed by JCAHO. According to the inspector, you are not signed up for a serum pregnancy test, which is a regulated analyte (this means you must report results back to the state). This is a type I recommendation. What must be done to bring the lab into compliance with the regulation?

2. You have just been surveyed by CAP. According to your inspector, your lab is not compliant in having all ground checks and safety checks done on all of your equipment in the department. Some are OK but others have not been checked in more than three years. How would you bring the lab into compliance with the phase II deficiency?

3. You have received a phase II deficiency on your laboratory because of lack of space. How would you address this problem? Remember, phase II deficiencies require documentation to clear the deficiency.

4. You have just completed your AABB inspection. Your inspector states that you are not compliant with your monitoring of the refrigerators for temperature fluctuations. In this instance you do not have remote alarms on the refrigerators. What can be done to bring the blood bank into compliance?

Chapter 38

Legal Considerations

Jane Hudson, Ph.D., MT(ASCP)SM, CLS(NCA)

OBJECTIVES

Upon completion of this chapter the learner will be able to

1. Identify the department of the hospital that should have the most information regarding personnel issues. *(Level I)*
2. Discuss legal issues pertaining to personnel. *(Level II)*
3. Discuss legal issues pertaining to the institution. *(Level I)*
4. Prepare a list of legal issues important to the laboratory. *(Level I)*
5. Analyze the legality of the situations in the case studies. *(Level III)*

TOPIC SUMMARY

An individual in a management position must be familiar with the legal parameters of the job. Laboratory legal considerations involve **personnel issues** and **job** or **institutional issues.** Legal considerations regarding personnel include issues such as job announcements, interviewing, hiring, termination, and leave (family, medical, maternity, or personal). Job or institutional legal considerations include issues such as confidentiality, following laboratory procedures, reimbursement policies, and specimen chain of custody procedures. Often the best source of personnel legal information is the Human Resource department of the hospital, so one should be sure to establish a relationship with that office and communicate with them when the need arises. Most hospitals employ legal counsel for consultation on difficult matters.

Personnel Issues

Each institution has regulations regarding posting of job vacancy announcements. These regulations include length of time a job must be posted and where it must be posted. Some jobs may be posted in-house, whereas others may require a larger search procedure. Once the announcement has been posted, the job description becomes a critical document for job applicants. In the job description the institution states all the requirements of the job (see Chapter 4 on job description). Once the announcement and job description are established, the institution is committed to complying with the details stated in these documents. Therefore, the employer should spend time in proper preparation of these documents.

Once the job has been posted and the job description made available to potential employees, then the applications are received and the candidates for interview are selected. During the interview certain questions are prohibited. For example, in order to determine whether a candidate will be able to meet the attendance requirements, one should state the demands of the job and inquire as to whether the candidate believes that he or she can meet the demands. One should *not* ask a question regarding the candidate's marital status or child-care arrangements. Another area of questioning that is prohibited is citizenship; however, the candidate must supply evidence that he or she can work in the United States. Questions regarding arrests, foreign languages spoken, height and weight, disability, credit status, date of birth, religious affiliation, property ownership, age, type of military discharge, personal finances, and memberships are also prohibited, unless the matter is directly related to performance of the job. Remember the proof that the topic is directly related will be the responsibility of the employer if challenged, so the manager should be sure that the topic *is* related. Certification applies to many laboratory positions and the question may be asked as to what certification the candidate has obtained; however, care must be taken not to indicate a preference for a particular certification because there are equivalent certifications such as National Credentialing Agency for Laboratory Personnel, Inc. (NCA) and American Society for Clinical Pathology Board of Registry (ASCP Board of Registry). Legally, one cannot discriminate if the certifications are equivalent. The manager should be familiar with laws such as Title VII of the Civil Rights Act, the Age Discrimination in Employment Act, the Rehabilitation Act of 1973, and the Americans with Disabilities Act.

Once the interviews have occurred, the best candidate is selected and the job offer made. It is important that the terms of the offer be exact and that the verbal offer and written job offer agree. After the candidate accepts the job, the employee now is impacted by many workplace legal stipulations such as collective bargaining, wage, hours, leave, termination, sexual harassment, and so on.

The laboratory is recognized as a collective bargaining unit by the National Labor Relations Board (NLRB) established under the National Labor Relations Act (NLRA) of 1935, and laboratorians can organize as a separate unit from other areas of the hospital. If the employees are employed in a collective bargaining situation, the manager must be familiar with the terms of the collective bargaining agreement and abide by the agreement. The laboratory is also governed by the federal wage and hour law, Fair Labor Standards Act (FLSA) regarding overtime, and the Equal Pay Act (EPA) regarding equal pay for equal work. The laboratory is required to pay time and a half for hours more than forty hours per week. But many laboratories use the 8/80 rule, which allows the employee to work eighty hours in a two-week period, with time and a half paid only on days that the employee works more than eight hours. The 8/80 rule allows the seven on seven off scheduling as well as other flexible scheduling. These hourly stipulations do not apply to the "salaried" employee, who is paid for the job, not by the hour. Usually only administrative personnel are salaried."

Other important federal regulations involve medical, maternity, and family leave. The Family and Medical Leave Act (FMLA) was originally designed to allow the employee who has been on the job for at least one year to take up to twelve weeks unpaid leave for specific reasons without loss of employment. Recently, there has been debate regarding the payment of this leave. Since federal and state regulations change often, the laboratory manager should always consult with the Human Resource office, because this office is responsible for obtaining the knowledge to keep the hospital in compliance with current laws. The manager can be held personally liable for errors made regarding FLSA and FMLA, and in some cases for errors made regarding other laws. Therefore, it is critical that the manager be aware of each applicable law.

Sexual harassment is a legal consideration for the laboratory. The institution should have a policy regarding sexual harassment, and all employees should be familiar with the policy. There should also be procedural steps for an employee to follow if a sexual harassment situation exist.

Termination of an employee must also be implemented in a legal manner. Usually three warnings, one verbal and two written, are given prior to termination in hopes that the employee behavior can be modified. If the employee's presence in the work environment is considered to be a danger to other employees or patients, the employee may be removed immediately. (Please refer Chapter 5 on Employee Interview and Selection, Chapter 6 on Employee Evaluation, and Chapter 7 on Employee Correction and Discipline.)

Institutional Issues

Many institutional issues exist, but one of the most important with respect to the clinical laboratory is the issue of confidentiality. For a health-care institution to exist, patients must be assured of confidentiality. In 1996, the Health Insurance Portability and Accountability Act (HIPAA) was enacted, and one of the purposes of the act was to protect patient confidentiality. Standards have been published governing electronic transmission and use of protected health information (PHI). HIPAA is extensive and essentially requires that *all* patient information be protected, that employees have access to patient information only on a "need to know" basis, and that no patient's information be disclosed without the patient's consent and authorization. The security standards, which will address areas such as equipment, facility, and technical security, will be published in the near future. Penalties for HIPAA violations vary according to whether the violation was intentional or accidental. Most institutions have instituted or are in the process of instituting detailed policies and procedures regarding this issue. In addition, the American Society for Clinical Laboratory Science professional code of ethics states that patient privacy is the expected conduct for the profession. Breach of patient confidentiality can result in institutional discipline as well as legal recourse.

Another important issue for the health-care institution is established procedures, such as those found in a procedure manual. Procedures must be followed at the workbench. If the employee does not adhere to institutional procedures and a patient is harmed, again, institutional discipline as well as legal recourse may occur. Often the laboratorian is asked to handle a specimen, the results of which may be used in legal proceedings; therefore, detailed documentation of specimen chain of custody is needed. Strict procedural adherence is required

The laboratory manager must be aware of the reimbursement policies established by federal agencies and insurance companies, and the manager must adhere to these policies to avoid fraud charges. Compliance is critical to the laboratory and the health-care institution in which the laboratory is located. Violations of reimbursement policies can result in severe negative consequences for the laboratory and in some cases the laboratorian. Therefore reimbursement policies and procedures should be carefully monitored by the laboratory manager. Many institutions have established a compliance officer within the laboratory just to deal with compliance issues. In addition to reimbursement issues, the Compliance Officer may deal with accreditation issues (e.g., JCAHO, CAP, OSHA, CLIA), issues relating to the Emergency Medical Treatment and Active Labor Act (EMTALA), and other compliance program issues such as conflict of interest policies, fair billing policies, ethical policies, and so on.

Even in the most careful laboratories, errors may occur. Errors should be handled quickly and with honesty. Dr. George Lundberg (1977) suggested that the laboratory should have a process to evaluate any possible errors to determine liability. Most laboratories address actions in the case of errors as a part of the quality management process.

BIBLIOGRAPHY

Desmond, Susan Fahey. 2002. *Employee relations manual for supervisors.* New Orleans, La.: Phelps Dunbar LLP.

Liebler, Joan Gratto, and Charles R. McConnell. 1999. *Management principles for health professionals.* 3d ed. Gaithersburg, Md.: Aspen Publishers.

Lundberg, George D. 1977. *Managing the patient-focused laboratory.* Oradell, N.J.: Medical Economics Company, Book Divison.

Peterson, Edward J., Jr. 2003. *What every student should know about compliance and HIPAA regulations.* Presentation at the Clinical Laboratory Educators' Conference, New Orleans, La., March.

Varnadoe, Lionel A. 1996. *Medical laboratory management and supervision.* Philadelphia: F. A. Davis.

INTERNET RESOURCES

American Medical Association. <www.ama-assn.org/ama/pub/category/4610.html>

Phelps Dunbar, Counselors at Law. <www.phelpsdunbar.com/site/html/publications/newsltr.htm>

U.S. Employee Laws. <www.mapnp.org/library/legal/emp_law/emp_law.htm>

QUESTIONS

1. The department of the hospital that should have the most information regarding personnel issues is _____. *(Objective 1, Level I)*

2. Two important documents relating to job vacancies that should be carefully prepared are _____ and _____

(Objective 2, Level II)

3. Illegal interview questions, unless related directly to the job, include *(Objective 2, Level I)*
   a. arrest record
   b. martial status
   c. number of children
   d. religious affiliation
   e. all of the above

4. Identify and justify a job situation in the laboratory when one might be asked about their arrest record. *(Objective 2, Level II)*

5. The laboratory is recognized as a _____ by the NLRB. *(Objective 3, Level I)*

6. Institutional legal issues are *(Objective 3, Level I)*
   a. confidentiality
   b. reimbursement procedures
   c. specimen chain of custody
   d. a and c only
   e. all of the above

EXERCISES

Completion of the exercises will enhance your knowledge of legal considerations. *(Objective 4, Level I)*

1. Interview the institutional legal counsel or the Human Resources department manager to determine the legal issues that most often arise.

2. Interview the administrative technologist to determine the most troublesome legal issues.

CASES

Analyze the following cases and formulate answers regarding the legality of the situation. *(Objective 5, Level III)*

1. A technologist, who has worked for many years, has a short-cut method for a particular procedure. This is not the method approved in the procedure manual. Would this employee be liable if a patient result was reported incorrectly? If so, would the employee be liable personally? Would the institution be liable?

2. On an employment interview, the candidate voluntarily states that she has five children and that she is a single mom. Should the interview be terminated because a legal issue has surfaced? What should the administrative tech do with this information?

3. A laboratory is operating in a physician clinic that houses more than 100 physicians. One of the nurses brings a urine specimen to the laboratory for a pregnancy test ordered by her physician employer. The urine sample happens to be from this nurse. Later the same nurse returns to the laboratory and requests the pregnancy test results. Should the results be given to the nurse? Why or why not?

4. An announcement states the need for a certified medical technologist/clinical laboratory scientist. The job description states that the individual must hold a specific certification from a specific agency. A candidate holds equivalent certification, but not the one specified. Can the employer deny employment based on the lack of the specific certification?

5. A pregnancy test is run by the technologist, and although it was positive, the technologist accidentally misread the test and reported it as negative. As a result of the test report, a D&C was performed on the patient, and a very young fetus was aborted. Is the technologist liable?

Chapter 39

Consulting

Jane Hudson, Ph.D., MT(ASCP)SM, CLS(NCA)

OBJECTIVES

Upon completion of this chapter the learner will be able to

1. Define *consultant*. *(Level I)*
2. Identify skills needed in consulting. *(Level I)*
3. Discuss at least four issues that need to be addressed if one decides to start a consulting business. *(Level II)*
4. Analyze the consultant role of the medical technologist/clinical laboratory scientist after attending a hospital-wide committee meeting or interviewing a medical technologist/clinical laboratory scientist with a consulting business. *(Level III)*
5. Create a marketing brochure. *(Level III)*
6. Create a proposal for specific laboratory services. *(Level III)*
7. Propose solutions for the case studies. *(Level III)*

TOPIC SUMMARY

Often the medical technologist/clinical laboratory scientist acts as a consultant, which can be defined as an expert who is called on for advice. A consultant must be able to gather, analyze, and provide information of a current and future nature. Some of the information will be beyond the scope of the employer's vision. Ability to share information is critical to the consultant's success. The consultant will critique the project, provide options, and perform or oversee performance of the project or aspects of the project. Therefore, the consultant must have research, data-management, education, analytical, communication, and technical skills. Lambert (1997) and Frings (1999) provide a detailed discussion of the role of the consultant.

Consulting is a part of your job as a medical technologist/clinical laboratory scientist and as a manager. The job can no longer be viewed as technical only, because the analytical phase is only one part of the responsibility to our clients, who are both the patients and the health-care providers. We must be involved in the preanalytical phase and the postanalytical phase of our work. In the preanalytical phase, the consultant advises the health-care provider regarding the appropriate test method, the proper specimen to be obtained, the cost of testing, and the parameters of each method. In the postanalytical phase, the consultant decides suitability of the results and provides information regarding alternative or additional testing and the predictability of the results. As you can readily see, the medical technologist/clinical laboratory scientist is involved already in consulting, but not necessarily called by that name.

Because we are consultants, how can one develop better consultant skills? First, **technical preparation** is required so that one has the technical competency necessary to serve the clients. Case histories involving clinical relevance are an excellent tool for enhancing one's ability to relate to the overall picture. Experience is also invaluable in technical preparation. Second, one must develop the **ability to consider a large volume of information and to synthesize** this material so that it is concise, organized, and understandable. Situations, such as preanalytical, analytical, and postanalytical outcomes assessment or management problems, that require analyzing and interpretation, can increase our skills in this area. And third, **knowledge of the literature and current happenings** to adequately predict the future is needed. **Ability to "think outside of the box"** in order to develop option diversity is required. Networking through professional organizations as well as avid reading of professional literature is essential to discover options. Fourth, **communication skills** can be enhanced by studying and practicing the art of oral (verbal and nonverbal) and written communications. And last, **basic marketing, self management, and business skills** can be learned through continuing education activities, literature analysis, and internships with others who are presently consultants. At the entry level to the profession the medical technologist/clinical laboratory scientist should have a basic introduction to skills needed for consulting. One interested in career advancement in the profession will continue to increase their knowledge and experience regarding these skills.

If one decides to start a consulting business, general issues that should be addressed are scope, liability, capital, publications, and marketing. For specific jobs, a proposal and a contract including fees must be developed. A brief discussion of each of these aspects follows:

Scope: It is important to establish the mission for the consulting business. Decide the purpose for the consulting business. Will the business be involved in advising and/or performing the tasks? Will the consulting business deal with only specialized topics, or will the business be broader in scope? Who will be the client? Some may choose to start with a limited mission and expand the mission as the consulting business grows.

Liability: Should the business be incorporated? Will incorporation limit personal liability? What about professional liability insurance or product liability? What is needed, and where does the business obtain the insurance? Is a license needed? Consultation with a lawyer might be necessary.

Capital: Will capital be required to start the consulting business? If so, what will capital fund? Where can one obtain the capital? What is the interest if money is borrowed? Some individuals may choose to borrow money or write a grant, in which case a business plan including the mission, owners of the business, prospective clients, need for the business, historical data regarding the particular business, marketing strategy, and present and future financial projections will be needed. Frings (1999) provides an excellent discussion of the business plan in his book.

Publications: What publications will be needed—business cards, stationary, brochures, and so on? Developing the business cards, stationary, and brochures regarding the business are critical, as these will be the initial impressions for a possible client. The publications should be of good quality and professional appearance. The information contained in the publications should be adequate, be concise, catch the client's attention, and be informative. Development of good publication materials may take some time, and proofing by another party is often beneficial.

Marketing: Now that all the general issues have been addressed, one must ask who the client is. Once the client is identified, the consultant may gain access to the client pool through professional organizations, similar businesses, referral, networking, and so on. Marketing never ceases; it is a continuous process.

Proposal (for the specific project): What should be in the proposal submitted to the client? The proposal should be a step-by-step list of activities that will be performed and the resources needed. It should also list a time table and cost for each activity. Last, but very important, is to tell your client what benefit will be derived from your consultation.

Contract (the final document delineating the terms of the agreement): What should the contract include? There are many aspects to the contract, and consultation with a lawyer might be beneficial. Generally, contracts include consultant's duties, items provided by the consultant and the client, cost, payment method, who owns work produced, deadlines, terms for termination, and so on. The contract is a very important document, and the major emphasis should be communication of the terms of the consultative activity. This also can be used as a legal document, so care should be taken in the preparation.

Fees: What fees need to be charged? Fees should adequately cover the costs associated with the consultation activity and provide income for the consultant and for reinvesting in the business. Decide how the fees will be billed—daily basis, performance basis, or fixed basis. The client must feel that your fees are competitive and are justified by the work to be done. Fees are a critical step in selling your services, so be sure to carefully justify your fees.

This brief discussion of consulting should provide a general awareness of the topic. Several good sources on the "how to" of the business side are suggested in the bibliography.

BIBLIOGRAPHY

Davis, Brenta G., Diana Mass, and Michael L. Bishop. 1999. *Principles of clinical laboratory utilization and consultation.* Philadelphia: W. B. Saunders.

Frings, Christopher S. 1999. *How to start and maintain a consulting practice.* Washington, D.C.: AACC Press.

Lambert, Tom. 1997. *High income consulting.* London, England: Nicholas Brealey.

Varnadoe, Lionel A. 1996. *Medical laboratory management and supervision operations: Review, and study guide.* Philadelphia: F. A. Davis.

INTERNET RESOURCES

American Society for Clinical Laboratory Science. <www.ascls.org/jobs/consulting.asp>

Consulting Academy. <www.consultingacademy.com>

QUESTIONS

1. The consultant is an expert who is called on for _____ or _____ advice. *(Objective 1, Level I)*

2. Skills needed in consulting are *(Objective 2, Level I)*
   a. _____
   b. _____
   c. _____
   d. _____
   e. _____
   f. _____
   g. _____

3. List and discuss at least four issues that need to be considered prior to establishing a consultant business. *(Objective 3, Level II)*

EXERCISES

Completion of the exercises will enhance your knowledge of consulting. *(Objective 4, Level III, Objective 5, Level III and Objective 6, Level III)*

1. Attend a hospital-wide committee meeting with the laboratory department representative. Summarize individually or as a group the consultative role of the medical technologist/clinical laboratory scientist. Include how consultation is done, who the consultant is, why consultation is done, who benefits from consultation, how the laboratory representative prepared for the consultation activity, and what skills are necessary for the representative to serve in this capacity.

2. Interview a medical technologist/clinical laboratory scientist who has established a consulting business to determine how the individual started the business, the need for the business, the skills needed to be a consultant, the advantages and disadvantages of establishing one's own business, the legal requirements of establishing a business, interaction with clients, and so on. Share your findings with the class.

3. Review the laboratory marketing brochure or the marketing brochure of the consultant that you interviewed. Select a laboratory-related or nonlaboratory-related consultant activity that interests you and develop a brochure for the consultant activity.

4. Review literature regarding development of a business proposal. You may use literature review, a specific business proposal from your laboratory (e.g., marketing proposal), or a specific business proposal from the consultant that you interviewed. After you have reviewed a proposal, perform the following: You have been asked whether the laboratory can handle the business of a small private laboratory that does CBCs and RPRs. Develop a proposal for the owners of the small private laboratory regarding the services your laboratory can offer.

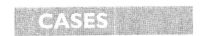

For each of the following cases, analyze the situation and propose a solution to the questions.
(Objective 7, Level III)

1. As the laboratory representative, you have just been asked to serve on a committee to develop and evaluate biological waste disposal recommendations for the entire hospital. As a medical technologist/clinical laboratory scientist, you have the expertise in biological safety. What things would you do to prepare for your role on this important committee?

2. You established a consultant business to assist doctors' offices with quality control documentation and other CLIA requirements, but no one has called you, even though you have distributed your business card to many of the prospective clients. The business card looked sharp with color and a nice picture. Included on the card was your name in bold letters, your credentials, and the name of your consulting company. Why do you think you have not received any calls?

3. You decide to start a consultant business advising local physicians regarding specimen requirements for "send out" testing. Most of the local physicians use a local, private reference laboratory for their "send out" tests. After a good publicity campaign regarding your consultant business, you do not have any request for your services. What could the problem be?

4. You have been asked to help a physician's office develop their procedure manuals. How would you develop this into a consulting business?

Chapter 40

Establishment of a Continuing Education Program

David Thrash, B.S., MT(ASCP), CLS(NCA)

OBJECTIVES

Upon completion of this chapter the learner will be able to

1. Define *continuing education*. *(Level I)*
2. State the number of contact hours required by the National Credentialing Agency (NCA) to maintain certification. *(Level I)*
3. List six variables that must be considered when implementing a continuing education program. *(Level I)*
4. Define *external client*. *(Level I)*
5. Define *P.A.C.E.®* *(Level I)*
6. Convert contact hours to continuing education units. *(Level II)*
7. Create an evaluation plan for a continuing education program. *(Level III)*
8. Convert continuing education units to contact hours. *(Level II)*
9. Create a proposal for a continuing education activity. *(Level III)*
10. Choose the continuing education activity that is the best buy for a specific situation, given a case with information regarding possible continuing education activities. *(Level III)*

TOPIC SUMMARY

Continuing education is a term that we hear almost every day of our professional life, whether we are a doctor, lawyer, insurance salesman, cook, teacher, or a medical technologist/clinical laboratory scientist. Schwabbauer (2002) states that continuing education includes educational activities not normally associated with an academic degree. Continuing educational activities include attending professional society workshops and seminars, attending employer sponsored seminars, completing journal or magazine articles with self-assessments, and so on. Certain variables must be considered when implementing a continuing education program (CEP) for clinical laboratory scientists (CLS) and clinical laboratory technicians (CLT). These include establishing a need, establishing a task force to implement the CEP, working within a required budget, researching different types of CEP, issuing credits, and monitoring the effectiveness of the CEP. A discussion of each variable follows.

Establishing a Need

Why does a CEP need to be established? Just as each institution establishes normal ranges for a complete blood count (CBC) from a random sampling of the population, each institution should establish its own need for a CEP. Most health-care institutions require its employees to obtain a specific number of continuing education units (CEU) or contact hours (CH) of continuing education each year. Failure to meet this requirement may result in disciplinary action. Some of these institutions may offer continuing education to its employees at no cost. Other institutions may not have the operating budget to provide no-cost continuing education to its employees; thus it is the responsibility of the health-care employee to obtain and pay for it. Required or not, every health-care professional should stay abreast of current health-care issues. In this day and age, Americans live on an information superhighway where, with a few computer strokes, a diagnosis of a disease may be made. However, there are drawbacks to accessing this information, because it may be outdated, antiquated, or guidelines may have changed since the original post date. For this reason, it is imperative that health-care professionals seek ways to stay abreast on current health issues that are of importance. Continuing education will enhance the ability of the professional to produce accurate and reliable results. Some of the factors that impact the employee's desire to participate in the educational process include the dynamic nature of healthcare, incentives, and job satisfaction. Those who choose to discontinue their education once they have secured a job will be "left in the dust" (Earhardt 1998). In other instances, certifying agencies require demonstration of continuing education to maintain certification. The National Credentialing Agency (NCA) for laboratory personnel currently requires thirty-six contact hours or 3.6 CEUs earned in the past three years to maintain NCA active status. Certain states, such as California, Tennessee, Louisiana, and Florida, have passed legislation implementing mandatory continuing education requirements for all laboratorians to maintain licensure. The employer may identify an educational need during the annual or competency evaluations and set a goal regarding desired performance. Or the employee may identify educational goals on the annual evaluation to enhance their professional status. The need for continuing education activities is dependent on employer demands, the knowledge explosion, the employees' level of job satisfaction, and certification and licensure requirements.

Establishing a Task Force to Implement a CEP

Once the manager of the clinical laboratory has established a need for continuing education, a task force is formed. The task force is usually composed of the education program leader or clinical coordinator for a specific department and at least two members of the technical staff. The goal of the task force is to review the availability of funds (budget), research different types of CEPs, determine the needs of the employees (time, location, length, and certification requirements), as well as a format for issuing credits for participation in a CEP.

Working within an Established Budget for a CEP

The next question is "How much money do I have to spend?" Cost is the number one obstacle that must be overcome when tackling the implementation of a CEP. Medical institutions today are faced with decreased reimbursement from regulatory agencies such as Medicare and Medicaid. This in turn leads to budget cuts. In order to keep the institution operating efficiently and to pay employee salaries, clinical departments will cut excess spending where necessary. The first item to suffer a decrease in funds is almost always CEPs. With limited or nonexisting funds, numerous methods for providing continuing education are available. These may include using volunteer speakers (who require no monetary reimbursement), obtaining sponsorship monies through professional organization grants and scholarships, or obtaining sponsorship monies through research and development projects (Earhardt 1998).

Because other health professionals within your organization also need continuing education, look for opportunities to sponsor and promote external client education programs. Clients may be physicians, nurses, patients, or anyone living in your community. Some examples of external continuing education programs may include hosting community health fairs, providing ongoing educational classes on health-related issues for the public, or providing educational updates for the staff. This may or may not be a revenue source for supporting the continuing education needs of the laboratory.

Researching Different Types of CEPs That Meet the Required Budget

After establishing a budget, researching different types of CEPs is the next most important aspect. Experts recommend that at the beginning of each year one should decide how required hours are to be met, either monthly, quad-annually (once every three months), biannually (once every six months), or annually (once a year). The style of learning as well as access to a variety of delivery methods, such as home study, didactic lectures, Internet courses, audioconferences, national or regional conferences, or workshops offered by state, regional, or national conferences, should also be considered. Organizations, such as the National Laboratory Training Network (NLTN) sponsored by the Centers for Disease Control (CDC), have been created specifically to provide continuing education courses to individuals and institutions with small operating fees.

Membership in a professional society, such as the American Society for Clinical Pathology (ASCP) or the American Society for Clinical Laboratory Science (ASCLS), is one of the best buys around for obtaining continuing education. Membership benefits usually include a journal or newsletter with home-study or self-study continuing education articles that can be completed at one's own pace (Guterl 1998).

Issuing Credits for Completing a CEP

After you have researched, budgeted, planned, and implemented a CEP for your institution, the education officer must award credits for completing the CEP. Organizations such as ASCLS choose to award P.A.C.E.® (Professional Acknowledgment of Continuing Education) credits in all laboratory disciplines with credit varying according to time spent in the activity and the type of activity. The American Society for Clinical Pathology (ASCP) chooses to award CMLE (Continuing Medical Laboratory Education) credits to all participants in the field of medicine, laboratory medicine, and forensic pathology. Whichever format, all clinical laboratorians receive credit in the form of CEUs, CHs, CMLE, and semester hours. One CH or one CMLE is equivalent to 0.1 CEUs. One hour of a course that awards CEUs is worth 0.1 CEUs. One semester hour, awarded upon completion of a college level course, is equal to fifteen CH or 1.5 CEUs. Another collegiate term is one-quarter hour, which equals ten CHs or 1.0 CEUs (*ADVANCE* CE Directory 1998).

Monitoring the Effectiveness of the CEP

The type of continuing education offered determines the method of feedback you will need to evaluate the success of a CEP. If an external speaker is used for continuing education purposes, three to four objectives should be submitted prior to the session as to what will be conveyed to the audience. The speaker is then rated on a scale of one (poor) to five (excellent) by the participant to determine how the fulfillment of each objective is viewed. Questions that might be asked are

- Was the presentation clear and concise?
- Was the facility conducive to learning?
- Was the topic discussed of a direct value to my current job?

Most institutions will prefer a simpler approach for determining success, such as an informal survey. This also serves as an effective method for determining feedback. A generic questionnaire may be formulated asking questions such as

- Was the CEP offered beneficial?
- What type of knowledge has been gained by participation?
- What is the preferred source(s) of continuing education?
- What could be done to make the presentations more effective?

Other questions such as "What cost(s) was incurred by the employee for obtaining continuing education?" may be asked if your health-care institution does not cover the costs for a CEP.

At first, there may not be an overwhelming response for a CEP, but as the laboratorian participates and becomes more comfortable with continuing education activities, acceptance of the CEP will increase. Regardless of the method for obtaining continuing education, the cost incurred, or response received, the need for laboratory professionals to stay updated on new methods in the field of clinical laboratory science is of vital importance to the public at large (Samant et al. 1998).

BIBLIOGRAPHY

ASCLS In-Service Reviews in Clinical Laboratory Science. 2000. *Lysosomal Storage Disorders.* Birmingham, Ala.: Oakstone Medical Publishing.

Bixenman, Helen. 1999. NCA recertification questions answered. NCA Clipboard. The Official Newsletter of the National Credentialing Agency for Laboratory Personnel. Vol. 5, no. 1, pg. 2.

Earhardt, Patty. 1998. No funds for continuing education: Try these creative solutions. *ADVANCE for Medical Laboratory Professionals* 10, no. 7: 22–24.

Guterl, Gail O. 1998. Choosing CEU sources takes planning, time, funds. *ADVANCE for Medical Laboratory Professionals* 10, no. 7: 17–20.

Samant, Madhuri, William N. Bigler, and Donna Lynce. 1998. Survey shows high approval rating for mandatory CE in California. *ADVANCE for Medical Laboratory Professionals* 10, no. 7: 25–26.

Schwabbauer, Marian. *Personnel regulations.* Virtual Hospital: The Clinical Laboratory Improvement Act (CLIA) and the Physician's Office Laboratory. Retrieved April 2, 2002, from <www.vh.org/Providers/CME/CLIA/Personnel Regulations.html>

Third Annual Continuing Education Resource Directory. 1998. *ADVANCE for Medical Laboratory Professionals* 10, no. 7: 28.

INTERNET RESOURCES

Virtual Hospital.
<www.vh.org/Adult/provider/pathology/CLIA/Personnel Regulations.html>

QUESTIONS

1. According to Schwabbauer, what is the definition of continuing education? *(Objective 1, Level I)*

2. How many contact hours does the NCA require per year to maintain certification? *(Objective 2, Level I)*

3. List six variables that must be considered when implementing a CEP? *(Objective 3, Level I)*
   a. _____
   b. _____
   c. _____
   d. _____
   e. _____
   f. _____

4. Who are external clients? Name two examples of external client education programs? *(Objective 4, Level I)*

5. Define P. A.C.E.® *(Objective 5, Level I)*

6. Convert fourteen contact hours to CEUs. *(Objective 6, Level II)*

7. If you wanted to evaluate the effectiveness of a CEP in your institution, how might you go about doing this? What might be some of the questions asked? *(Objective 7, Level III)*

8. Convert 1.0 CEUs to contact hours. *(Objective 8, Level II)*

EXERCISES

Completion of the exercises will enhance your knowledge regarding establishment of a continuing education program. *(Objective 9, Level III)*

1. Interview (in person, by telephone, or by computer) the education program leader (or education manager) at a local or affiliated hospital to find out what steps were taken in choosing continuing education, which variables were the most important in selecting, and what is the outcome. This may be accomplished as an individual activity or group project. Reports of findings should be shared.

2. Survey the laboratorians and determine continuing education needs of the group. Then investigate ways to provide the continuing education needed. Create a proposal to present to the administrative technologist documenting the need for the continuing education, how the continuing education activity might be provided, the cost of the activity, credit to be awarded upon completion of the activity, and how evaluation will be accomplished.

CASES

For the following case, choose the most cost effective method for providing the continuing education. *(Objective 10, Level III)*

1. The date is June 1999. Your institution has implemented a policy that requires employees working in patient areas, such as nursing, laboratory, physical therapy, and so on, to have at least twelve contact hours by his or her seniority date. The manager of the laboratory, Ima Qutee, has come to Jena Rachun, the education officer, and stated that there is only $775 in the laboratory's budget for continuing education. Ima Qutee also states that the budgeted fiscal year began in May 1999 and will end in April 2000. Ima, with time on her hands, researched a few items to give Jena an idea of what she might implement. These are listed below. Ima tells Jena that she may use one or more of these item or try to find something on her own.

   Internet courses—$50/person/per course
   (Total laboratory technical support—thirty. Ima states that this would be a good choice because most of the computers in the lab have an Internet Service Provider (ISP) allowing each employee to use their own sign-in account. Ima continued to say that if no time was allocated at work to participate, most employees could participate on their own time and pace if they had access to a personal computer)

   Teleconference—$95/teleconference
   (Ima feels this is a good idea, because the teleconferences may be videotaped and viewed by employees on their own time. Ima states that the employees would write a one-page summary of the topic to receive from 0.1 to 0.2 CEUs, depending on the length of the teleconference.)

   Audiocassettes—$375/ for one-year subscription
   (Two audiocassettes, six posttests, and the answers are furnished once per month for one year. The posttests may be submitted back to the original continuing education provider at no costs for P. A.C.E.® or CLME credit. Ima feels this is a good idea, but a drawback is that only six persons from the lab may participate to receive P. A.C.E.® or CLME credit. But Ima tells Jena that copies of the posttest can be made available so that all can participate.)

   Jena likes these ideas but decides to research, with the help of two hematology technologists, more options. The group finds the following items:

   Magazine subscription—$0–65/twelve months
   (The group thinks that this may be a good idea because continuing education articles with posttest are furnished in each issue. Jena discovered one magazine in particular that offers a free subscription to laboratory personnel. Continuing education articles with posttests are published in each issue. The only drawback is a posttest processing fee of $18 that is required from the participant to officially earn the CEUs. The education officer could develop an evaluation system for any articles read and award in-house CEUs.)

   External speakers—$95/one 2-hour lecture
   (The group thinks that this may be a good idea because the speaker could be videotaped and viewed by each employee at their own pace. The group feels a posttest could be devised and administered to the participants to earn credits from 0.1–0.2 CEUs, depending on length of topic.)

Regional conferences—$50/ASCLS member; $80/ASCLS nonmember
(The group feels that this might be a good idea. A few employees could attend the conference and then share what they had learned in an informal type question-and-answer session.)

Of the previous continuing education items, which three might be the best buy for the money budgeted, and why?

Chapter 41

Construction and Delivery of an Instructional Unit

Claudia Miller, Ph.D., MT(ASCP), CLS(NCA)

OBJECTIVES

Upon completion of this chapter the learner will be able to

1. Identify characteristics to consider when establishing the target audience. *(Level I)*
2. List the advantages and disadvantages of the teaching strategies discussed in this chapter. *(Level I)*
3. List the advantages and disadvantages of the flip chart, printed material, overhead projector, and LCD projector. *(Level I)*
4. Identify three criteria to be included in the objective. *(Level I)*
5. Identify and define the three domains of educational objectives. *(Level I)*
6. Differentiate the use of a goal versus an objective. *(Level III)*
7. Determine the appropriate teaching strategy for the instructional unit. *(Level II)*
8. Evaluate written objectives using established criteria. (Level III)
9. Construct a unit/lesson plan including goals, objectives, teaching strategies, and media use. *(Level III)*
10. Construct educational objectives in three domains and at different taxonomic levels. *(Level III)*
11. Critique a presentation determining various ways the material might have been presented. *(Level III)*
12. Analyze the case studies and propose solutions. *(Level III)*

TOPIC SUMMARY

The construction of an educational unit and its delivery are necessary competencies for the laboratory professional. Clinical laboratory students, in-services, changing methodologies, and other situations require that new information be offered in the most effective manner possible. Use of concise, measurable objectives, dynamic teaching strategies, and supportive media make the learning experience positive and enjoyable.

Audience

The instructor must know the audience or target population. By being familiar with the characteristics of the learners, the instructional unit can be constructed for optimal results. A **lesson plan** that includes goals, objectives, teaching strategies, and media can enhance the learning process if the needs of the learners are considered. Educational level, prior knowledge, previous experience, and biases are student characteristics that should be considered. An instructional unit in red cell morphology would be different if it were being taught to a high school student rather than to a clinical laboratory science student.

Educational Objectives

A **goal** is an achieveable statement of broad direction. It allows the instructor to target the purpose of the educational unit and provides the base upon which measurable objectives are constructed. An **objective** is a specific statement of what the learner is expected to know or to be able to do after a period of instruction; it is totally learner based.

Construction of objectives allows the instructor to plan the unit of instruction. The selection of a teaching strategy, material to be used, media support, and evaluation technique are made easier by these clear statements of expectations. With objectives, the learner has a guide that enables him or her to focus on relevant points during instruction, to read for pertinent points, and to complete assignments. Objectives are a crucial part of any type of instruction.

Mager (1997b) and Gronlund (1995) are two educators who have set the foundation for the construction of educational objectives. There are three questions that educational objectives must address:

- What does the instructor want *the student* to do at the conclusion of the unit?
    Example: Demonstrate the method for counting and calculating platelets.
- Under what conditions should the learner accomplish the objectives?
    Example: Using the Neubauer chamber
- What is the criterion that signifies achievement?
    Example: Results must be obtained that are within 40,000 plts/mm^3 of the technologist's results.

The completed objective should read: Using the Neubauer chamber, demonstrate the method for counting and calculating platelets by producing results that are within 40,000 plt/mm^3 of the technologist's results.

Sometimes the conditions under which the learner accomplishes the objective is implied or absent; other situations may not need published criteria. It is always better to include as much information as possible to assist the learner to reach the desired outcome.

Example: Perform microscopic analysis of a random urine (it is not necessary to write "using a microscope")

Example: Group and type a unit of blood for transfusion (it may not be necessary to add "with 100% accuracy")

If the criteria or conditions for a group of objectives are the same, they may be listed at the beginning of the objectives.

Example: At the end of the lecture, the learner will achieve the following. Achievement will be met when a minimum score of 75% is earned on the examination covering this material.

1. State the steps involved in the production of thyroid hormones.
2. Trace the feedback mechanism for thyroid hormones.
3. Differentiate between subclinical and clinical hyperthyroidism and hypothyroidism with regards to clinical symptoms, causes of disease, and treatment.
4. Compare the three types of thyroid cancer: include demographics, laboratory results, and tumor markers.

The instrument must determine the learner's competence in a visible and measurable manner.

Example (measurable): Correlate clinical signs with laboratory data eighty-five percent of the time.

Example (measurable): Compare the methodologies for determining total and direct bilirubin.

Example (not measurable): Develop an understanding of mediation in the workplace.

Example (not measurable): Realize the importance of keeping a clean workplace.

Objectives are divided into three domains or categories—cognitive, psychomotor, and affective. Each domain has taxonomic levels that are arranged in hierarchical order from simple to complex. The manner in which these levels are communicated to the learner is by use of measurable verbs that are specific for each taxonomy level.

Bloom addresses the cognitive domain. This area is concerned with intellectual outcomes; it is knowledge based and ranges from simple recollection to high level skills. The levels are as follows: *knowledge, application, analysis, synthesis,* and *evaluation.* Simpson incorporates motor skills in the psychomotor domain. The levels are as follows: *perception, set, guided response, mechanism, complex overt response, adaptation,* and *origination.* Krathwohl's affective domain of objectives includes interests, attitudes, appreciation, and the development of a value system. It is the most difficult area for which to construct objectives and their subsequent measurement. The levels of affective objectives include the following: *receiving, responding, valuing, organization,* and *characterization by a value or value complex.*

Many times an objective will overlap domains. Psychomotor objectives may require cognitive competence in order to be performed. Likewise, the affective domain may enter into a psychomotor domain objective.

Example: Perform phlebotomy using multiple tubes and in compliance with established laboratory policy.

> Cognitive: The learner must know the steps to venipuncture and the order of draw.
>
> Psychomotor: The learner must actually perform the successful draw.
>
> Affective: The learner must interact and communicate with the patient.

The taxonomies may be collapsed for ease in writing objectives. For example, six cognitive levels become three general areas—Levels I, II, and III.

Level I—Recall

Level II—Application

Level III—Evaluation

The objectives in this book are written in this simplified manner. Clinical laboratory certification examinations also incorporate three general taxonomic levels. Psychomotor levels condense into

Level I—Observation

Level II—Performance

Level III—Troubleshooting/problem solving

Affective domain levels are harder to reduce. They are usually condensed as

Level I—Exhibition of a behavior/value due to an established rule

Level II—Exhibition of a behavior/value due to personal development

The manner in which these levels are communicated to the learner is by use of measurable verbs that are specific for each taxonomic level. Table 41–1 lists examples of verbs that can effectively be used in the construction of objectives.

General verbs such as *know* and *understand* are poor choices for writing objectives, because these verbs cannot be measured. If these or comparable verbs are used, the degree of competence must also be included in the objective to make it measurable.

TABLE 41–1. Sample Verbs

COGNITIVE	PSYCHOMOTOR	AFFECTIVE
Level I:	**Level I:**	**Level I:**
define	demonstrate	comply
identify	prepare	obey
list	set up	attend
name	select	observe
Level II:	**Level II:**	**Level II:**
compute	smear	appreciate
relate	titrate	internalize
calculate	perform	question
use	measure	justify
Level III:	**Level III:**	
analyze	troubleshoot	
compare	develop	
correlate	create	
differentiate	change	

Example (poor): Understand the metabolism of bilirubin.

Example (better, but lengthy): Understand the metabolism of bilirubin; include origin, pre- and post-conjugation states, conversion to waste products, and disease states.

Example (better and easier to interpret): Trace the metabolism of bilirubin from origin to elimination from the body. Correlate bilirubin results with disease states.

It is imperative that educational objectives be written at varying taxonomic levels that are consistent with the target audience. If progression to a higher level is desired, use of lower taxonomy verbs will not let the learner achieve that end. It is acceptable to start a unit of instruction with lower level verbs and continue to increase the verb complexity until the level of competence or desired outcome is reached.

Example: Define creatinine. (Recall—Level I)

> Calculate a creatinine clearance. (Application—Level II)
>
> Utilizing BUN and creatinine values, determine the renal status of the patient. (Evaluation—Level III)

Teaching Strategies

Teaching strategies differ depending on the topic, setting, and learner. A topic such as reading Gram stains is confusing if a lecture is the only way it is being taught. Some individuals learn best through auditory methods, others, by visual enhancement. The presenter must be aware if the learner is confused so that alternative methods can be utilized or additional assistance offered.

The setting is also important. A **laboratory** portion is a necessary part of the curriculum of a parasitology course. Pictures in the textbook can be used as a guide; however, observing wet mounts or prepared slides provides the appropriate resources for the learner. Accompanying lectures bring the unit together for maximum benefit.

The **lecture** is most frequently used in presenting an educational unit. It is used to give timely information, summarize material, and supplement other types of instruction. Lectures are effective when the number of learners is considerably large.

If the material is available in printed form, the lecture is not needed; learners can read the same information in a shorter period of time. When measures of knowledge (examinations) are used, the lecture has been shown to be as effective as any other type of instruction. However, when retention, transfer of knowledge, and problem solving are desired, other types of instruction may prove beneficial.

Very often lecturers try to include vast amounts of material in the time allotted; it is important to prepare a lesson plan that includes an outline and educational objectives. This preparation keeps the instructor on track and allows the learners to reap maximum benefits from the presentation.

Demonstration is also a method used in the clinical laboratory that teaches skills, procedures, or techniques. It is usually used in conjunction with another method of instruction. The drawback for the demonstration method is the limited number of learners who can be accommodated. The demonstration should always be followed very closely by having the learners participate in controlled practice.

Discussion involves the exploration of a single topic, problem, or question by a group of learners. It is a learner-centered method and is not used as frequently as lecture and demonstration. Discussion is an effective way to build increased levels of thinking and to develop the affective domain. It is not useful for imparting of new information.

Role-playing develops human relation skills and provides a concrete basis for discussion of a topic. It involves situations in which the learners adapt to the roles to which they have been assigned. Nonparticipants may function as observers. Because it is possible for role-playing to expand into areas other that those assigned, the instructor must maintain control at all times.

Media Support

The selection of media to support the instruction is very important. Media carry the message and help the instructor get information to the learner. The number of learners, the size of the room, and the teaching strategy must be considered.

A **chalkboard** or **flip chart** may hold the attention of the learners and is good for the discussion technique. It allows for a building of ideas in a graphic form, but learners may be confused if the information placed on the chart does not match the verbal communication directly.

The **overhead projector** is still the most popular method for imparting information in the lecture format; however, electronic programs and the LCD projector are rapidly replacing it. The overhead projector is easy to use and saves on class time when overheads are prepared before the instruction. It allows visual learners to track with the auditory part of the instruction. Disadvantages include lack of instructor eye contact with the learners and providing too much information that forces the learner to copy frantically and not listen to the presentation.

The **LCD projector** and electronic programs allow for colorful visuals and movement of information into the screen. Care must be taken not to make the fields too busy with decorations. Also, there is always the problem of the technology failing. It is a good idea to have duplicate 35-mm transparencies/slides or overhead acetates for emergencies.

Printed material (e.g., charts, diagrams, and tables not found in the textbook) should accompany each unit of instruction. It should not contain the instructor's lesson verbatim and should leave space for the learner to make notes. The outline and the objectives should be attached to the printed handouts.

The medical technologist/clinical laboratory scientist must teach. This teaching may be directed toward students, new employees, nurses, physicians, other health care professionals or patients. Through the activity of teaching, one communicates information from the laboratory critical for quality patient care. Because the laboratorian must be an effective teacher, knowledge and skills in preparing an instructional unit enhances the teaching activity and allows more effective and efficient communication of the information.

BIBLIOGRAPHY

Gronlund, N. 2000. *How to write and use instructional objectives.* 6th ed. Englewood Cliffs, N.J.: Merrill.

Mager, R. F. 1997a. *Making instruction work or skillbloomers.* 2d ed. Center for Effective Performance, Atlanta, GA.

Mager, R. F. 1997b. *Preparing instructional objectives.* 3d ed. Center for Effective Performance, Atlanta, GA.

INTERNET RESOURCES

Humboldt State University. <www.humboldt.edu/~tha1/bloomtax.html>

University of Washington. <http://faculty.washington.edu/krumme/guides/bloom.html>

QUESTIONS

1. Two of the four characteristics to be considered when investigating a target audience are *(Objective 1, Level 1)*

   a. _____

   b. _____

2. List at least one of the advantages and disadvantages of each of the following teaching strategies. *(Objective 2, Level 1)*

Strategy	Advantage	Disadvantage
Lecture		
Discussion		
Demonstration		

3. List at least one advantage and one disadvantage when using media support. *(Objective 3, Level 1)*

Media	Advantage	Disadvantage
Flip chart		
Printed material		

Overhead projector

LCD projector

4. What are three criteria that must be addressed in writing an objective? *(Objective 4, Level I)*

   a. _____

   b. _____

   c. _____

5. Identify and define the three domains of educational objectives. *(Objective 5, Level I)*

   a. _____

   b. _____

   c. _____

6. Identify the domain of these objectives. *(Objective 5, Level I)*

   a. Compare the intrinsic and extrinsic pathways in coagulation.

   _____

   b. Operate the hematology instrument to determine the hemoglobin and hematocrit of the patient.

   _____

   c. Maintain a professional attitude in the workplace.

   _____

7. Differentiate the use of a goal versus an objective and give an example of each. *(Objective 6, Level III)*

8. The goal of the instructional unit is for the student or employee to develop Gram stain skills. What is/are the appropriate teaching strategy(ies)? *(Objective 7, Level II)*
   a. laboratory
   b. lecture
   c. demonstration
   d. role play
   e. a, b, and c
   f. all of the above

9. The goal of an instructional unit is for the student or employee to interact professionally with patients. What is/are the appropriate teaching strategy(ies)? *(Objective 7, Level II)*
   a. laboratory
   b. lecture
   c. demonstration
   d. role play
   e. a, b, and c
   f. b, c, and d

10. Evaluate the following objective. *(Objective 8, Level III)*

    Following a discussion regarding different patient responses to the venipuncture procedure, the student will demonstrate understanding.

    a. good objective; no changes required
    b. poor objective; use of the word *understanding* is not measurable
    c. poor objective; "95% of the time" should be added
    d. poor objective; the discussion teaching technique is inappropriate

11. Evaluate the following objective. *(Objective 8, Level III)*

    Following a demonstration and discussion regarding the materials necessary for performing a phlebotomy procedure, the student will assemble all the required materials accurately.

    a. good objective; no changes needed
    b. poor objective; practice is needed in addition to demonstration and discussion
    c. poor objective; need "95% of the time" added
    d. poor objective; "required materials" is too vague

EXERCISES

Completion of the exercises will enhance your knowledge of construction and delivery of an instructional unit. *(Objective 9, Level III, Objective 10, Level III, and Objective 11, Level III)*

1. Construct a ten-minute presentation to be taught to preclinical laboratory students; include goals, objectives, teaching strategies, and media.

2. Write two objectives for each domain. One objective should be at the basic level, the other, at a higher level. Exchange papers with another student and perform peer review of the project.

3. Critique a presentation of any type. Determine various ways in which the same material might have been presented.

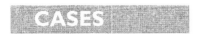

Analyze the following case studies and propose solutions. *(Objective 12, Level III)*

1. As a clinical laboratory science faculty member, you have a student who always has a puzzled look on her face when you are teaching. You feel that she doesn't understand the topic. What should you do to accommodate her? How should you teach the rest of the class?

2. You are a new clinical laboratory science graduate who has been assigned to teach operation of a new instrument to a technician who has twenty years of experience. How would you handle your assignment? What preparation would you make? What strategy would you utilize?

3. You are a clinical laboratory science student who is going to recruit for your program. You have to go to a high school and teach urinalysis in a forty-five-minute period. How would you approach this project? Are there are special considerations for this audience? What style of teaching would you select?

Chapter 42

Measurement and Evaluation Strategies for an Instructional Unit

Claudia Miller, Ph.D., MT(ASCP), CLS(NCA)

OBJECTIVES

Upon completion of this chapter the learner will be able to

1. Differentiate between measurement and evaluation. *(Level I)*
2. Define reliability and validity as it relates to construction of measurement instruments and subsequent evaluation. *(Level I)*
3. Differentiate between norm-based and competency-based education. *(Level I)*
4. Distinguish between formative, diagnostic, and summative levels of education. *(Level I)*
5. Identify the advantages and disadvantages of each type of cognitive measurement instrument; include any guidelines for construction. *(Level I)*
6. Summarize the use of item analysis in reviewing cognitive measurement and evaluation. *(Level I)*
7. Identify the advantages and disadvantages for each type of psychomotor instrument; include any guidelines for construction. *(Level I)*
8. Identify evaluation difficulties in observer techniques. *(Level II)*
9. Identify special guidelines to be used when constructing affective domain instruments. *(Level I)*
10. Evaluate and revise measurement instruments for the cognitive domain. *(Level III)*
11. Relate an objective to a corresponding question. *(Level II)*
12. Select, construct, and apply appropriate measurement instruments for the affective domain. *(Level III)*
13. Identify and apply solutions to the evaluation difficulties. *(Level II)*
14. Construct an affective domain evaluation instrument student rotation. *(Level III)*
15. Perform item analysis. *(Level II)*
16. Select, construct, and apply appropriate measurement instruments for the psychomotor domain. *(Level III)*
17. Analyze the case studies and propose solutions. *(Level III)*

TOPIC SUMMARY

Appropriate measurement and evaluation development must follow construction of an instructional unit. It can be used for competency checks of students and new or experienced employees. The terms **measurement** and **evaluation** are often used as synonyms, yet they are totally different processes. Measurement is concerned with the application of an instrument or instruments (i.e., a tool produced to measure intended outcomes, e.g., an examination) to collect data for some specific purpose. Evaluation is the process of appraisal with specific purposes or aims in mind. Both are necessary processes.

There are two problems in instrument construction. The first is to determine what to measure and the second is to determine how to measure it. There is a relationship between what the learner is required to do and what the educational unit undertook to teach him to do. The measurement instrument must achieve this purpose. If a unit is constructed to teach proper Gram staining technique, a written cognitive measurement may not be appropriate.

Instruments should be **reliable,** showing consistent measurement from test to test and over multiple times. In addition, they should be **valid,** measuring relevant tasks. If an instrument is reliable only, the problem is usually in the construction of the unit. The unit is taught the same time after time, and learners perform well; however, it lacks validity. If an instrument is valid only, the lack of consistency with the instruction is most likely at fault. One common example is the multiplicity of bench instructors. One student may receive thorough instruction in operating the chemistry equipment; another may not. The evaluation instrument is not flawed. It lacks reliability because of the difference in instructors.

There are two basic ways of interpreting learner performance on measurement and evaluation instruments. **Norm-based education** describes performance in terms of position in a group of peers. Each learner is compared with the other. Grades may be curved, with the learner making the highest grade earning an "A" even if the grade itself is below the usual passing level. Most high school and higher education courses follow this method.

Another way of observing achievement is to describe performance in terms of a specific behavior; this is **competency-based education.** Learners are evaluated against established competencies; they are not compared with each other. In true competency-based education, the learner has as much time as needed to achieve the goal. Entry into a profession requires that the learner achieve competencies. Most clinical laboratory science education is structured on a modified competency-based model. The difference is that there are time constraints in clinical education; a learner cannot take all semester to learn to make feather-edged microscopic slides for hematology.

A reliable and valid measurement instrument is constructed from the educational objectives for a particular unit. An **objective** is a specific measurable statement of what the learner is expected to know or to be able to do after a period of instruction; it is totally learner based. There are three questions that educational objectives must address.

- What does the instructor want *the student* to do at the conclusion of the unit?
- Under what conditions should the learner accomplish the objectives?
- What is the criterion that signifies achievement?

Objectives are divided into three domains or categories—cognitive, psychomotor, and affective. Each domain has taxonomic levels that are arranged in hierarchical order from simple to complex. The manner in which these levels are communicated to the learner is by use of **measurable** verbs that are specific for each taxonomy level. The taxonomies may be collapsed for ease in writing objectives. Objectives were discussed in detail in the previous chapter.

The development of the learner during the clinical education demands that different types of instruments be used for appropriate evaluation. It is important that the evaluator and learner recognize what level of evaluation is in progress. Categories are as follows:

- Formative—evaluation of learning progress during instruction
- Diagnostic—evaluation of learning difficulties during instruction
- Summative—evaluation of learner achievement at the end of instruction

The measurement and evaluation instruments used for these categories should reflect the level at which the learner is involved. Preclinical classes should concentrate on basic material (formative). The measurement instrument and the related evaluation should be based on lower level objectives. A learner in a preclinical or basic hematology class might only be evaluated on recognition of normal red and white blood cells. If there was difficulty in reaching this competency, additional instruction, practice, and evaluation would be necessary (diagnostic). When the learner reaches the clinical rotation, higher taxonomic levels must be addressed. Evaluation of the recognition of abnormal differentials would be required. In addition, the learner would probably be expected to correlate findings with a clinical diagnosis (summative).

Choosing the Instrument

It is imperative that the appropriate instrument be chosen for each behavior measured and evaluated. Objectivity, relevance, efficiency, and specificity must be considered when selecting a technique. If the affective domain objective—works effectively as a team member—is to be evaluated, a multiple choice examination will not be the correct measurement instrument.

It is always helpful if the instructor makes a blueprint of the proposed measurement/examination. The plan specifies the characteristics desired in the finished product. It ensures that the examination will measure the instructional objectives and course content in a balanced manner. Domain, quantity of questions, question's agreement with the objectives and taxonomic level should be included. This tabulation allows for ease in revision; items can be replaced with those that are identical in taxonomy and domain.

Cognitive Domain Measurement

The **short answer** and **completion** measurements both supply examination items that can be answered by a word, phrase, number, or symbol. A question is asked in the short answer item; the completion item consists of an incomplete statement with a space following for the answer. Suggestions for constructing short answer/completion examinations include

- keep the answer brief
- be original and direct
- follow the question with a blank equivalent in length to the desired answer

Essay questions should be used primarily for the measurement of those learning outcomes that cannot be measured by objective test items. An essay allows the evaluator to observe not only information but the learner's organization. It gives an indication of ability to synthesize and analyze. However, essays will only sample small content areas. In addition, it is difficult to obtain objectivity, and the essay results in excessive time spent in evaluating. Before scoring, the evaluator should list the areas/topics that must be covered in the response. Multiple evaluators are highly recommended.

Suggestions for constructing essay examinations are as follows:

- Avoid entirely if outcomes can be measured by objective instruments.
- Construct questions that call forth the particular outcomes desired.
- Be clear and concise, leaving no question as to what is desired from the learner.
- Indicate a time limit for each question.
- Avoid optional and/or extra credit questions.

Oral measurements are extremely beneficial during the formative and diagnostic periods. There is personal contact and a more relaxed atmosphere. Multiple assessors add objectivity. There is, however, inadequate standardization. Often irrelevant factors such as telephone calls interfere with the process. This method is also costly in the time used by the working professionals at a clinical site. The evaluator should be prepared to give an immediate evaluation that is objective and supportive.

If oral measurement is to be used formally in clinical education, then the evaluator must identify the level of the learner. Questions for a learner in the first weeks of a rotation would be expected to cover more basic information than one in the last week. Having a set of the objectives available at each rotation station is a valuable reference resource for bench evaluators.

True/false measurements, if utilized at all, should only be present during the formative period. These measurements must be free from ambiguity and irrelevant clues. Statements should be specific, positive, simple in structure, and equal in length. Learners have a 50/50 chance of guessing the right answer. If a learner correctly answers the question as "false," there is no assurance that the "true" response is known. Learners should be instructed to change any false statement into a true one. Many times students who have the ability to solve higher taxonomic level problems do not perform well on this measurement.

Matching examinations have limited usefulness. Matching is really a modification of a multiple-choice test; it is easier to construct, because all the author has to do is place one correct answer for each term and shuffle the choices. Matching can be appropriate for Level 1 outcomes used in the formative period. The author of matching measurements should remember to

- use only homogeneous material in a single exercise
- include an unequal number of items in each column and write specific instructions for answering
- keep the list brief
- place responses in logical order
- place all items for each matching unit on the same page
- avoid implausible choices

The **multiple-choice** examination is very versatile and can measure from the most simple to the most complex. There is ease in scoring, and it can be administered to large groups. These measurements are difficult and time consuming to construct. However, it is the measurement used most frequently in clinical programs, and it is the format for certification examinations.

If not written appropriately, cues can appear and an unprepared learner can guess the correct answer. When constructing these items, the problem must be stated in the *stem* (first part); all the *choices* (alternatives/distracters) must be plausible and relevant. Following are guidelines for editing multiple-choice items:

- Item refers directly to an established objective.
- There is only one correct answer.
- Language is direct, relevant, and devoid of excess wording.
- Stem contains as much of the problem as possible.
- Problem is stated in positive terms; if necessary to use a negative, the negative is capitalized, boldfaced, or underlined.
- Alternatives are similar in form and length.
- All alternatives are grammatically correct with the stem; each choice must combine with the stem to make a sentence.
- Alternatives are plausible and attractive to the lower achiever.
- Alternatives are arranged in logical order, for example, normal values or answers to math problems.
- Alternatives such as "none of the above" and "a and b" are rarely used and, if used, are absolutely necessary because no other plausible alternatives can be supplied.

Item Analysis

Item analysis is an effective tool that examines the agreement of the learner's answers with the acceptable responses for specific items on a measurement instrument/examination. If utilized for norm-based evaluation, the process is long and cumbersome. It is based on the separation of questions as they are answered by higher and lower achieving groups. A modified method can be used for competency-based/professional education. Competency-based measurements demonstrate the type of learning achieved. It is not based on separation of measurement items as they are answered by higher and lower achieving groups like the norm-based method.

Item analysis for professional education can be performed in various ways. One method is to list how many questions were answered incorrectly. Tabulation should be question/item specific and include the incorrect answer choices and the number of students involved.

If more than fifty percent of the class answers incorrectly, the item should be examined as to its reliability and validity. Questions to be answered about each item might include the following:

- Is there a related objective?
- Was the information stressed during instruction?
- Is the answer on the answer key correct?
- Is the item clear; should it be rewritten if used for another class?
- Should the item be included in the measurement instrument or discarded?

Psychomotor Domain Evaluation

Utilization of cognitive instruments to measure learning outcomes in psychomotor areas is difficult and inappropriate. Learning outcomes can be evaluated by

- observing the learner as he or she performs and describing his or her behavior
- Judging the quality of the product resulting from his or her performance
- Asking him or her for a self-report on performance

Observational methods seem to be the best way to measure and evaluate psychomotor performance.

Practical examinations are commonly used to evaluate a learner's psychomotor ability. Previously tested patients' samples are given to the learner so that substances such as antibodies, bacteria, or abnormal cells can be identified. This is a method that closely approximates actual laboratory work. It is mandatory that the criteria for grading a practical examination be published and given to the student at the time of administration. Each learner's practical examination must be evaluated using the same standards.

Anecdotal records are a short narrative of daily observations of the learner's performance. If an inaccurate record is kept, bias may result. This is not a freestanding evaluation tool. It is to be used to supplement and validate other observations. This is a good method to use during the formative period, but because the same individual must always record, it takes a great amount of time and may not be appropriate for the clinical portion of the education.

The **critical incident** evaluation is similar to the anecdotal record. It asks the evaluator to observe behavior that is necessary for competency in the profession. It records antecedents to and consequences of behavior. It is simple to construct but may be subjective, time consuming, and difficult to score. It is valuable for use in the diagnostic period.

Self-evaluation is difficult for the student to provide. This method offers awareness of present abilities and limitations. It also allows the learner to understand ramifications of procedures and bear the consequences of each decision. It prepares the learner for working in the profession; however, it needs an experienced guide/mentor. It should not be used for the summative evaluation.

Simulations concretely represent reality for a specific purpose. They allow for the evaluation of application of relevant knowledge and skills in a manner appropriate to the task. Simulations may be paper and pencil, audiovisual, simulated patients/role-playing, mannequins, or computer generated.

Role-playing involves the use of real situations that pose a problem. It is an effective technique for allowing learners to develop certain skills before applying them in a real life situation. Utilized within a group, it helps the other observer learners indirectly develop their skills. It is used best in the formative and diagnostic stages.

Difficulties in Observational Techniques

A prepared list of statements relating to performance of tasks is a **checklist,** which is often used with observational evaluations. It evaluates the skills and attitudes of the learner and usually consists of the type and number of procedures a learner is expected to perform. There is space for the evaluator to mark whether a particular test was done. Other details that might appear are whether the procedure was done according to laboratory policy; done, but did not meet criteria; never performed; and not observed. Feedback to the learner is immediate.

It is imperative that if a checklist is to be used as a measurement instrument then grading criteria be published. The learner should know what needs to be done to earn a passing grade or what constitutes unacceptable performance.

Usually a checklist is only used to keep track of a learner's progress. It is used in conjunction with a **rating scale.** The checklist is a set of defined traits on which learners are judged. The scale associated with each trait allows an indication of the extent to which the student possesses the trait. Five categories are usually utilized; the middle one would be the equivalent of an average "C" student. There should always be a space for evaluator and learner comments. The form should be signed by both the evaluator and learner.

The main limitation of this type of instrument is that there can be possible misuse resulting in a consequent decrease in objectivity, especially if there are multiple evaluators. It is mandatory that the use of the instrument be explained to every individual who will be involved with its administration.

Objectivity is extremely important in evaluation methods that use one of the observational techniques. Several errors can occur.

- Bias—evaluators tend to evaluate all students the same. Generosity error occurs at the high end of the scale; the evaluator is usually trying to avoid confrontation from the learners. Severity error places all learners at the bottom of the scale Central tendency error avoids both ends of the scale and makes every learner average.
- Halo—the evaluator rates on the general impression of a learner, which affects all evaluation characteristics. If the evaluator likes the learner, all areas will be marked very high; if the learner is not liked, all areas will be low even if that learner has earned a better evaluation. This error differs from the bias because each learner is evaluated differently.
- Logical—similar ratings are given for areas perceived to be related. An example would be giving a learner an excellent evaluation for the psychomotor domain because he always earns the highest mark on the cognitive examinations.

Proper design and use of measurement instruments followed by communication with those individuals who will be using them can eliminate most of these errors.

Affective Domain Evaluation

Instruments used in the evaluation of professional behavior in the affective domain are also based on observational techniques. Rating scales, anecdotal records, and critical incidents are useful in performing this task. Special attention must be paid to the construction of the affective domain objectives so that their outcomes are measurable. This category is probably the most difficult evaluation to perform.

Because subjectivity may be a problem when evaluating the affective domain behaviors, it is important that the objectives be checked for certain points. The desired behavior must

- match the competencies of the profession
- be appropriate for a learner
- not embarrass or punish the learner
- be objective, observable, and measurable
- belong in the affective domain

Guidelines to be followed when performing affective domain evaluation include

- publish the objectives.
- monitor the students before evaluation.
- confront any problems.
- offer assistance to the student.
- determine the severity of a problem before evaluation.

It is sometimes difficult for a student to adapt to professional behavior during the formative period.

Guidance and mentoring play an important role in developing the learner's professional behavior. Affective evaluations should be used at the end of the formative and throughout the summative stages.

Measurement and evaluation strategies for an instructional unit provide the feedback required to assess whether instruction has been effective. The goal of an instructional unit is to enhance the learner's knowledge and/or behavior. One can not ascertain whether the goal of an instructional unit has been met without proper measurement and evaluation strategies. Therefore, these strategies are critical to documenting the accomplishment of the goal for both the learner and the instructor.

BIBLIOGRAPHY

Beck, S., and V. LeGrys. 1996. *Clinical laboratory education.* 2d ed. Dubuque, Iowa: Kendall/Hunt Publishing Company.

Gronlund, N., and R. Linn. 1990. *Measurement and evaluation in teaching.* New York: Macmillan.

Neufeld, V., and G. Norman, eds. 1985. *Assessing clinical competence.* New York: Springer.

INTERNET RESOURCES

National Council on Measurement in Education. <www.ncme.org/pubs/emip.ace>

QUESTIONS

1. Differentiate measurement and evaluation. *(Objective 1, Level I)*

2. Define reliability and validity as it relates to construction of a measurement instrument. *(Objective 2, Level I)*

3. What is the difference between norm-based and competency-based education? *(Objective 3, Level I)*

4. Define formative, diagnostic, and summative levels of education as it relates to clinical education. *(Objective 4, Level I)*

5. List at least one advantage and disadvantage of each type of cognitive measurement instrument. *(Objective 5, Level I)*

Instrument	Advantage	Disadvantage
Essay		
True/False		
Matching		
Multiple Choice		

6. Summarize the value of item analysis. *(Objective 6, Level I)*

7. List at least one advantage and disadvantage for each type of psychomotor instrument. *(Objective 7, Level I)*

Instrument	Advantage	Disadvantage
Anecdotal record		
Checklist		

8. Discuss evaluation difficulties when using observational techniques. *(Objective 8, Level II)*

9. Summarize guidelines to be used when constructing affective domain instruments. *(Objective 9, Level I)*

10. Evaluate this multiple-choice question. *(Objective 10, Level II)*

    Indirect bilirubin will be increased in
    a. any disease in which the liver, as a large organ, is not working properly
    b. hemolytic disease
    c. the indirect portion is never elevated
    d. hyperparathyroidism

    a. good question
    b. ineffective question because of stem
    c. ineffective question because of distractors

11. The objective reads *(Objective 11, Level II)*

    List the reagents in the Sternheimer-Malbin stain.

    The question reads

    What color are hyaline casts when stained with Sternheimer-Malbin stain?

    Evaluate the relationship between the objective and the question.
    a. The relationship is clear; the question should be used.
    b. There is no agreement between the objective and the question; the question should not be used.

12. A technologist has a certain student baby-sit for her on the weekends. She evaluates this student at the highest level on the clinical rating scale. This is the highest evaluation the learner has ever received. What might be the evaluation problem? *(Objective 13, Level II)*

13. Every learner who is evaluated by the microbiology supervisor receives a "C" grade. What might be the evaluation problem? *(Objective 13, Level II)*

EXERCISES

Completion of the exercises will enhance your knowledge of measurement and evaluation strategies for an instructional unit. *(Objective 10, Level III, Objective 14, Level III, Objective 15, Level III, and Objective 16, Level III)*

1. Construct an affective evaluation instrument for a student rotation in blood bank.

2. Design a practical evaluation for mycology.

3. Review a multiple-choice examination and revise questions that do not meet the criteria for effective questions.

4. Perform a modified item analysis on an examination. Report your findings to the class.

5. Determine alternative ways of measuring and evaluating a student's psychomotor abilities in phlebotomy.

CASES

Analyze the following case studies and propose solutions. *(Objective 17, Level III)*

1. Learners perform below the national mean in chemistry on the national certification examination. What steps should be taken in analyzing this occurrence?

2. There is a technologist in immunology who always gives the students an "A" for the final grade in this rotation. What should be done to ensure objectivity in evaluation?

3. Another technologist in hematology is always complaining about "students who aren't as dedicated as we used to be." Her evaluations reflect this belief. What can be done about her allegations? If they are true, what should be done; if exaggerated, how can the technologist's perspective be changed?

4. A clinical laboratory technician student receives an evaluation in microbiology that he states is unfair. He says he thought that he was doing fine. What steps must be taken to solve this problem?

ANSWERS FOR QUESTIONS AND CASE COMMENTARIES

Chapter 1, Professionalism

ANSWERS FOR QUESTIONS

1. Profession—vocation with a body of knowledge defining the scope of the profession, code of ethics to advocate standards of excellence, professional society to promote dignity and social standing, certification agency for entry into the profession, and accreditation agency to establish educational criteria.

   Professional—one who practices the profession.

   Professionalism—providing quality in the total scope of practice.

2. ASCLS—developed body of knowledge and code of ethics.

   NCA—responsible for a national certifying examination.

   NAACLS—establishment of standards for medical technology/clinical laboratory science educational programs.

CASE COMMENTARY

1. There are perhaps several ways to approach this case. The physician is not behaving in a professional manner, and it is difficult to communicate while one is acting in this manner. Therefore, the first step would be to put the interaction on a professional basis by defusing the situation. One might say, "I regret you are having such a difficult time receiving your test results as I know you are seeking the best care for your patient. Could you give me some specific details so that I can help you address this situation?" Once the situation is defused, the problem can then be addressed. It is important *not* to react to this physician but to take control of the situation and *act*.

2. The major criterion to be considered is what is best for your client. The client may be the patient, the physician, or both. In some cases the client may prefer the less expensive, less accurate method, and in other cases the client may prefer the more expensive, more accurate method. Perhaps this testing procedure would be best as a "send out test" so that your client may select the appropriate method for a specific medical situation. The professional would base the decision on patient care quality, although cost may be a factor in deciding whether the test should be done "in house." Communications with the client regarding the differences in the two methods is a professional responsibility.

Chapter 2, Professional Ethics

ANSWERS FOR QUESTIONS

1. Medical ethics is the study of conduct and moral judgment relating to the practice of medicine.

2. Duty to the patient includes providing quality services through a high standard of practice and protecting the patient's privacy.

    Duty to colleagues and the profession includes dignity, honesty, integrity, reliability, good communications, and cooperative relationships with other professionals in order to provide quality care for the patient.

    Duty to society includes a commitment to the well-being of the community and complying with relevant laws and regulations.

3. B. Honesty is not listed as an ethical principle. Justice, autonomy, veracity, fidelity, and beneficence—nonmaleficence are listed as the ethical principles.

4. Deontological—right and wrong are inherent, action is independent of consequences, means are more valuable than end results.

    Teleological—end results are more valuable than means, action should be taken that produces the most benefit.

CASE COMMENTARY

1. The ethical problem could be identified as one of ethical dilemma because some individuals would benefit from the testing, yet the cost would be great. The ethical approach, either deontological or teleological, would depend on your viewpoint. There do not seem to be any practical alternatives. The item regarding contribution to the general well-being of the community from the Code of Ethics addresses this case. Interestingly, this case can be compared to the debate that occurred regarding testing all blood units using the HIV antigen test in addition to the antibody test.

2. The ethical problem could be identified as ethical distress or locus of authority. The ethical approach, either deontological or teleological, would depend on your viewpoint. Please note that you are answering the question "Should you insist upon drawing the blood?" and have not addressed the legal issue of whether you can actually draw the blood. No one should draw blood on a patient unless the patient's permission is given. Practical alternatives might include informing the physician and allowing the physician to interact with the patient. The Code of Ethics refers to preserving the dignity and privacy of patients and may apply to this case.

3. The ethical problem may be ethical distress, ethical dilemma, or locus of authority. The ethical distress and locus of authority exist because it is the responsibility of the physician to inform the patient regarding results, not the responsibility of the laboratory personnel. In many cases, it may be illegal or against hospital policy for the laboratory personnel to provide testing results unless approved by the physician. Therefore, if you read this case as "Should you tell the patient?" you have certain ethical problems to address. However, the question is "Do you believe the patient should be told the results?" This presents a different question, and the ethical problem would be ethical dilemma. The ethical dilemma is whether the patient should be told in this situation. If the patient is told the truth, the

patient may take drastic actions. The ethical approach, either deontological or teleological, to the ethical dilemma would depend on your viewpoint. There are really no practical alternatives because the patient is requesting the information. However, the patient's statement regarding life with cancer should be shared with the physician, so that the physician could be sensitive to the patient's attitude when presenting the information. Seeking to establish cooperative and respectful working relationships with other health professionals and preserving the dignity and privacy of patients, both found in the Code of Ethics, apply to this situation.

4. The ethical problem could be identified as ethical distress, ethical dilemma, or locus of authority. Ethical distress is the barrier regarding providing confidential information to an individual other than the patient. Ethical dilemma is what happens if I give information, what happens if I do not give information, and how is the friend and perhaps the public affected by the decision. And locus of authority is who has the authority to provide the information. Basically, all the ethical problem types could be involved. The ethical approach will depend on your viewpoint. There are no practical alternatives for this situation as the law (Health Insurance Portability and Accountability Act—HIPAA) is very specific that confidentiality of the patient is required. If a laboratorian knows a patient personally, it would be best to allow someone else to perform the test in order to avoid this conflict of interest. The Code of Ethics strongly addresses this in the pledge to preserve the dignity and privacy of patients. However, the contribution to the general well-being of the community in the Code of Ethics may be cited if the disease is communicable. It may be interesting to think of this case as strep throat and then determine your reactions. Then think of this case as HIV and note your reactions.

5. The ethical problem could be identified as ethical distress or ethical dilemma. In this case, the supervisor is a barrier presenting ethical distress; however, in deciding what to do, the individual may experience an ethical dilemma because actions may involve going above the supervisor or deciding to do nothing. The ethical approach would depend on your viewpoint. There are many practical alternatives, including talking with the coworker yourself, remaining at the job and doing nothing, terminating employment, or going to the next supervisor level. Sections of the Code of Ethics that apply to this case are maintain and promote standards of excellence in performing and advancing the art and science of my profession, uphold and maintain the dignity and respect of our profession, seek to establish cooperative and respectful working relationships with other health professionals, and contribute to the general well-being of the community.

Chapter 3, Resumé

ANSWERS FOR QUESTIONS

1. A. The purpose of a resumé is to get an interview.
2. Two resumé format styles are chronological and functional.
3. The chronological format is used to list the accomplishments in chronological order and no special skills or accomplishment should be emphasized. The functional format style is used to emphasize a special skill or accomplishment.
4. The cover letter should include the following:
   - Your name and a return address.
   - The employer's name, title, and address.

- Should be written to a specific person.
- Include in the first paragraph the reason you are writing, the position you are applying for, and how you heard about the position.
- Include in the second paragraph the reason you are interested in the position or the company, why you are qualified, and relate these to the employer's needs.
- Include in the last paragraph an appreciation for the employer's time in reviewing the cover letter and resumé. Request an interview or a meeting to discuss the position further. Include a contact phone number.
- In closing the letter be sure to add the word *Enclosure* two spaces below your signature.

CASE COMMENTARY

1. Under Campus Address heading, which includes 3333 Cliff View Ct., do not abbreviate Court. Court should be spelled out. Spell out Mississippi throughout the resumé rather than using abbreviation. Omit the Personal Data section. Under the section Background, the word American is misspelled.

2. Omit the word *resumé* in the title; you could increase the font of the title to enhance the heading. Boldfacing the category titles Career Objectives, Education, and so on would offset and enhance the overall appearance of the resumé. Consider changing the resumé format to a chronological style rather than centering all of the information. The high school award does not need to be included in the resumé. Spell out the names of the organizations ASCLS, MSCLS, ASCP, and the title MLT. The Reference section does not have to be included on the resumé.

Chapter 4, Job Description and Job Advertisement

ANSWERS FOR QUESTIONS

1. The job description document not only defines and provides a baseline for the performance tasks of the employee, but it defines the employee's interactions with people and how the position is integrated into the entire organizational scheme.

2.
   a. Title of the organization
   b. Job title
   c. Position summary
   d. Essential functions and duties
   e. Authority level
   f. Internal/External relationships
   g. Working conditions
   h. Qualifications and experience required
   i. Certification and/or licensure required

3. The job description is the basis for the advertisement, the interview, hiring, orientation, and evaluation. The job description is a way for the organization to clarify its expectations to the employee.

4. A. Name of the organization, position title, qualifications/experience required, and certification/licensure requirements.

CASE COMMENTARY

1. The first section of the advertisement is good. In the second and third paragraphs changes would include:
   a. A medical technologist/clinical laboratory scientist is certified not registered. Certification means someone has taken and successfully passed a national examination. Registration means simply your name is on a list somewhere. Many people confuse this because of the name "Board of Registry." However, when one passes the "Board of Registry," they are certified.
   b. Listing only one certification examination limits your ability to consider other candidates with equivalent certifications. It is also illegal to specify one specific certification when others are considered equal. Therefore, "CLS(NCA) or equivalent" should be used.
   c. The salary is not listed in the advertisement.
   d. The advertisement says call, but does not give phone number. Only an e-mail address is provided. If one really wants the candidate to call, a phone number should be listed.

2. This appears to be a communication problem. The employee received only a simplified job description and only very basic orientation; therefore, the employee does not appear to know what job performance is expected. The manager is expecting a higher level of performance. Remember, the job description makes the organization clarify the job expectations and is used to communicate to the new employee those expectations. To correct this situation and prevent it from happening in the future, the manager should carefully review and develop a detailed job description, share the job description with the new employee, and use the job description to develop the orientation list. If the employee is fully informed regarding the job and its expectations, then poor performance should be avoided.

Chapter 5, Employment Interview and Selection

ANSWERS FOR QUESTIONS

1. E. The employer's goals for the interview are to verify written information, evaluate the candidate's skills and personality, and ask questions to clarify information.

2. A. Establish social contacts. Candidate's goals for the interview include providing additional information; assessing the job, institution, and the individuals that will be colleagues; determining the benefit package; and asking clarifying questions.

3. E. Candidates should not make anonymous phone calls or make major changes to the previous submitted resumé.

4. E. All of the above. The candidate should make available a list of three references with relevant contact information, refrain from negative comments about past employers, make eye contact, and answer all questions completely and truthfully.

5. D. Appropriate dress would not include sandals or a tongue ring.

6. Professional maturity might be judged by listening carefully to how one has performed in the past given certain situations or posing situations and asking how the candidate would solve the situation.

7. E. It is illegal to ask age, religious, financial, or pregnancy questions unless these questions have a documented relevance to the job.

8. E. Components of the thank-you letter should include interview date, the position interviewed for, reemphasis of skills, and any additional information.

CASE COMMENTARY

1. Questions from the evening supervisor might include
    - In what area(s) do you most prefer to work?
    - In what area(s) do you least prefer to work?
    - Do you have a problem being designated as in charge on a rotational basis when the shift supervisor is off duty?
    - Where do you see yourself in two years? In five years?
    - Do you have a problem with performing phlebotomy draws when the supply of phlebotomists is low or when asked to do so?
    - Do you have a problem working weekends and holidays?
    - Do you see yourself as a team player? Why do you feel this is vital as a rotating technologist on this shift?

2. Reasons for the question may be to determine if the candidate meets the criteria for the position, if the candidate did homework in preparation for the interview, whether the candidate recognizes his or her abilities, or to identify areas for personal growth. Strengths may include ability to work well with other personalities or work as a team player, ability to set an example, ability to think and act in a positive manner, being goal oriented, thriving on challenges, adaptability, and ability to multi-task well. Limitations might include not having enough time to read all the current professional literature or balancing an intense desire to accomplish the work quickly and effectively with taking personal time for lunch. Note that the limitations state strengths.

3. Reasons this question might be asked would include to determine if the candidate fit the criteria for the position, the goal orientation of the candidate, the vision of the candidate, if the candidate and current supervisory personnel would be complementary, and length of employment plans. Responses might include "I would like to be working here and plan to have developed into an effective, respected supervisor with whom the staff feels comfortable. I would also like to be capable of making immediate decisions related to staffing and emergency response. I plan to have proved my value to this company by setting goals and attaining those goals for the benefit of the company and my colleagues."

4. This question should have no bearing on the candidate's ability to perform in the position. The question is inappropriate and probably is asked because the interviewer is concerned that children might inhibit one from doing the job. The candidate could respond by acknowledging the demands of the job and stating his or her ability to meet the demands of the job.

Chapter 6, Employee Evaluation

ANSWERS FOR QUESTIONS

1. E. The evaluation instrument should be related to job description, performance standards, and the reward system.

2. D. Vroom's expectancy theory includes
   a. the employee must expect (perceive) that high effort will lead to high performance.
   b. the employee must expect (perceive) that effort will lead to outcomes.
   c. the employee must have a preference for the outcomes.

3. a. Knowledge of the job
   b. Proximity to the person being evaluated
   c. Skill and training to conduct the evaluation
   d. Time to dedicate to the evaluation process

4. The most common reward is money; however, other rewards may include promotion, professional leave for attendance at workshops, flexible shifts, work assignment, reserved parking space, and so on. In order for the reward to motivate, however, the employee must have a preference for the reward.

5. When the employee first starts the job, the manager is in a telling mode that involves detailed task instructions and not much discussion regarding the quality of performance. As the employee matures, the manager assumes a selling role that involves task instructions, but now discussing quality of the performance. The next role for the manager is the participating role that involves minimum task instruction and much encouragement regarding the quality of the performance. The ultimate role that the manager would like to assume with all employees is the role of delegating, which involves little task instruction or quality of performance encouragement, because the employee is performing the job with quality and needs no instructions. Evaluation is needed at each phase of the employee's job development in order to assist the employee in moving to the next level. It is critical in the first phase to identify an employee who does not have the ability to perform the job. Even when the employee has reached the phase in which delegation is used, the employee must be evaluated and receive feedback on the performance to sustain performance.

CASE COMMENTARY

1. The new employee was not evaluated on a continuous basis during the probation period. Because everyone was friendly, the employee probably felt that she was doing a good job. This situation could have been avoided by periodic formal evaluations during the probation period. If the new employee had realized that her performance was not satisfactory, there would have been time for correction during the probationary period, and termination might have been avoided.

2. The problem is that the employee is receiving poor evaluation; however, no action is taken. Other employees in the department might view this lack of action as a signal that poor performance will not be addressed. They might feel that because poor performance is acceptable, they do not have to perform either. This situation is difficult because the laboratory manager is not participating in the evaluation process. The department supervisor might talk with the laboratory manager and explain the morale problem that no action could have

on the department. The department supervisor and the laboratory manager should decide whether the evaluation process is working. If the process is not working, they should decide how it could be changed. This situation puts the department supervisor in a very challenging position because the supervisor is honestly evaluating the department employees, yet is being undermined by the laboratory manager.

3. This evaluation process is performed as recommended. To encourage continuation of this excellent performance, the manager might decide to reward the individual. A variety of rewards are available and should be used not just with this new employee but with all employees.

Chapter 7, Employee Correction and Discipline

ANSWERS FOR QUESTIONS

1. E. The goal of the correction plan should be to salvage the employee and enhance the effectiveness of the institution.

2. The steps in the correction procedure are as follows:
   1) The first step is to talk with the employee informally to understand the situation, identify causes, and assist the employee in solving the situation.
   2) The second step is to issue a verbal warning that involves identifying the problem and performance that is needed, offering assistance, and keeping formal notes on the conference.
   3) The third step is a written warning that states the problem and the performance that is needed to demonstrate that the employee has overcome the problem. This is signed by the manager and the employee.
   4) The fourth step is a second written warning, sometimes accompanied by a suspension period. The employee is put on notice that any further occurrences of the problem will result in dismissal. The written warning is signed by both the manager and the employee.
   5) The fifth step is dismissal.

CASE COMMENTARY

1. You have already performed the first step by documenting and confronting the employee with the unacceptable behavior. At this point you may wish to treat your communications as informal. The employee has been honest with you regarding the problem of attendance, and perhaps you can direct the employee to individuals who might help find a less expensive child care situation. In addition, you might wish to consider scheduling options that would address the problem. However, the employee must understand that the behavior cannot continue. If the behavior is corrected, then be sure to praise the employee for attention to the problem. If the problem is not corrected, then the second step is to issue a verbal warning and keep notes on the conference. The third step is to issue a written warning that states the problem and states the performance needed. Signatures are obtained from both the manager and the employee. The fourth step is to provide another written warning with the information that if the problem occurs again, the employee will be dismissed. Upon occurrence of the problem again, the employee is dismissed. Please note that this is an attendance

problem and lack of attendance is a behavior that should be handled just like other problems in the laboratory. Of course, there should be a clearly written attendance policy that all employees are given the first day of work or perhaps even during the job interview.

2. As the manager, you are not dealing with the drug problem, but with the behavior resulting from the drug problem. You suspect a drug problem but have no proof; therefore, it is better at this point to deal with the behavior of poor performance. The same procedure as listed in #1 would be followed. Note: many hospitals have a drug testing policy, thus the manager must be familiar with the drug policy and carefully follow the procedure outlined in the policy.

3. The manager should take immediate action in this case. When one is threatened, especially with a weapon, the manager should call security and have the employee removed from the premises immediately. The manager does not follow the step as in #1 in a threatening situation.

4. The same steps as in #1 should be used starting with step 2.

5. Again the same steps as in #1 should be used; however, realize that this is secondhand information. You would need to document this behavior in order to take action; therefore, you would want to alert the evening shift supervisor to carefully observe the situation. Once documented you would proceed with the steps as in #1. This may be viewed as endangering patient care by the hospital and immediate dismissal may be possible. You should be familiar with your hospital policies regarding immediate dismissal.

Chapter 8, Celebrating Diversity

ANSWERS FOR QUESTIONS

1. Diversity may be summarized as a business's response to swift sociological and cultural changes. Internally, it is a means of providing employees an environment where they feel valued by and contribute to an organization. Externally, the organization is adaptable and perceptive about changes occurring in world markets.

2. According to Lebo (1996) diversity is needed in the workplace in order to increase competitiveness, increase the effectiveness of quality management, decrease employee turnover, and reduce cost. Decision making is enhanced by a more varied group because more ideas and approaches are present. Also, the diverse group reflects the consumer. If diversity is celebrated within the laboratory, employees feel comfortable in the workplace and are empowered to do their best. These factors reduce turnover and reduce cost.

3. Diversity issues include age, gender, nationalities and origin, religion, physical or mental challenges, sexual orientation, and so on.

4.
   a. Mature workers are ages fifty-five and older and constitute twenty-one percent of today's workforce.
   b. Baby boomers are ages thirty-nine to fifty-four and constitute fifty-two percent of today's workforce.
   c. Generation X workers are ages nineteen to thirty-eight and constitutes twenty-six percent of today's workforce.
   d. Generation Y workers are ages eighteen and younger and constitute less than ten percent of today's workforce.

5. a. The Glass Ceiling Commission is chaired by the Secretary of Labor.
   b. It is appointed by the current U.S. President.
   c. Its purpose is to work to identify "glass ceiling barriers" (those invisible and artificial barriers that prevent qualified individuals, such as women and minorities, from advancing into positions of responsibility).

6. Culture may be defined as customs, values, and traditions.

7. A few examples of cultural barriers include eye contact, gestures, and personal space. Asian colleagues may never look you in the eye when talking. As Americans, we may take this as a sign of shyness or that the person does not like us. In actuality, the Asian person is showing you respect by not looking you in the eyes, as this is a sign of disrespect in their native land. Also, in the United States, we normally vigorously shake the hand of our colleague as a sign of goodwill and character. The Native American population may consider this a sign of aggression. Personal space should also be considered when confronting colleagues. Usually in the United States a comfort zone of about eighteen inches is expected when talking to someone else. Mexican Americans tend to stand closer, as this is a sign of the importance of what is being said by the speaker (Dunlap 2001).

8. No.

9. a. The Age Discrimination in Employment Act was established to protect individuals who are forty years of age and older.
   b. This act simply states that
      1) an individual may not be terminated from his or her place of employment simply for growing old
      2) the recruitment of future employees should not be limited only to younger applicants
      3) denial of benefits to older employees is prohibited.

10. A. The hiring of handicapped persons

CASE COMMENTARY

1. The administrative assistant chief technologist may be breaking at least two job discrimination laws. First, he or she may be discriminating against Laser Jett based on his color, which is strictly prohibited by the EEOC. Second, he or she is in violation of the Age Discrimination in Employment Act.

   This is not an acceptable practice. If job discrimination laws are being broken protecting rights of job applicants, Laser Jett may file a complaint. This may lead to an investigation, which may cost the organization large amounts of money in litigation fees, not to mention money that may be paid out if lawsuits are filed by Laser Jett or by former job applicants. If it is determined by the EEOC that there are in fact unfair hiring practices, the institution may lose local, state, and federal funding.

   Because of Laser Jett's age, the administrative assistant chief technologist may have thought that he could have been in need of medical benefits within the next couple of years. He may have thought that going with the younger candidate would save the organization money in the long run by not having to pay health-care expenses.

2. The tech from Greece probably suggested the hemoglobin F and A_2 analysis because she has seen a variety of hemoglobinopathies in her previous experience in Greece. She recognized

the signs and symptoms of the patient. She is probably more able to relate to this case because of her cultural background and experience. She definitely increases the laboratory's effectiveness because she has a broader background in hemoglobinopathies and would naturally consider more possibilities than possibly the tech who had not had this background.

3. Hiring this individual will make your department more marketable within and outside your particular healthcare setting. If a patient who spoke only Spanish were to come into the laboratory or the ER, he or she would have difficulty communicating with English-speaking technologists. By having a technologist who can speak Spanish, he or she could communicate with the patient and then translate this information to the laboratory, doctor, and other members of the healthcare team. In addition, if you have doctors within the area who primarily speak Spanish, then your outreach program may be enhanced by a Spanish-speaking tech's participation.

4. Age is the diverse factor here, and each age contributes expertise to the situation. For example, the older tech seems capable of performing a CBC by older methods, because these are probably the methods the tech first used. However, the older tech may not have the expertise with the computer. Thus, the younger tech seems capable of consulting with the doctor on the computer assistance. The diverse ages allow your laboratory to serve more clients.

Chapter 9, Change

ANSWERS FOR QUESTIONS

1. C. Change is defined as anything that is different from what has been routinely done.
2. B. Change is not usually viewed as enjoyable.
3. The process that drives change may be diagrammed as follows:

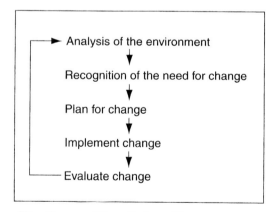

The Process That Drives Change

CASE COMMENTARY

1. Because this is a mandatory change, the manager is responsible for providing information to the employees regarding the necessity of the change. The manager should tell the employees of the change and share information as to why the hospital administration has made this decision. The manager might intercede with the hospital administration regarding the purchase of scrubs and the timing of the change. If there is any flexibility, employee needs should be considered.

2. The manager might decrease resistance to this change by explaining the problem with the present back-up system and asking employees how the system might be revised to solve the problem. This would include the employees in the change process, and a solution might be presented other than the one proposed by the chief technologist.

3. The first step would be to analyze the environment. What is happening now? Is there a problem that is causing this question? The second step would be to analyze the data that you have collected. If indeed it appears that having the nurses collect the blood would be more efficient, then the third step, planning for the change, should occur. In the planning stage, in-service education may be required for the nursing staff on the procedure for collection and the processing of the blood to the laboratory following phlebotomy. This will enable the nursing staff to ask questions and develop more confidence in performing a new task. After everyone is familiar with the procedure for the change, step 4, implementing the change, can occur. As the change is implemented, it should be monitored and, step 5, evaluated. After a period of time, the evaluation data should enable you to analyze the environment (step 1) and start the process again.

4. You have already analyzed the environment and recognized a need for change. Now you must plan for the change, implement the change, and evaluate it. Again, this is an excellent opportunity to involve the employees by identifying the problem and asking for possible solutions. The employees may have more information that, when added to your information, might provide a different solution than you otherwise would have implemented.

Chapter 10, Stress Management

ANSWERS FOR QUESTIONS

1. a. Eating balanced meals
   b. Exercising at least three times per week
   c. Getting plenty of sleep
   d. Participating in relaxation or family activities

2. OSHA holds employers legally accountable for job-related illnesses including stress-related problems.

3. Groups of work-related individuals comprise a work team, such as individuals working in the hematology department in a large hospital laboratory or the entire day shift in a small laboratory. These individuals must work together effectively without tension in the group. Therefore, a good way to diffuse group tension is for the group to interact outside of the work situation.

4. Professional Stress Management Program

   I. Stress
      A. Definition
      B. Causes
   II. Importance of physical health
      A. Nutrition
      B. Exercise
      C. Sleep
      D. Relaxation
   III. Importance of mental health
      A. Identification of personality traits
      B. Methods to change certain personality traits
   IV. Goal setting
      A. How to
      B. Problem solving
      C. Time management
   V. Social skill improvement
      A. Conflict resolution
      B. Assertiveness
      C. Social ties

CASE COMMENTARY

1. One way to address the stress within this group might be to arrange recreational activities, such as bowling, cookouts, and so on. If the group members related pleasantly outside of the work environment, it could alleviate barriers created at work, lead to better teamwork, productivity, and work environment, and ultimately eliminate some of the work-related stress for the employees. If this did not reduce the stress within the group, you would proceed with the steps in the stress management program.

2. This problem seems to be one that is stress related. Obviously, the stress of a new position, in addition to the family stressors, have overwhelmed the individual. One strategy would be to allow the individual to step down from the supervisor position permanently. You could also allow the individual a week off to attend to some of the stress factors with the family. Or you might chose to provide the individual with an assistant on the job or remove some of the responsibilities of the job, if possible, until family stressors were under better control.

Chapter 11, Professional Writing

ANSWERS FOR QUESTIONS

1. Accurate business communications are necessary because written documents represent you to the professional community and serve as documentation of your communications. As official documents, the recipient may file your letter, e-mail, report, or proposal for future referral. Your signature, initials, or e-mail address signify that the document has your approval and exists as a record of your opinions, statements, ideas, results, or ideas.

2. E. The phone number is not a part of the letter.

3. D. The credentials of the sender is not a part of the memo.

4. The purpose of a report is to provide information on a definite topic or results from a specific project.

5. The purpose of a proposal is to set forth a plan of action submitted for acceptance by an individual or group.

6. One of the following:
    Clinical Laboratory Science published by the American Society for Clinical Laboratory Science
    Laboratory Medicine published by the American Society for Clinical Pathology
    Journal of Clinical Microbiology published by the American Society for Microbiology
    Transfusion published by the American Association of Blood Banks
    Clinical Leadership and Management Review published by the Clinical Laboratory Management Association

7. The format for scientific journal articles includes the following parts:
    a. Abstract
    b. Introduction
    c. Material and methods
    d. Results
    e. Discussion or conclusion

8. Peer review is important for submissions to professional journals because peers, or persons in the same profession, share the goal of providing quality continuing education and news of discoveries for members of the organization and for readers of the journal.

9. A journal article is submitted to the publication editor. The editor of the journal will send copies of the article to two or three volunteers who serve on the editorial board of the journal. These volunteer peer-reviewers assess the article and recommend acceptance or rejection of the article based on the journal's standards, purpose, and audience. Articles that are recommended for publication are frequently returned to authors with editorial recommendations for improvement. The author may make the suggested changes or explain why the change would not enhance the article. The author signs an agreement with the journal's publisher to assign copyright to the publisher. After an article is accepted for publication, the author will receive the final copy of the article, or page proofs. Page proofs display the article as it will appear in the journal. It is the author's responsibility to check the page proofs for accuracy.

10. A. The purpose of an abstract is to provide a mechanism to introduce preliminary or completed research results to the professional audience quickly.

11. Corrections for letter.

August 13, 2002 — *Move date*

Sandy Johnson — *Capitalize "J." Move inside address over sender's information*
Software specialist
SOFTWARE.com
5960 Bryson Street
Baltimore, MD 21110

Jody Blue
Laboratory Information Officer — *Correct spelling of officer and information*
County Hospital — *Correct spelling of Hospital*
Red Creek, MD 21900

Dear Ms. Blue:

SUBJECT: Software demonstration on August 12, 2002, at County Hospital, Red Creek, MD
More accurate description of visit

Sample of a rewrite
Note use of more formal language than original version.

Thank you for your review of SOFTWARE.com demonstration materials. I appreciate your comments. I believe SOFTWARE.com can design a product that will be useful in your laboratory. I will contact you when the custom software is completed. I hope you will visit our exhibit at the ASCLS meeting. I look forward to working with you in the future.

Sincerely, — *More appropriate for business letter*

Sandy Johnson

Letter Corrections

CASE COMMENTARY

1. A proposal is the best type of communication for requesting an instrument and will provide the administrator with more detailed information. Prepare a proposal that includes a statement of purpose, a statement of the problem, the solution—including facts about the current situation and how a new instrument would provide a solution, and a brief conclusion.

2. A report should have been prepared. A financial report contains specific facts and figures necessary to evaluate the financial status of the department. Note: An administrator should make clear his or her expectations concerning a document. It would not be unusual for an administrator to provide a format for a detailed report.

3. A proposal should be prepared. The proposal should include a title, benefit for the institution, the cost, the proposed date for implementation, method of notification of employees, background information, and, if they support your proposal, sample dress codes from other laboratories.

4. The fastest means is submission of an abstract to propose a presentation at a scientific meeting. The smaller the meeting, the easier it is to have an abstract accepted. Larger meetings may have more stringent criteria for acceptance but will have a larger number of attendees. The method of communication that will reach the greatest audience is a journal article. However, journals often have a significant lag time between preparation and submission of a manuscript and publication. Many journals will accept for publication manuscripts that contain previously presented information from a poster or oral presentation. The best approach may be to submit an abstract for a presentation at a meeting and follow that with preparation of an article for publication in a journal. Note: Other options for consideration also exist, although these methods are not directly considered in this chapter. One may make use of a professional society's list to contact members, or one may create a Web page to promote an idea. Both may be excellent mechanisms for disseminating information.

5. The poster title should be in a large font, and other written material should be readable from a distance of four feet. Include colored charts, tables, diagrams, and photographs. Hint: Prepare one-page summarized handouts for participants who view your poster. Include contact information (phone, address, fax, e-mail) on the handout.

Chapter 12, Communications and Interpersonal Relationships

ANSWERS FOR QUESTIONS

1. C. Five purposes of communication are Informative, Affective, Imaginative, Persuasive, and Ritualistic.

2. Primary routes of communication are verbal, nonverbal, and paraverbal.

3. Paraverbal is how we say what we say.

4. Barriers to communication include the following:
    1) Nonverbal barriers include body language, eye contact, eyes rolling or shut, and so on.
    2) Verbal barriers would include using words that were unfamiliar to a person due to nationality or race.
    3) Paraverbal barriers include things such as the tone being too high, speaking too fast, the pitch being too high, and the volume being too loud or too low.
    4) Environmental barriers include temperature of the room, proper dress, proper use of cologne or perfume, neatness and cleanliness of hair, and so on.
    5) Overcommunicating is a barrier in which too much communication at any one time is given.
    6) Undercommunicating is not giving enough information for the person to understand what you want him or her to do or understand.
    7) Communicating at inappropriate times, such as when the person is busy doing another task or talking to someone else.

5. Four styles of communication are the following:
   1) Concrete sequential—likes to focus on ideas or tasks, thinks methodically and predictably, slow to adjust to change.
   2) Abstract sequential—prefers learning from logical presentation of ideas, relies on logical impersonal analysis, creates theoretical models from a wide range of information, is slow to decide, is less concerned with people than ideas.
   3) Concrete random—prefers learning from trial and error, relies on experience-based information, makes decisions based on finding solutions, is quick to decide, is a risk taker, relies more on people than technical analysis for information.
   4) Abstract random—prefers learning from lots of free-form ideas, is an intuitive thinker, balks at structure, likes to generate new ideas.

6. Intrapersonal communication is communication with one's self. Interpersonal communication is exchanges with other people.

7. Sources of conflict include
   1) scheduling
   2) communication breakdown
   3) staffing problems or solutions
   4) costs or financial issues
   5) pressure
   6) personality
   7) inadequate interpersonal skills
   8) expectation of others
   9) administrative skills

8. E. Advantages of excellent communications include the following: helps to change an organization by getting all employees aligned, speeds up the decision process, creates proactive behavior, and improves all working relationships.

CASE COMMENTARY

1. Verbally she agreed to work the shift. The nonverbal response, turning her back and stomping away, let the supervisor know she was not happy about working and was really saying no to being asked. How we say what we say is the paraverbal part of communication. In this case, the tone of her voice also let the supervisor know she was not happy about working even though she gave a positive response to the question. Her response was more passive aggressive. She said she would work but her nonverbal and paraverbal responses were aggressive. The supervisor should meet with the employee in the office, away from other employees, to discuss her response to your request. She should be told that her response, even though she agreed to work, was not appropriate—that you appreciate her working, but her response told you that she really did not want to work the weekend. The supervisor should ask her why she responded the way she did. Other questions that might be asked include was there a reason she could not work or did she know of someone else who might need or want the overtime.

   There are several ways to ask someone to do something for you. In this particular case, it probably would have been better to call the employee into the office and ask her in a different way. You could start out asking if the employee had plans for the weekend, and if she did could she change them easily. The employee, most of the time, feels that a negative response cannot be given to a supervisor. A supervisor must remember that all employees have lives away from the job, and we should take that into consideration when requesting someone to work or to do anything that might affect their lives outside the job. This style of communication would indicate open communications and show respect for the employee.

2. This is a classic barrier to effective communication. The manager should never communicate important changes in procedures or policies when the employees are busy doing something else. When they are busy concentrating on their daily tasks, they cannot assimilate all of the information you are giving them. The manager should always make sure that they are able to absorb the information correctly.

A solution to the problem would be to have a meeting with all of the staff at a time when they are not busy. This could be done more than once to enable all employees to attend. Make sure that you outline the policy and that you cover the same information in each of the meetings. You also should give them a copy of the policy and let them take it and read it later, so that they can fully understand the policy. Also, have a question and answer period during the meeting to allow them to ask questions. If you are not really familiar with the policy, you might want to include someone from Human Resources to help with the explanation and to answer questions.

Chapter 13, Motivation

ANSWERS FOR QUESTIONS

1. Motivation is the factor that inspires a person to act.

2. **Maslow's Hierarchy of Needs**

    Maslow identified physiological and safety needs as basic physical needs that would motivate if not satisfied. Satisfaction of physical needs is required before higher level social needs, such as esteem and love, will motivate. If the physical and social needs are satisfied, motivation will occur as a result of growth needs, such as self-actualization. Therefore, the hierarchy of needs are the following: physical needs—social needs—growth needs.

    Herzberg's Two-Factor theory

    Herzberg identified two factors: 1) the basic needs, hygiene factors, that correspond primarily with Maslow's physical and social needs, and 2) motivators, that correspond primarily with Maslow's growth needs. Herzberg's theory differs from Maslow's theory in that Herzberg indicates only the growth needs motivate, and there is no hierarchy in that unsatisfied needs could occur in both the hygiene and motivator areas at the same time.

    Vroom's Expectancy theory—(Adapted)

    The theory can be expressed as

    $E_I \times E_{II} \times$ Net Preference = Motivation

    The independent variables are 1) the individual's expectation (perception) of the probability that high effort will lead to high performance (E_I), 2) the individual's expectation (perception) that high performance will lead to outcomes (E_{II}), and 3) the individual's preference for the outcome (net preference).

3. C. Net preference problem

4. A. Maslow's theory. The insurance need would be a physical need according to Maslow and a hygiene factor according to Herzberg. Hygiene factors do not motivate.

5. E. Hygiene factor and physical need. Body fluid protection precautions would be a safety need.

CASE COMMENTARY

1. According to Maslow's theory, more money would motivate. However, according to Herzberg's theory, money is a hygiene factor and would not motivate. An EII problem would be identified using Vroom's theory, and money would have to be provided to motivate the individual.

2. According to Maslow's theory, the manager has satisfied all the physical, social, and growth needs. Activities that provide more growth needs, such as self-actualization, would probably be required to motivate the individual. The same is true of the Herzberg theory, because the manager is operating in the motivators level. According to Vroom's theory, the net preference would have to change to motivate this manager.

3. In example #1, the only motivator would probably be money because this would be an urgent issue for the employee and the family of the employee. In example #2, the hospital administration might provide additional advancement, and the net preference would change positively if the advancement was desired by the manager. Do you have other ways you believe the individuals could be motivated?

4. The problem according to Vroom is an EII problem. To increase their motivation, the manager might have the administration reward them for some work accomplishments. This would increase the employee trust in the reward system. Be very careful though, because if the administration rewards an individual that does not deserve the reward, then the reward will not be viewed by the other employees as a reward.

5. Seek for rewards within the manager's control. For example, designating someone employee of the month with a party and perhaps a designated desired parking space. Work assignment adjustments, continuing education opportunities, flexibility in scheduling, and so on are some items that could be within the manager's control to use as rewards.

6. According to Vroom, the problem is an E_I problem. The employee does not believe that he can do the job. Retraining including having an experienced sympathetic phlebotomist accompany him to the nursery several times and providing a mentor for the probation period might increase his ability and confidence. Of course, if at the end of the probationary period the individual still cannot perform, the manager would have to consider termination. As a manager you want to do all you can to salvage the individual if possible because the laboratory has a monetary investment in the recruitment expense, training time expense, and expense of allowing decreased productivity for this individual during the probation period. Also, on a humanitarian level, you would like to see all your employees succeed.

Chapter 14, Leadership

ANSWERS FOR QUESTIONS

1. E. Leadership is employing management skills, people skills, and vision to accomplish the work of the organization.

2. a. Tannembaum and Schmidt theory describes a leadership style continuum from authoritative to democratic.
   b. McGregor's X theory relates to the authoritative leader, whereas the Y theory relates to the democratic leader.
   c. Blake and Mouton described five types of management situations: 1) the impoverished management characterized by a low concern for people and production, 2) the authority-compliance management characterized by a low concern for people but a high concern for production, 3) the middle-of-the-road management characterized by medium concern for people and production, 4) country club management characterized by high concern for people but low concern for production, and 5) the team management characterized by high concern for people and production.
   d. The Hersey-Blanchard theory is based on the maturity of the follower. The ultimate goal of the leader is to motivate the follower to advance in job knowledge and responsibility.
   e. Fiedler indicated the style used by the leader may vary according to the situation, with a very favorable or very unfavorable situation requiring a task-oriented leader and a moderately favorable or moderately unfavorable situation requiring a relationship-oriented leader.

3. Position authority and personal authority.

4. B. Departmentalization will route the work to several departments, and the number of tests for the technologists to control will be less.

5. The leader's authority would be divided into the different departments, and the leader would have to delegate to supervisors of the departments, because it would probably be impossible for the leader to supervise all the work.

6. The group operating is the informal group. The manager might decide to use the informal communications by sharing information with the individuals in the group so that accurate information could be communicated.

7. If the situation is very bad or very good, the group will usually accept a leader with an authoritative leadership style; however if the situation is neither very bad nor very good, the group will usually want a leader with a democratic leadership style.

CASE COMMENTARY

1. a. Delegating situation
   b. Telling situation
   c. Delegating situation
   d. Selling situation

2. a. The leader should not interfere with the employee.
   b. The leader should tell the employee how to do the job.
   c. The leader should take the employee back to the participating situation by asking the employee for a reason for the performance. Then the leader should work to help the employee move back to working with proficiently in the delegating situation.
   d. The leader should continue to observe the performance and comment on performance.

3. Using the Getzels and Guba theory, the leader should observe the personality and need-dispositions of the potential supervisor to determine whether these matched the role and expectations of the position.

4. Very good management situation: the best leadership style would probably be democratic or participatory, but any style could be accepted. A difficult situation: an autocratic leadership style might be the best. For most people, the style would change depending on the situation; therefore, one would agree with Fielder.

5. In the Blake and Mouton model, in a good management situation the best leadership style would probably be the team management style. In a difficult situation, the authority-compliance management style might be the best.

6. In designing the laboratory, the following issues must be addressed: Decentralization—allows decisions to be made closer to the work, but there is less control by leader; Departmentalization—allows for more specialization, but there is more isolation of the work and possibly workers; Unity of command—provides for only one boss but if boss is inefficient, then unit will be inefficient; Scalar principle—provides for organized communications, authority, and responsibility, but inhibit communications, which may dilute authority and responsibility; Exception principle—allows the worker to do the work without having to check on every step but can be a source of errors; and Delegation of Authority—disburses the workload so more can be accomplished, but the leader may have to accept that tasks may not be done the way the leader wishes. As the designer of the laboratory, one must consider efficiency and effectiveness and the leader of the laboratory must be selected carefully, as the leadership style must match the design of the laboratory or the design must be changed.

Chapter 15, Team Building

ANSWERS FOR QUESTIONS

1. C. forming, storming, norming, performing

2. Suggestions for early stages of team development follow:
   - Have the team work together on short-term challenges. This allows for the process of working together, talking to each other, and building relationships.
   - Have team meetings outside the work environment. Team social events or parties are great ways to allow members the opportunity to socialize without the pressures of work-related tasks.
   - Have the team research traits of successful teams. This will encourage these traits in your own team members.
   - Engage in team development exercises. A team development exercise is one that focuses on developing positive images of team members.

3. Benefits include 1) team members are empowered to do the work, 2) shared responsibilities relieve individual stress of employees, 3) a sense of ownership develops when employees are involved in decision making, 4) a sense of accomplishment develops when employees learn more about the overall work process, 5) communication barriers are brought down when the employee is allowed to freely contribute ideas, 6) staff retention increases when employees are more satisfied with their jobs, and 7) productivity of staff is increased.

4. A. Employees as a group solving work issues

5. Major characteristics of a quality circle follow:
   - The program centers around management having a simple desire to build up their employees.

- The program is not mandated by management but is strictly voluntary.
- All employees need to be involved—input is desired from all of the people.
- Group effort is the focus, not individual effort.
- Both the employees who participate and management should be trained so that techniques are there for employees to choose from to avoid frustration.
- Each person helps the others grow.
- A creative environment will develop when members and management encourage and support any and all ideas.
- All tasks that the team takes on must relate to their work.
- All team members need to develop an attitude of partnering for the benefit of improving the quality of their work.
- Rewards are normally not monetary, but include items such as patches, hats, T-shirts, certificates, and so on—all members of the group will be recognized.
- There are team leaders who are selected by the team members and they serve in a facilitating role to guide the team through its initial development stages.

6. Benefits of quality circles include
   - increased productivity
   - increased communication from team member to team member and from team to management
   - decrease in the number of errors
   - a more positive environment
   - increased quality of patient care
   - increased job satisfaction

7. Relevant team-building points worthy of remembering as a manager follow:
   - Keep a checklist of the motivators and refer to the list regularly to ensure that all these motivators are being utilized systematically to keep the interest and enthusiasm of the employee at a high level. The list of motivators, other than money, might include such items as increasing the level of responsibility of the member, honoring the individual publicly or with a change in title or work space, designating a parking space for a set period of time, giving an employee of the month award, and so on.
   - Verbalize performance expectations. It is also important to put these expectations in writing and relate the individual performance to the goals and objectives of the laboratory. Ensure that the staff stays informed about the successes as well as the setbacks that the laboratory is experiencing. It is important to communicate future plans or projects of the lab to all staff as these plans are developed and allow for staff input when possible. Allow staff members the control over the work they do, and they will develop ownership in the organization. This will give rise to increased interest in the company as a whole, and they will try much harder to do a good job.
   - Praise the staff for their hard work. A phrase that is most effective and a memorable motto is to remember to praise employees in public and discipline them in private.
   - Encourage both personal and professional growth in employees.
   - Have an open-door policy, and make certain that you appear approachable to staff when conflicts arise that they need to discuss. Keep in mind that a good laboratory manager will not fly off the handle or take matters too personally. A good manager will not allow a few problems to overshadow a positive outlook. It is important to consider an employee's feelings.
   - Remember to hire people that are smarter that you—this truly shows that you are a wise manager.
   - If you want to know what motivates your employees, simply ask them.
   - Value the minds of employees as resources.
   - Manage like you have no authority whatsoever. Lead by the quality of your ideas.

- Find the squeaky wheels and don't jump so quickly to oil them. A great idea may surface.
- When listening and collaborating with an employee, seek to understand and not just to find agreement.
- Encourage employees to bring solutions with their problems or concerns.

CASE COMMENTARY

1. The first step is to determine the exact problem. The problem seems to be that each department is only concerned about the work in the individual department, and there is no responsibility for the total laboratory performance. The question is *why* does this situation exist? This situation could be due to several factors. It could be due to isolation of the individuals structurally, and you might investigate the layout of the laboratory. Structural modifications might be necessary. This situation could be due to lack of recognition of the expectation that employees are to assist one another. Good communications by the manager could alleviate this problem. Or this situation could be due to individuals only being familiar with individuals in a particular department. You might have all the laboratory employees meet outside the work environment to allow them to socialize without the pressures of the work environment. Hopefully, this would build relationships and thus a desire to assist each other. You also might develop a short-term challenge to allow them to work together and build relationships. You could assign the informal leaders to investigate ways effective teams operate and make suggestions to you as to how the laboratory work could be more effectively handled by the group. Perhaps the administrator could be encouraged to give awards for total laboratory performance, thus encouraging them to work together.

2. Good communications are essential in this situation. As manager, you might want to hold a meeting for all the laboratory employees to discuss the situation. Getting the employees involved would empower them to make recommendations and suggestions as to how the team would handle the situation. It also would allow the team to address the situation as a responsibility of the entire team. The manager should approach the situation positively, using this as an opportunity for the team to be creative. Involvement of the team would perhaps increase the satisfaction and productivity of the staff and avoid frustration. If the laboratory is too large, team leaders could be used to accomplish the goals of one large meeting. Rewards should be developed for the entire team when the creative ideas are accomplished and the situation is handled. After successfully solving this situation, the laboratory team would be experienced and more willing to address any new situations that occur.

Chapter 16, Conflict Management

ANSWERS FOR QUESTIONS

1. disagreements

2. Avoiding—avoid the issue. Lose-lose approach—neither side is satisfied.

   Accommodating—adapt to the circumstances of the issue. Lose-win approach—one side is satisfied, but the other is not.

   Compromising—each side gives up something. Lose-lose approach—neither side is satisfied.

Forcing—one party exerts power over the other party. Win-lose approach—one side is satisfied.

Collaborating—working together to solve the issue. Win-win approach—both sides are satisfied.

3. a. forcing
   b. accommodating
   c. collaborating

CASE COMMENTARY

1. The conflict is between Nurse Precise and Phleb. Phleb is working hard, but he is the only phlebotomist. Nurse Precise has learned to expect her results at 3:00 P.M. As manager, you might begin by investigating the situation to be sure that Phleb is performing his job in an efficient manner and that Nurse Precise must have her patient's blood drawn at exactly 3:00 P.M. Assuming that Phleb is working as efficiently as possible and Nurse Precise must have the blood drawn at 3:00 P.M., then you might rearrange the phlebotomy schedule giving Phleb some help—this would be an accommodating approach. If, however, Nurse Precise did not need her blood drawn at exactly 3:00 P.M., then you might want to use the compromising or collaborating approach to solve the situation.

2. The conflict is that Rumor, Idle, and Chatter are not following the fire evacuation procedure. As the manager, you are responsible to ensure that all procedures are enforced. Therefore, you have no other alternative but to use the forcing approach in this situation for the safety of the employees. There is no time to discuss this situation, the employees must simply abide by the procedure.

3. The conflict is between the hospital administrator and the lab personnel regarding the dress policy. As manager, the hospital administrator is your superior, therefore, this might be a good time to use the accommodating approach and have all laboratory personnel avoid jeans. At a later date, you might wish to use collaborating with the hospital administrator to establish some days that jeans might be worn so that your employees realize that you did present their views on dress. There is another problem though, and that is one of a lack of dress policy. As a manager, do your homework and be prepared to present a reasonable dress code policy when the opportunity arises. Remember, you have earned credits by accommodating immediately, which perhaps can be used in the future to address the laboratory personnel's wishes regarding dress.

4. The conflict is confusing in this case. The conflict appears to be between you and Ms. Friendly because you have been told she is not doing her job. But this is a situation that needs clarification. As manager, you need to gather more facts, thus the avoiding approach might be the best first approach. Perhaps the conflict is between Mr. Guy and Ms. Friendly. Mr. Guy could be hurt because Ms. Friendly is now spending her time with Mr. Handsome. If you investigate and find out that Ms. Friendly is not carrying her share of the workload, then you might choose to use forcing or collaborating depending on the situation. However, if Ms. Friendly is carrying her share of the workload and the department is productive, then perhaps you will choose to continue the avoiding approach because this seems to be a personal matter between the participants. However, interpersonal situations can decrease the productivity of a section. If the productivity is being adversely impacted, then staffing changes may be necessary, which could be considered the forcing approach.

5. The conflict is between the individuals working in Chemistry and the individuals working in Hematology. This case calls for a collaborative approach to reach the best solution for each department, the lab and the client. If collaboration fails, then compromise might be used. The collaborative approach would give you and the department personnel a chance to come up with a solution neither of you has considered. The compromise approach would allow each department to receive part of their request. For example, the shared tech could alternate between the departments.

Chapter 17, Telephone Etiquette

ANSWERS FOR QUESTIONS

1. Proper telephone etiquette is important to the laboratory operation because it conveys to customers that their concerns can be handled in a competent and professional manner.

2. Basic telephone etiquette rules when answering a call include the following: be polite—even if the other party is not polite; if you have to put someone on hold, be honest and tell them approximately how long it will be; avoid a speakerphone when possible; be helpful; listen carefully; know your laboratory; be interested; whenever possible avoid voice mail, and when voice mail is necessary be sure to return calls quickly.

3. Basic telephone etiquette rules when making a call include the following: be polite; identify yourself; remember that the other person may be busy, and when possible allow a call back; give full information on voice mail; politely ask that a speakerphone not be used if confidential information is to be discussed.

CASE COMMENTARY

1. If your laboratory manager is on the telephone when you need to ask her a question, it would be best, for you and for her, to leave and come back later. If you interrupt her conversation, she will probably be annoyed and most likely won't give you her full attention. Also, it would be rude to "hang around" until she hangs up.

2. The best action to take is to look the result up yourself. We are all in the business of patient care regardless of what department we are in at the time. You can never go wrong by making the welfare of the patient your first priority. If the nurse has a question about the result, the sample, and so on it would then be appropriate to transfer her call to the Chemistry department, making sure that someone in that department is aware of the STAT nature of the call.

3. If you suspect that you are on speakerphone and you think that you may possibly be discussing private or confidential information about someone, politely ask the other person to take you off of speakerphone so that there is no question regarding confidentially.

Chapter 18, Customer Satisfaction/Public Relations Program

ANSWERS FOR QUESTIONS

1. Anyone who is a recipient of an output of service is a customer, for example, patients, visitors, physicians and their staff, and other health-care providers.

2. RESULTS: Customers expect superior results from our product or service. They expect the product or service to be the best value for their money.

   RELATIONSHIP: Customers expect a relationship that is consistent with their value system.

   RESOURCE: Customers expect you to be a resource to help them solve a problem.

3. The facts that dissatisfied customers tell eight to ten people about their bad experience and that it costs five times as much to attract a new customer than to keep an existing one should be used in the argument.

4. There are several strategies that can be used by the health-care manager to be sure the customer is satisfied with the service provided.
   a. Hire service-savvy employees. This is done by using certain criteria when conducting the interview. Look for eye contact, a smile, the tone of voice, the way he or she speaks, the handshake, and the use of certain words such as *please* and *thank you*.
   b. Establish high standards of customer service. Does your staff serve customers in a consistent manner? Establish service standards that clearly tell your staff what you expect of them when they are serving customers. Include these standards in your job description and appraisal tools.
   c. Help your staff hear the voice of the customer. Give your staff the tools to work with and allow them to hear and deal with the customer's complaints directly. They must be able to take ownership of the process.
   d. Remove all barriers so that staff can serve the customer. The first person you need to change is yourself. What are your own motives and bias against action? If you are determined to remove barriers for staff, it is going to take work from everyone, including you.
   e. If possible, reduce anxiety to increase satisfaction. Any situation can cause anxiety for the customer. This may be waiting for an appointment, finding a parking place, answering insurance questions, anticipating news on the results of tests, or worrying about being on time for the appointment. Anxiety can cause a downward spiral for the customer, which may affect the employee. As caregivers, we can increase customer satisfaction by focusing on and preventing or reducing customer anxiety. Customers need to feel we are going above and beyond our normal responsibilities to reduce their anxiety.
   f. You need to help the staff cope better in a stressful atmosphere. Help the staff improve workspace to reduce stress. Involve the staff in creating a space that fosters calmness, efficiency, and comfort. Help them develop coping skills that will allow them to take better care of themselves during stressful times. Try to build a supportive work team that helps each other in stressful times in order to avoid getting caught in the downward spiral of anxiety.
   g. Always maintain your focus on service. Integrate your service focus into your everyday activities and routines.

CASE COMMENTARY

1. The customer in this case is the patient, patient's family, and the nursing staff. To address the problem, the manager first should investigate to see if what the nurses are saying is true. If it is not true, then following up with the nursing manager of the unit would be appropriate to let her know that perhaps their assumptions are not true in this particular case. However, if an investigation shows that the phlebotomist is not properly trained, then the phlebotomist should be pulled from this particular duty until retrained. This training should be under the direction of a more proficient phlebotomist and include not only written training and documentation but also documented observation of the phlebotomist performing the procedure correctly. It is most important in neonates or any other pediatric patient that the stick is done properly and with the least amount of trauma. As a part of your customer satisfaction program, the manager would constantly monitor satisfaction with the work of the laboratory via surveys, direct communication, and so on. To prevent this situation from occurring, the phlebotomy training program should be of such quality that a phlebotomist would never be approved to perform this task if they did not have the skills.

2. The physician group is the primary customer, and this situation must be handled carefully. The patient is the secondary customer in this situation. The manager must help the physician group understand that it is extremely important for the orders to be coded correctly. The physician group must understand that coding is not only required by Medicaid and Medicare, but also by independent insurance companies. Miscoding or no coding of the orders can constitute fraud under federal government guidelines and can potentially cause the funds to be pulled from the institution. Resolution of the coding problem is in the best interest of both the provider and the customer. The best people in the physician's group with which to start would be the office staff. This is usually where the coding occurs. The staff must understand the importance of proper and correct coding and its effect on the hospital's revenue and accreditation. They must understand that improper coding may affect the physician's practice if the federal government or insurance company feel that the office is committing fraud by either coding up or down to affect the reimbursement of funds. With care, this situation can be addressed and the provider, the customer, and the patient will benefit.

3. Before submitting the proposal, make sure you, as the manager, know the needs of the physician practice. You need to know what they expect from you, and you need to know what you can actually do for the practice. Listen to the customer. Do not promise the practice something you cannot do. Remember, you must have high standards of service. Other important initial questions to ask include the following:
    a. When do they need pick-up service and how many times a day?
    b. Do they need pick up seven days a week and on holidays?
    c. Do they expect you to supply them with the materials to do phlebotomy and other types of collection devices?
    d. Do they want to do the phlebotomy on the patients, or do they want you to provide a phlebotomist for them?
    e. Do they want to bill the patient, or do they want you to do the billing for them?

   (Note: on Medicare and Medicaid patients, you will probably need to do the billing.) When all of these questions are answered, you then must look at your competitors and derive a proposal that you and the physician practice can implement. By all means be realistic. Again, be reasonable and do not make promises or proposals you cannot keep. Your proposal and subsequent work should astonish the customer and surpass expectations in providing exceptional customer service.

Chapter 19, Clinical Laboratory Safety

ANSWERS FOR QUESTIONS

1. B. OSHA. The Occupational Safety and Health Administration

2. A. Telephone communications

3. An employer must make the information available to an employee within three working days of the employee's written request. Employers are obligated to provide training and education for employees who work with hazardous substances upon initial assignment to the work area and prior to a new assignment. Review training should be conducted for all clinical laboratory employees at least annually.

4. Components of the blood-borne pathogens plan are
    a. types of hazards employees may encounter
    b. education and training programs
    c. workplace safeguards
    d. barrier equipment
    e. medical surveillance

5. The risk of acquiring HIV from a needle-stick injury is about 0.3%, whereas the risk of acquiring HBV is 6–30%.

6. True. An employer must offer the Hepatitis B vaccine at no cost to its laboratory employees. The employee may decline the HBV vaccine but should sign the employer's declination form.

7. The components of a chemical hygiene plan (CHP) follow:
    a. Teach employees about the hazards of chemicals and instruct them in the use of PPE, safety devices and work practices, and measures to prevent or minimize exposure.
    b. The clinical laboratory safety officer or a chemical safety coordinator should be designated to provide ongoing chemical safety training for laboratory employees and to maintain the CHP.

8. A safety director has ultimate authority over the laboratory safety program, which includes the following duties:
    a. Oversee safety program and provide guidance to safety manager.
    b. Provide leadership for an effective safety program.
    c. Resolve problems involving employee and/or environmental safety.

    A clinical laboratory safety officer has responsibilities that include the following:
    a. Develop and maintain safety training manual.
    b. Keep director/manager updated on safety needs and safety conditions in the department.
    c. Conduct or coordinate safety training for supervisors. Assist with annual safety training of employees, as needed.
    d. Develop safe work methods and determine safety equipment needs.
    e. Document and maintain departmental safety training and accident investigation records.
    f. Conduct or coordinate periodic laboratory inspections.
    g. Represent the laboratory's interest on the facility's safety committee and/or coordinate activities for the laboratory safety committee.

9. The five types of hazards found in the clinical laboratory are
    a. biological
    b. chemical
    c. physical
    d. electrical
    e. radioactive

10. Safety precautions that could be implemented to address biological hazards include the following:
    PPE should be worn when handling biohazards, and established work practices must be utilized to prevent exposure. Work practices should also be instituted to keep "clean" areas contamination free. Hand-washing is the single most important method for preventing the spread of infection. Hands should be washed immediately
    - after contact with blood, body fluids, and contaminated materials
    - after removing gloves
    - before eating or smoking
    - before and after contact with patients
    - before leaving the laboratory, and before and after using the restroom

11. D. Barrier protection categories include engineering controls, personal protective equipment, and work practices.

12. The NFPA system consists of four small diamond-shaped symbols grouped into one larger diamond. The left diamond is blue and warns of a health hazard. The top diamond is red and warns of a flammable hazard. The right diamond is yellow and warns of a reactive-stability hazard. The bottom diamond is white and is used to indicate specific properties of the chemical, for example, its incompatibility with water or radioactive properties. Areas where hazardous chemicals are stored and used should be labeled with the appropriate warning symbols.

13. Biohazardous wastes should be segregated from noninfectious and chemical wastes. Biohazards wastes should be discarded into red/red-orange bags in leakproof containers that have the biohazards symbol on them. Biohazardous wastes must be incinerated or autoclaved to kill microorganisms, prior to disposal.

14. Medical records must be kept for thirty years, and safety-training records must be kept for three years after an employee has left the workplace.

CASE COMMENTARY

1. a. The following PPE should be worn when pouring and mixing chemicals, when cleaning chemical spills, and when working with chemicals:
        (1) gloves
        (2) goggles
        (3) lab coat
        (4) apron
    b. Hydrochloric acid manipulations should take place underneath a fume hood or in a well-ventilated area. The container should be stored in a safety cabinet, below eye level. The storage container must be compatible with the chemical, and only compatible chemicals should be stored together. Workers should have access to MSDS, prior to using the chemical.

      c. The spill should be cleaned up as soon as possible. Spills of HCl should be neutralized and absorbed with "spill kit" materials or other appropriate substances (see MSDS and laboratory protocol). Contaminated clean-up items should be disposed of in red biohazard bags or by other appropriate methods.

2. a. Yes, blood and body fluids from any patient should be assumed to be infectious for HIV, HBV, HCV, and other blood-borne pathogens.
   b. Yes, all workplace accidents/incidents should be immediately reported to the supervisor.
   c. The injured individual should seek prompt medical attention.

3. a. The first signs of fire (flames, smoke, burning smell) should immediately be reported according to the organization's protocol.
   b. Type C fire extinguishers (foam or dry chemical) may be used for electrical fires.
   c. Defective equipment should be unplugged immediately and labeled for maintenance. Contaminated parts should be disinfected prior to sending out of the lab for repairs or having personnel come to the lab to repair the instrument.

Chapter 20, Marketing and Development of an Outreach Program

ANSWERS FOR QUESTIONS

1. Marketing could be defined as determining what your client's needs are and providing products and services that meet and exceed those needs.

2. Competition from national laboratories, outpatient testing, and financial returns have promoted hospital marketing.

3. B. Interview physicians

4. a. Convenience of drawing stations for the patients
   b. Response time to supply requests
   c. Knowledge of staff with regard to tests
   d. Timely delivery of results
   e. Timely address and resolution of complaints or problems
   f. Turnaround time of results
   g. Pricing of tests

5. A. The anti-kickback statutes prohibit providing inducements, such as pricing below costs, to physicians in return for their Medicare/Medicaid patient business.

6. C. Stark legislation bars physicians from referring Medicare patients to laboratories in which the physician or their family members have a financial interest.

7. Two laboratory groups that have a major impact on the outreach program are technologists who are performing the testing and clerical staff who answer the phones.

CASE COMMENTARY

1. It is important that you immediately address the issue with the client. Thank them for reporting the problem, assure them that it will be addressed, and tell them that you will follow

up with them to see if there has been an improvement. Reinforce to the receptionist staff how important they are to the outreach program. They make the first impression with the caller, and it is important that they greet the caller with a positive attitude. It may be a good recommendation to make a phone etiquette course a part of their orientation and as a refresher course. Meet with the laboratory staff to share your concerns and to reinforce that they are an integral part of the outreach program. Without their skills and expertise, the program would not succeed. Remind them that each phone call they receive is an opportunity to promote the facility where they work and the outreach program by being concerned and helpful to the caller. Even though we never like to hear complaints, it is an important part of customer service to know what the problems are and to correct them. We would never know where we needed to improve if we were not given any feedback. The customer will stop complaining and look for another lab if we fail to follow up on complaints and correct them.

2. Your analysis reveals that
   - physician offices are not using your services. A survey of the physician offices should be done to determine their needs, what other outreach programs are providing, and pricing of present services. You might enhance the response by offering pizza or donuts to the offices responding. If you discover that you can meet the needs and offer a more competitive service at a reasonable profit, you could increase the business from these offices.
   - most hospitals will only be concerned in utilizing your outreach services for esoteric tests. You will need to determine the esoteric tests needed and whether your laboratory is capable of meeting this need and obtaining a reasonable profit.
   - the long-term care facilities are using your outreach program extensively; however, it is costly to provide a drawing station in each of the facilities and transport the specimens. If you increase your physician office business, your courier service will be more effectively used.
   - other possible market segments you should consider might include businesses that want employee testing, veterinary offices, and government agencies.

   You must consider the total outreach program and the client mix to determine whether a profit is possible.

3. Clients' needs change, so customer satisfaction needs should be determined and modifications continuously made if necessary. Also, constant communications with your customers are essential. The communication and customer satisfaction determinations could be continuously monitored with a full-time medical technologist/clinical laboratory scientist sales representative.

Chapter 21, Writing Procedures in the NCCLS Format

ANSWERS FOR QUESTIONS

1. E. All of the above. The procedure manual provides instructions for daily performance and serves as a communication resource and teaching tool.
2. B. National Committee for Clinical Laboratory Standards
3. GP2-A4 offers many suggestions to someone writing a procedure, whether it is a preanalytic, analytic, or postanalytic procedure. It discusses what sections should be included, what

sources may be used in preparing the procedure and how to reference them, how the procedure should be designed, and includes information about organizing the procedure manual, archiving and managing documents, using manufacturers' procedure manuals for automated procedures, and many examples of different types of procedures.

4. a. Title
   b. Purpose or principle
   c. Procedure instructions
   d. References
   e. Author
   f. Approval signatures
   g. Specimen information
   h. Test method
   i. Reagents and/or media
   j. Supplies
   k. Special safety precautions
   l. Equipment calibration and maintenance
   m. Quality control
   n. Calculations
   o. Expected values
   p. Interpretation of results
   q. Method limitations

CASE COMMENTARY

1. a. All necessary elements are present except for references. It is necessary to include any references that were used to write the procedure such as manufacturer's package inserts, NCCLS guidelines, or textbooks.
   b. (1) If the tech was not aware that a clotted sample should be rejected, he or she might use an improper sample, resulting in an inaccurate result.
      (2) Without realizing that newborns normally run a higher reticulocyte count than adults, the tech might inadvertently flag a normal result as high or incorrectly inform a nurse or physician that the count is high.
      (3) Without easy access to the formula for the final result, the tech will either have to figure it out on his or her own or take time to look it up in a reference.
      (4) If the technologist is not aware that the stain must be filtered prior to use and this step is skipped, the results would be slides that are difficult or impossible to read. Stain artifacts or precipitate on the slide might be mistaken for reticulum resulting in a falsely elevated reticulocyte count.
      (5) If the technologist doesn't realize that the stain/blood mixture should sit for fifteen minutes before making slides from it, the slides might be made too soon resulting in understained reticulocytes that are hard to see and possibly cause the count to be too low.
      (6) The lack of a current review signature indicates that the procedure hasn't been reviewed as often as required, and any changes in the procedure that may have occurred since the last review will not appear in the written procedure.
   c. There is no calibration step to this procedure, and no panic value is listed at this hospital for reticulocyte counts. The NCCLS guideline is just that—a guideline. It may not be exactly the same for every assay.

Chapter 22, Laboratory Budgeting and Finance

ANSWERS FOR QUESTIONS

1. A. Development of goals, budget assumption, forecast of expenses, and monitoring
2. The laboratory goals must be based on the organization's goals.
3. a. past earnings
   b. cash flow
   c. changes in state and federal laws
4. a. annual test volume
   b. revenue generated
5. Capital expenses are those expenses that add value (be assets) to the organization, and operational expenses are necessary to operate the organization and do not add value.
6. a. Replacement
   b. New Equipment
   c. Cost Reduction
7. a. Increased volume
   b. Vendor price increases
   c. Changes in policy and procedure
8. When calculating this cost, it is important to look beyond the mere cost of reagents, equipment, and technologist time. Many factors, such as cost of maintenance, salaries of support staff, nonmedical supplies (paper, pens, etc.), and travel and education, contribute to this bottom line. Many laboratories will even include the cost of telephone service, electricity, and water.

CASE COMMENTARY

1. Begin by calculating your reagent cost. You will note that the usage is different per assay. Most laboratories repeat assays that are positive—although you cannot bill for the repeat. Calculate by multiplying the cost per kit times annual usage. Add the costs, then divide by the number of billable drug screens.

	Cost per Kit	Annual Usage	Annual Cost
Amphetamine	$135.00	128	$17,280
Barbiturates	$130.00	125	$16,250
Benzodiazepine	$130.00	133	$17,290
Cocaine	$145.00	129	$18,705
Cannabinoids	$115.00	146	$16,790
		Annual Reagent Cost	$86,315

   - Annual reagent cost ($86,315) divided by billable drug screens (539 × 12 months) = $13.34.

   Equipment cost should be calculated over a five-year period—the same as the depreciation period. Divide the equipment cost by the number of drug screens you expect over a five year period. You may want to calculate into this any expected increase or decrease in utilization of this test. For this example, we will anticipate usage to remain the same.

- Instrument cost ($116,000) divided by annual usage (6468 × 5 yrs.) = $3.59. (539 × 12 months = 6,468 screens per year)
- Cost of service contract ($9,212) divided by annual usage (6,568) = $1.42.
- Annual medical supply ($205,874) divided by annual total billable tests (789,352) = $.26.
- Annual nonmedical supply cost ($51,722) divided by annual total billable tests (798,352) = $.06.
- Annual direct expense cost ($47,892) divided by annual total billable tests (798,352) = $.06.
- Annual travel & education cost ($22,171) divided by total annual billable tests (798,352) = $.03.
- Annual salary cost ($1,892,364) divided by total annual billable tests (798,352) = $2.37.

Total cost per billable drug screen = $21.12, the sum of all the calculations.

2. The lease option on instrument #1 is the most economical because it would cost the lowest total amount.

	Instrument 1		Instrument 2	
	Purchase	Lease	Purchase	Lease
Purchase Price	$87,750.00	$0.00	$78,000.00	$0.00
Service Contract	$60,600.00	$0.00	$65,240.00	$0.00
(annual cost × 4 yrs)	($15,150 × 4)	($0.00)	($16,310 × 4)	($0.00)
Reagent Pricing (5 yrs)	$411,081.25	$531,987.50	$435,262.50	$551,332.50

(Reagent cost × 265 samples/day × 365 [days per yr] × 5 yrs
Instrument 1 Purchase 0.85 × 265 × 365 × 5 = $411,081.25
Instrument 1 Lease 1.10 × 265 × 365 × 5 = $531,987.50
Instrument 2 Purchase 0.90 × 265 × 365 × 5 = $435,262.50
Instrument 2 Lease 1.14 × 265 × 365 × 5 = $551,332.50)

| **Total Cost** | **$559,431.25** | **$531,987.50** | **$578,502.50** | **$551,332.50** |

Total cost is the sum of purchase price, service contract, and reagent pricing.

Chapter 23, Fraud and Abuse

ANSWERS FOR QUESTIONS

1. Corrects and prevents
2. a. Development of written policies, procedures, and standards of conduct that promote the laboratory's commitment to compliance.
   b. Laboratories should comply with all OIG fraud alerts.
   c. Appointment of a compliance officer and other appropriate bodies.
   d. Development of effective training and education programs for all employees.

e. Development and maintenance of effective lines of open communications (hotline) with the compliance officer to receive complaints while maintaining the anonymity of complainants.
   f. Laboratories should have periodic compliance audits and other evaluation techniques.
   g. Enforcement of standards through well-publicized disciplinary directives.
   h. Development of procedures to respond to detected offenses and to initiate corrective actions.

3. Managers should oversee the day-to-day operations of the compliance program and must be readily accessible to staff to discuss and resolve compliance issues. They are asked to monitor the implementation of the compliance plan through performance of periodic audits of laboratory operations.

   The managers also carry the responsibility of educating and training their employees (individuals authorized by state law to order lab tests, phlebotomists, testing personnel, and coding/billing staff).

CASE COMMENTARY

1. a. The urinalysis cannot be billed more than once when it is only performed once. Claims for tests that were not performed due to laboratory accidents or insufficient specimens should not be submitted for payment. A laboratory should ensure that all claims for testing services submitted for reimbursement accurately and correctly identify the services ordered by the physician *and* performed by the laboratory.
   b. Educate employees, modify the format of requisition forms, change lab policy where the lab requisition will not be accepted unless accompanied with the proper specimen (especially for those specimens collected by hospital staff other than lab personnel), and use software with editing capabilities for medical necessity and billing accuracy.

2. a. Yes, laboratories can offer customized profiles to their physician clients as long as the tests ordered are medically necessary.
   b. Clinicians can abuse the panels and order unnecessary testing. Clients must sign a physician acknowledgment stating their understanding of the potential implications of ordering customized profiles that require constant monitoring and updating.

3. a. The medical technologist/clinical laboratory scientist is in compliance. Overpayment can occur when laboratories bill for individual tests that should have been grouped together (i.e., bundled) for payment purposes and billed at a lower rate. Therefore, chemistry panels may not be "unbundled" and each test billed separately. Correct application of coding and billing activities and review of claims are part of the medical technologist's job to avoid billing and bundling edits. The medical technologist/clinical laboratory scientist is not questioning the medical necessity of the testing.
   b. Train and educate clinicians and keep information updated and readily available. Annual notices should be sent to physicians and other individuals authorized by law to order tests setting forth the medical necessity policy and components of each laboratory profile.

Chapter 24, Workload Recording

ANSWERS FOR QUESTIONS

1. The primary use of workload recording is to measures employee productivity, which relates directly to staffing levels.

2. E. The CAP workload unit determines the amount of time required to perform a test, including the time for paperwork, phone calls, and so on, and separates workload reports into three sections of ordered tests, repeated tests, and quality control tests.

3. True. The adjusted patient days method is dependent on a ratio of inpatients to outpatients.

4. A commonly used workload recording method that considers the number of procedures billed on a daily basis is billable procedures.

5. The LMIP involves not only workload recording for labor per billable procedure, but also other expenses per billable tests and expenses for nonbillable tests. In addition, this program will compare the lab with peer groups based on size and complexity.

CASE COMMENTARY

1. The workload recording report that you would have been using should have indicated to you that your volumes were not adequate to increase your staffing without special permission from your supervisor. At 85% productivity you should be examining staffing to see where you might cut back to be able to reach the desirable 100% staffing index. This could be accomplished by reviewing your part-time hours to see if cuts could be made there without affecting your full-time employees. This should always be done before you are mandated to do so by your supervisor. If you do have a special project coming up, you would want to discuss adding the additional hours with your CEO/CFO/supervisor to get their approval before putting them in place.

2. This would be the time to approach your administrative supervisor about adding additional personnel on a full-time basis. With a consistent history in hand of staffing indexes in excess of 120%, you will be in a good position to argue the need for the added hours to avoid burnout, increased employee turnover, decreased employee morale, and placing your accreditation in jeopardy.

Chapter 25, Purchasing

ANSWERS FOR QUESTIONS

1. B. Purchasing is determining need, evaluating product, locating product and determining best value.

2. E. Items to be purchased include operational supplies, capital equipment, and services.

3. Greater efficiency in inventory control, stock rotation, and "buying power" of the organization is the advantage of using a central storeroom or warehouse.

4. a. applicability
   b. quality
   c. value

5. Contractual agreement is negotiated for a fixed rate for services over a period of time. Time and materials requires payment for services as needed and may include travel, labor, and parts.

6. D. The requisition is used to request supplies and so on, and it is completed by the requesting department.

7. B. The purchase order authorizes payment from the ordering institution.

CASE COMMENTARY

1. The number of blood agar plates seems to be adequate, but some are outdated, causing the shortage. Therefore, one should consider ordering more frequently to avoid this problem. Because this is a regularly ordered item, one should consider placing a standing order with shipments on specific dates. There are inventory tools for predicting precisely when to order, how much to order, and the base level needed. A good discussion of these tools is found in *Medical Laboratory Management and Supervision — Operations, Review, and Study Guide*.

2. The cost of the contractual agreement is $2,400/yr. And you have already paid $2,400 × 10 = $24,000 for 2 five-year contractual agreements. To sign another five-year contractual agreement would cost another $12,000. On the other hand, if you had a problem, the time-and-material arrangement with the autoclave would cost: travel $500; one night hotel $65; labor 5 hours travel × $100 = $500, plus actual time working on the autoclave, estimate 5 hours = $500, thus $1,000 total, plus parts. So one visit would cost approximately $1,565, plus parts. If there were two visits per year, the total cost would be approximately $3,130, plus parts.

    Considering that this autoclave is ten years old and the past history you have had with the autoclave, it would seem more cost effective to keep the contractual agreement, because the yearly cost for the contractual agreement is $2,400 and the estimated time and materials arrangement is $3,130, plus parts. The autoclave should be monitored for repair costs. When costs for parts excluded under the contractual agreement reach high levels, replacement of the autoclave should be considered.

    One aspect we did not address is the expertise of the biomedical team at your institution. If the biomedical team can do the same service and repairs as the technical service representative, then you would only be considering parts as an expense. In that case, you would recommend the time-and-materials arrangement.

Chapter 26, Employee Scheduling

ANSWERS FOR QUESTIONS

1. Six factors that impact scheduling are
   a. test menu
   b. education and experience of staff
   c. number of employees needed for test volume

d. number of emergency areas served
e. turnaround time expectations
f. level of test complexity

2. C. Number of employees, number of hours worked by each employee, and education/experience level of each employee impact the laboratory salary budget.

3. C. 31.25

   Billable test volume (5,000) × Standard Unit (0.5) = 2,500 divided by 80 hours in the fourteen-day period = 31.25

4. If all highly educated and experienced techs were used, then the salary dollars would be high; however, if one used a mix of experienced and less experienced, and highly educated and less educated, then the salary dollars would be less.

5. If the test volume decreases, the productivity will decrease and fewer hours should be scheduled. If the test volume increases, the productivity will increase and more hours should be scheduled.

6. D. 90.9%

   2,500 hours earned divided by 2,750 hours actually worked = 90.9% productivity.

7. Staff with increased education and experience would be able to work more independently, however, the salary dollars would be higher. Staff with less education and experience would require supervision, but the salary dollars would be lower. It is important to have a staff with various education and experience for cost containment, but at the same time be able to provide quality patient care.

8. E. Adequate coverage for the laboratory, fairness, personal preference, and opportunities for rewards are all important factors for employee morale and retention.

9. A large test menu would require more techs, and a high test complexity would require more experienced techs.

10. 3–4 weeks.

11. Examples of shift options include
    a. 7 A.M.–3 P.M., 3 P.M.–11 P.M., and 11 P.M.–7 A.M.
    b. seven days on, seven days off
    c. extended weekends

12. One should investigate whether the payroll is set to consider overtime as greater than forty hours per week or greater than eighty hours in a pay period. Any time an employee works more than forty hours for the forty-hour per-week payroll schedule, the employee is paid overtime. With the eight and eighty option, any time an employee works more than eighty hours in a pay period or eight hours in a workday, the employee is paid overtime.

13. Advantages of using PRN personnel are that these individuals can cover
    a. during vacations
    b. during holidays
    c. on scheduled days off

14. The manager (scheduler) should discuss schedule changes with employees. The primary factor is excellence in patient care and occasionally, even with good planning, the schedule must be changed.

CASE COMMENTARY

1. First, determine the number of employees needed for the anticipated workload increase. Apply the standard unit of 0.25 to determine the number of worked hours that the daily volume of 140 tests would justify.

    140 tests/day × 0.25 = 35 hours/day earned or 175 hours/week (M–F)

    Remember that it is easier and less painful to add hours to a schedule than it is to take them away. Add additional staff only if absolutely necessary and add them during the time frame during which the anticipated increase in volume is to occur. Add hours slowly and reevaluate regularly to determine if more are needed. The use of PRN employees in the hours after 3 P.M. could eliminate the hiring of additional full-time staff.

    Next, determine if the current staff mix on the schedule after 3 P.M. is appropriate for the test mix that is expected. Both Medical Lab Technicians/Clinical Lab Technicians and Medical Technologists/Clinical Lab Scientists can perform routine hematology and chemistry testing, and laboratory assistants can help in specimen processing. Clerical staff will be needed to perform test ordering in the computer. Remember the effect that the staff mix will have on the salary budget.

    Finally, calculate the current productivity. If it is below 100%, the current staff level may be able to absorb the workload without adding hours to the schedule. If it is above 100% already, additional staff will probably be needed.

2. The two things related to the schedule that can fix this problem are the number of employees scheduled and the time that each one reports for duty. It could be determined if the delays occur on a particular day of the week, and employees' off days could be scheduled around the busiest surgery days. If it is not an option to schedule more employees, then the employees that are scheduled could come in earlier to accommodate the surgery workload.

3. Various scheduling options that can be explored include the following:
    - Eliminate overtime by having adequate overlapping of the shifts. The new shift can start new tests while the outgoing shift completes work in progress.
    - Do not fill vacant positions and shift current employees to cover the schedule.
    - If vacant positions must be filled, evaluate the situation to determine if an employee with less experience and/or education can perform the duties of the position.
    - Ask for volunteers who would like to reduce their hours while remaining in the same payroll class (e.g., full-time, part-time, PRN).
    - Reduce hours worked by PRN staff and ask full-time staff to cover them while adhering to a "no overtime" plan.

4. It is extremely important for a manager to demonstrate loyalty to all employees, especially faithful, long-term employees.
    - Determine if the time needed at home is during the hours that the employee normally works. If so, the employee may be able to change shifts with another employee temporarily.
    - Work longer hours but fewer days per week. For example, instead of five 8-hour shifts, she could work four 10-hour shifts or three 12-hour shifts during the week.
    - A full-time weekend shift could be an option if the employee is able to work long hours.
    - Work earlier hours in the day and leave early.
    - The employee, if able, could reduce her hours while maintaining her current employment status. Some facilities consider sixty-four hours per pay period as full-time status; the employee could reduce her hours from eighty hours to sixty-four hours and still keep her insurance benefits.
    - Reduce hours worked and use vacation hours to supplement her worked hours to total the number of hours needed for the pay period.

Chapter 27, Evaluation of New Test Methods—The Comparison Study

ANSWERS FOR QUESTIONS

1. Method validation

2. Simply stated, it refers to an assessment in which a number of patient samples are analyzed by both the test method and comparative method.

3. Comparison studies will point out any differences there may be in results due to differences in reagents and methodology from one system to the next. In addition, comparison studies will also point out any differences there may be in therapeutic ranges due to differences in the sensitivities of reagents being compared.

4. a. A need has been determined for this new methodology.
   b. Requirements have been determined for this new methodology.
   c. A review of the current literature available on this new methodology has been solicited.
   d. The manufacturer has provided training with the new methodology.

5. a. What is the cost per test?
   b. What is the turnaround time?
   c. What reagent storage facility is required?
   d. What is the availability and skill of laboratory staff needed?

6. Normally, new analytical methods come into being to increase precision or accuracy over current methods to reduce reagent costs or to measure a new analyte.

7. The Food and Drug Administration (FDA)

8. D. Submit experimental data.

9. a. Precision—tests the reproducibility of an assay method.
   b. Accuracy—tests the agreement between the mean estimate of a quantity (measured by a new method) and its true value (measured by a reference method).
   c. Analytical sensitivity—is a measure of the lowest concentration of analyte in a sample that can be accurately measured.
   d. Analytical specificity—represents the degree of assay interference from drugs or other chemicals present in the specimen.
   e. Diagnostic validity—compares the ability of a new assay method (test method) to accurately diagnose/predict the presence or absence of disease with that of an established method (reference method).

10. D. New reference levels, estimated date of change, and any other changes

CASE COMMENTARY

1. The results of your investigation should be shared with the physicians who are requesting the new method. Just looking at the research, it appears that the old test method may be adequate; however, the physicians may need the higher specificity and sensitivity. If they need the higher specificity and sensitivity on all of their patients, you would try to justify to the hospital administration a need for the change. However, if they did not need the higher specificity and sensitivity, you may be able to convince them that the present method was

adequate. If they needed the higher specificity and sensitivity on only a few of their patients, then you might consider offering them the new method on a send-out basis. It appears that the new test would cost the patient more; therefore, it possibly could be used as a follow-up method in special cases.

2. a. You should determine a need for the D-Dimer assay before proceeding. Because you are the only health-care facility within a 100-mile radius of two larger health-care facilities, you should first interview physicians, especially those in the emergency department, to determine either if this test will be performed daily on patients who present with symptoms of deep vein thrombosis and/or pulmonary embolism or if these patients will be transferred to one of the nearby larger medical facilities. If it is determined that a need does exist within your institution for the D-Dimer test, then you may proceed further.

b. Normally, before a new test or assay is marketed, it has received FDA approval and the manufacturer should supply this information to the buyer. But this isn't always the case. So it is a good idea to check to see if a specific test has indeed received FDA approval. With the possibility of adding the D-Dimer assay, new equipment and test kits will need to be purchased. It is generally a good idea to determine the cost per test for the D-Dimer assay, the materials management required for this assay, as well as the expertise needed by the technical staff in performing this assay. Also, training on the new instrument should be supplied by the manufacturer either in house to all technical staff or off site to a member of the technical staff designated by the laboratory manager. Normally, training criteria is decided by the manufacturer and buyer and written into the capital equipment contract before purchase.

c. First of all, you should solicit responses not only from the physicians, as stated before, but also from the technical staff in the laboratory. Ultimately, they will be the ones who will be performing the test. If currently understaffed, the addition of the D-Dimer test may increase the workload of the laboratory personnel, thus requiring the need for more technical help. It would also be a good idea for you to perform your own research on the assay being considered for addition to your laboratory test menu. This may be accomplished by reading articles contained within professional journals as well as by contact with other institutions that currently have this test in use.

d. Because this will not be a comparison study, but rather a new procedure for your laboratory, you must formulate a procedure based on NCCLS format. (See chapter 21 on writing procedures in the NCCLS format for more details.)

Chapter 28, Quality Control

ANSWERS FOR QUESTIONS

1. Quality control (QC) is the process by which one monitors analytical procedures in order to ensure the accuracy and precision of test results and thus the validity of patient results prior to their reporting.

2. Internal QC involves
   1) establishing the mean and standard deviation for the QC material, verifying the accuracy and precision of the control material, and establishing acceptable statistical limits for each analytical method using that control material.
   2) assaying the QC material concomitantly with patient samples and verifying that the control material results fall within the acceptable limits prior to accepting or rejecting a given assay run (test analysis).

3) monitoring control results over time for changes in precision (random error) or accuracy (systematic error) using prescribed methods and then addressing the problem, when one exists, by finding and correcting the source of error and reanalyzing the patient and control samples.

External QC involves
1) the comparison of a lab's assay results from unknown test samples with the mean results of those obtained on the same samples by other labs.
2) the comparison of a lab's assay results from unknown test samples with those obtained by an external agency using a reference method. This is often part of a proficiency testing program.

3. a. Accuracy:
   A measure of how closely a test result agrees with the "true" value for that sample.
   b. Precision:
   A measure of how closely repeated measurements of a sample (replicates) agree with each other.
   c. Reliability:
   A measure of both the accuracy and precision of a method.
   d. Mean:
   The average of all data points in a data set calculated by: $\bar{x} = \dfrac{\Sigma x_i}{n}$
   e. Median:
   The middle data point of all the data points arranged in numerical order.
   f. Mode:
   The most frequent number or value found in a data set.
   g. Range:
   The difference between the high and low values of data points in a data set.
   h. Variance:
   A mathematic representation of the dispersion or degree of tightness of data points around the mean or peak in a data set.
   i. Standard deviation:
   A mathematic representation of the dispersion or degree of tightness of data points around the mean or peak in a data set.
   j. Confidence intervals:
   Refers to the limits (high and low values) between which a specified proportion of the data points in a data set will fall. In a data set with normal distribution 68%, 95%, and 99%, confidence intervals (CI) will have the following ranges:

   $68\% \text{ CI} = \text{mean} \pm 1 \text{ SD}$
   $95\% \text{ CI} = \text{mean} \pm 2 \text{ SD}$
   $99\% \text{ CI} = \text{mean} \pm 3 \text{ SD}$

   k. Coefficient of variation:
   The standard deviation divided by the mean and multiplied by 100 to obtain a percentage.
   l. Trend:
   A small but steady and continuous change of the control values in one direction. If left unchecked, the control values will go off the chart over time. Trends often indicate reagent or calibrator deterioration or gradual instrumental failure.
   m. Shift:
   A change of the mean for the control material. The new mean is continuous, but different from the original mean. This can reflect the resetting of an instrument, a small but consistent flaw in the instrument, or a change of lot number of control material.

n. Central tendency:
Represents a large group of data points that are equal to or very nearly the same as one data point (cluster of data points) and are represented by a peak on a frequency diagram.
o. Normal distribution:
Implies that there are approximately the same number and distribution of data points to either side of the peak (symmetrical spread of data points around the peak).
p. Skewed distribution:
Refers to the asymmetrical spread of data points around the peak.
q. Imprecision:
Measurements do not closely replicate, and the standard deviation will be larger.
r. Westgard rules:
A set of criteria by which one can monitor test performance and accept or reject the run.
s. Random error:
Error occurring on a unique sample or without any defined pattern.
t. Systematic error:
Error that is present in all samples and affects those samples approximately equally.

CASE COMMENTARY

1. Mean = 140.6   Median = 140   Mode = 138

No, they do not represent a Gaussian distribution, and therefore you should reject this control. Instead you should contact the manufacturer and ask for a new lot number of control.

Explanation: To determine the mean, one should first determine the sum of all the data points (i.e., add them) and then divide that value by the number of data points in the data set.

Sodium mmol/L

145	135	143	146
151	136	137	133
148	142	134	140
138	146	141	138
140	138	139	142

$$\bar{x} = \frac{\Sigma x_i}{n}$$

where: $\bar{x}$ = mean.

x_i = individual value.

Σ = sum of.

n = number of values or data points

Sum of the data points = 2812

Mean = 2812/20 = 140.6 mmol/L

To determine the median value and the mode, one should first rank the data points (arrange them in order of increasing numerical value). The median is the middle data point. The mode is the most frequent data point found in the data set.

Sodium Value mmol/L

145	135	143	146
151	136	137	133
148	142	134	140
138	146	141	138
140	138	139	142

Sodium Order

133
134
135
136
137
138 most frequent (mode)
138 most frequent (mode)
138 most frequent (mode)
139
140 middle (median)
140 middle (median)
141
142
142
143
145
146
146
148
151

Because the mean, median, and mode are not the same, one does not have a Gaussian distribution (normal distribution), and one should reject the control.

2. Method A:

   Mean = 100 mg/dL   Median = 100 mg/dL   Mode = 100 mg/dL   SD = 2.53

   Method B:

   Mean = 99.95 mg/dL   Median = 99 and 100 mg/dL   Mode = 105 mg/dL   SD = 6.56

   No, Method B does not exhibit a normal distribution. Method A is more precise.

   Method A is more accurate. You should chose Method A for your laboratory.

   Explanation: The mean, median, and mode are determined in the same manner as in question 1. Method A has the same value for the mean, median, and mode and therefore represents a data set with a Gaussian distribution (normal distribution). Method B does not exhibit a Gaussian distribution because the mean, median, and mode do not have the same value.

   Precision is a measure of how closely repeated measurements of a sample (replicates) agree with each other. It is determined by calculating the SD for the replicates. The lower the SD, the more precise the assay is. To determine the SD, one first determines the variance and then takes the square root of it.

Glucose mg/dL Method A				Glucose mg/dL Method B			
100	105	101	99	107	100	93	99
102	98	104	96	110	105	91	94
101	97	99	103	89	108	111	92
100	98	102	101	102	98	96	104
99	95	100	100	95	97	105	103

Number of Values Minus One = 19

Sum of the Squares = 122

Number of Values Minus One = 19

Sum of the Squares = 818.9

To determine the sum of the squares, one should first calculate the difference between each individual value and the mean for all the replicates in the data set. Then one should square each difference and sum those squares.

Method A			Method B		
Values	Value – Mean	(Value – Mean)²	Values	Value – Mean	(Value – Mean)²
100	100 – 100 = 0	0	107	107 – 99.95 = 7.05	49.7
105	105 – 100 = 5	25	100	100 – 99.95 = 0.05	0.0025
101	101 – 100 = 1	1	93	93 – 99.95 = –6.95	48.3
99	99 – 100 = –1	1	99	99 – 99.95 = –0.95	.90
102	102 – 100 = 2	4	110	110 – 99.95 = 10.05	101.0
98	98 – 100 = –2	4	105	105 – 99.95 = 5.05	25.5
104	104 – 100 = 4	16	91	91 – 99.95 = –8.95	80.1
96	96 – 100 = –4	16	94	94 – 99.95 = –5.95	35.4
101	101 – 100 = 1	1	89	89 – 99.95 = –10.95	119.9
97	97 – 100 = –3	9	108	108 – 99.95 = 8.05	64.8
99	99 – 100 = –1	1	111	111 – 99.95 = 11.05	122.1
103	103 – 100 = 3	9	92	92 – 99.95 = –7.95	63.2
100	100 – 100 = 0	0	102	102 – 99.95 = 2.05	4.2
98	98 – 100 = –2	4	98	98 – 99.95 = –1.95	3.8
102	102 – 100 = 2	4	96	96 – 99.95 = –3.95	15.6
101	101 – 100 = 1	1	104	104 – 99.95 = 4.05	16.4
99	99 – 100 = –1	1	95	95 – 99.95 = –4.95	24.5
95	95 – 100 = –5	25	97	97 – 99.95 = –2.95	8.7
100	100 – 100 = 0	0	105	105 – 99.95 = 5.05	25.5
100	100 – 100 = 0	0	103	103 – 99.95 = 3.05	9.3

Variance is:

$$s^2 = \frac{\Sigma(x_i - \bar{x})^2}{n - 1}$$

where: s^2 = variance

Σ = sum of

x_i = individual value

$\bar{x}$ = mean

n = number of values or data points

Variance (Method A) = 122/19 = 6.42

Variance (Method B) = 818.9/19 = 43.1

And the standard deviation is the square root of the variance or:

$$s \text{ or } SD = \sqrt{\frac{\Sigma(x_i - \bar{x})^2}{n - 1}}$$

where: s or SD = standard deviation

$\sqrt{}$ = square root of

Σ = sum of

x_i = individual value

$\bar{x}$ = mean

n = number of values or data points

SD (Method A) = 2.53

SD (Method B) = 6.56

Method A is more precise than method B because the SD for method A is less than the SD for method B.

Accuracy is a measure of how closely a test result agrees with the "true" value for that sample. This is determined by comparing the mean of repeated testing values with the true value determined by a reference method such as gravimetric analysis. In this case there is a reference value of 100 mg/dL ± 3 mg/dL. Method A is slightly more accurate than method B because it has the exact mean value as that listed for the reference value, whereas method B does not. Method A also fits the target value for assay precision better. Because method A exhibits Gaussian distribution and better accuracy and precision than method B, one should select method A.

3.

Prostatic Acid Phosphatase ug/L:			Prostatic Acid Phosphatase U/L:		
Mean	**SD**	**%CV**	**Mean**	**SD**	**%CV**
2.84	0.40	14.08	1.61	0.06	3.73
21.56	0.89	4.13	8.20	0.05	0.61

The kinetic assay has a lower %CV and therefore is the better test.

Explanation: The coefficient of variation (%CV) is a ratio of the SD to the mean for a given method. It allows one to compare two or more analysis methods with very different means. Assays with low coefficients of variation are more precise than assays with high coefficients of variation. To calculate the %CV, one should divide the SD by the mean and multiply the quotient by 100.

$$\%CV = \frac{(SD)}{\bar{x}}(100)$$

where: %CV = coefficient of variation

SD = standard deviation

$\bar{x}$ = mean

Thus for the mass assay one would have the following results:

Level 1 %CV = (0.40/2.84) × 100% = 14.08%
Level 2 %CV = (0.89/21.56) × 100% = 4.13%

The kinetic assay would give the following results:

Level 1 %CV = (0.06/1.61) × 100% = 3.73%
Level 2 %CV = (0.05/8.20) × 100% = 0.61%

Because the kinetic assay has a lower %CV at both levels it is the better assay.

4. The 95% confidence interval for this batch of control is 3.2 – 4.0 mmol/L. The chart indicates a continuous increase of potassium values from day 13 through day 20. This represents a trend. You should check your calibrator and reagents by using a new bottle and then a different lot number of each. Then you should check your instrument.

Explanation: The 95% confidence interval equals the mean plus and minus two SDs. Thus for a control with a mean of 3.6 mmol/L and an SD of 0.2 mmol/L one would have the following:

2 SD = 2 × 0.2 mmol/L = 0.4 mmol/L
mean + 2 SD = 3.6 mmol/L + 0.4 mmol/L = 4.0 mmol/L
mean – 2 SD = 3.6 mmol/L – 0.4 mmol/L = 3.2 mmol/L
95% confidence interval = mean +/– 2SD = 3.2 – 4.0 mmol/L

The plot of the QC data is as follows:

Day	Potassium mmol/L	Day	Potassium mmol/L
1	3.5	11	3.7
2	3.4	12	3.9
3	3.8	13	3.8
4	3.6	14	4.0
5	3.7	15	4.2
6	3.4	16	4.5
7	3.3	17	4.6
8	3.9	18	4.6
9	3.6	19	4.8
10	3.5	20	4.9

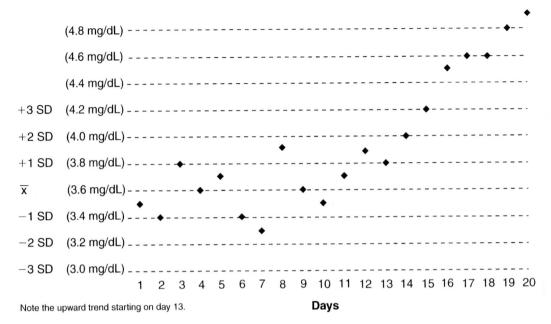

Note the upward trend starting on day 13.

5. The assay value for day 5 is a violation of the 1_{3s} rule. This suggests a random error. Do not release the patient data. Instead repeat the assay and if the control is now in limits then you may release this patient data. If it is not in limits then you should investigate the source of the error. The assay value for day 6 is a violation of the 2_{2s} rule. This indicates a systematic error. Do not release the patient data. Instead, one should investigate the source of the error.

Explanation: The following is a plot of the QC data for the laboratory.

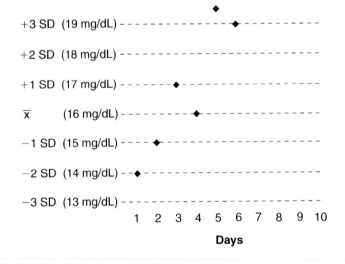

On day 5 there is a one control that lies outside the mean +/− 3SD, in violation of the 1_{3s} rule. On day 6 there is a second control value (2 consecutive control values) that lies outside the mean + 2SD and both controls are in the same direction (i.e., both are + 2SD or both are −2SD). This is in violation of the 2_{2s} rule.

6. Sources of errors would include 1) sample mix up; 2) defective QC material due to shipping conditions, storage conditions, or improper manufacturing; 3) unreliable instrumentation or defective reagent(s); and 4) transcription errors, math, and/or dilution errors. One should review the lab reports to rule out transcription, math, and/or dilution errors. One

should retest the proficiency testing QC sample (one should save a portion of this when initially assaying it) to rule out random error or a sample mix-up (mix-up between two proficiency specimens or with a clinical specimen). One can then ask the external agency to send another proficiency sample that the lab assays to rule out improper shipping or storage conditions. If the target values represent a reference assay value, one can inquire as to the mean and SD obtained by other labs participating in the proficiency testing program. If these values are in agreement with your lab's values, then the problem could be with the initial specimen manufacture. One should also investigate the possibility of defective/unreliable instrumentation by splitting samples and assaying them simultaneously on the lab's instrument and a new instrument at a neighboring lab.

Chapter 29, Quality Management

ANSWERS FOR QUESTIONS

1. Quality is a value. Quality is how we do our work. Quality is doing the right things right and making continuous improvements.

2. B. Information, choice, participation, coordination of transitions, and knowing preferences.

3. The patient ultimately evaluates the quality of health care provided by the professional.

4. Accessing is the process of acquiring the information, communicating with a knowledgeable provider, getting an appointment, or entering a care site.

   Assessing and diagnosing include clinical (hands-on), laboratory, radiologic, and other diagnostic processes.

   Planning includes strategic/quality plans and the patient/family plan of care.

   Treating includes drugs, procedures, counseling, teaching, and care in support of patient oxygenation, circulation, behavior, perception, mobility, nutrition, elimination, and immunity.

   Reentering is the process of an informed patient moving to another level of care, site of care, agency, or provider relationship.

   Evaluating is the process used to determine whether interventions were effective and helpful to the patient and family served.

5. C. Complexity includes mistakes and defects, breakdowns and delays, inefficiencies, and variation but not cost controls.

6. One way to reduce variation is standardization: getting everyone to use the same procedures, materials, equipment, and so forth. Another way is to study the process as it now operates, look for potential sources of variation, and gather data to see if these factors do affect the output. Statistical process control is a useful tool for reducing or eliminating variation. Statistically designed experiments are often helpful.

7. James O. Westgard has applied concepts and techniques of quality management to the medical laboratory. Westgard delineates a quality management framework that involves quality laboratory processes, quality control, quality assessment, quality improvement, quality planning, and quality goals. Westgard points out that quality assurance is the outcome of this whole quality management process rather than being a component in the process. Westgard suggests that these components work together like a feedback loop. Quality planning is

concerned with establishing and validating processes that meet customer needs. Selection and evaluation of new methods and instruments are examples of quality planning. Quality laboratory processes are the policies, procedures, personnel standards, and physical resources that determine how work gets done in the laboratory. Quality control and quality assessment measure how well the work is getting done. When problems are detected, quality improvement determines the root causes, which can then be eliminated by implementing effective changes in quality laboratory processes.

8. a. What are we trying to accomplish?
   b. How will we know that a change is an improvement?
   c. What changes can we make that will result in improvement?

9. a. personal mastery of the clinical competencies required to practice clinical laboratory science
   b. a mental "big picture" of the health-care delivery system and a close-up view of the processes that make it happen
   c. a working definition of quality from the perspective of what matters to the patient
   d. team skills that allow for team learning and contribution to improvement initiatives
   e. tools and techniques for active participation in process improvements to eliminate error and waste

CASE COMMENTARY

1. As the laboratory manager you must investigate the complaints. Is it true that the inpatients have received breakfast late waiting on the phlebotomy team or is this just something the patients are being told to hide inefficiencies on the part of another unit of service such as dietetics or nursing services? If you find after investigating the situation that patients are indeed waiting on the phlebotomy team, then you will need to evaluate the phlebotomy schedule and the phlebotomy team. A part of your investigation might be to ask the phlebotomy team to meet with you to discuss the situation. Often the individuals doing the work will be familiar with and offer good solutions to a situation. Perhaps the team needs to begin phlebotomy earlier in the morning or perhaps patients that are non per os (NPO) until the blood is drawn can be scheduled first in the morning phlebotomy rounds. There may be multiple causes for the situation and multiple solutions. The manager should use problem-solving techniques to discover the best solution. Remember, quality happens when we meet or exceed customer requirements, and it is the patient who evaluates the quality of health care received. This situation would represent a delay type of complexity.

2. Yes, this situation is a problem, and it does address quality. A quality management program seeks to eliminate errors prior to their occurrence, but if an error has occurred, the program seeks to discover the reason and keep the error from occurring again. A flow chart should be prepared showing every step in the process from the preanalytical step to the analytical step to the postanalytical step. The flow chart should indicate what is done in each step and who is responsible. Once the flow chart is prepared, the actual procedure starting with the preanalytical step should be examined. As the entire process for prothrombin times was investigated using the accepted protocol indicated on the flow chart, it was revealed that the nursing staff who are collecting the blood are either underfilling or overfilling the blood tube, thus causing a problem with the anticoagulate to blood ratio. However, when the tubes are received in the laboratory processing center, the on-job-trained laboratory assistants are not noticing this error; therefore, they are withdrawing the plasma and sending it on to the coagulation department for the analysis. The analysis is done correctly; however, the preanalytical phase of this prothrombin time test process is in error. Inservice education for the

nursing staff and the on-job-trained laboratory assistants is indicated, and the situation should be monitored to be sure the problem is corrected. This type of situation would represent an error type of complexity.

Chapter 30, Problem Solving

ANSWERS FOR QUESTIONS

1. E. Steps in problem solving are 1. define the problem, 2. create scenarios, 3. implement solution, 4. examine resolution, and 5. reflect (on problem/solution).

2. Define problem — The first order of business is to determine if a problem exists and what it is exactly.

   Create scenarios — As an individual, brainstorm the potential approaches that might be considered with regard to the specified conclusion. Then discuss with others affected by the problem what they might consider the desired outcome to the problem.

   Solution implementation — Choosing the most appropriate answer to the problem is not always easy. If at all possible, test the solution on an individual or small group before allowing full-scale implementation.

   Examine resolution — Consider the following questions when examining the resolution. Is the resolution effective? Are there any new conflicts that have developed since the resolution? What might be the most effective part of the solution? Is the fix permanent or temporary? Does more work need to be done to completely resolve the problem?

   Reflection — After a period of time, reconsider the original conflict. Look at the possible resolution scenarios developed.

CASE COMMENTARY

1. Many problems exist in this case, which stem from basic communication deficiencies in various forms: electronic, verbal, and written. The bottom line for most health-care professionals is to see that each patient receives timely and effective treatment. Delays in reporting results are counterproductive and unacceptable.

   Resolution should focus on getting the missing results onto the patient charts as soon as possible. The approach may be as simple as activating a default manual system designed to prevent this type of problem or resubmitting the results through the network. Other possible scenarios may range from moderately complex to extremely involved. Options range from manually entering the patient results to getting the hospital information system (HIS) department to coordinate resolution efforts. A short-term solution may require laboratory personnel to copy all of the results and deliver them to the nursing stations for posting to the patient's charts. A combination of multiple solutions may provide the best outcome for long-term management.

   Contingencies to consider when designing the best resolution may include but are not limited to the following questions.

   Is the HIS department aware of the problem?
   Has the electronic communication problem been corrected?

If the problem has not been fixed, what is the estimated time for repair?

When were the last results were posted? How many results are missing?

Will additional personnel be needed to correct this problem?

Once resolved, the problem and resolution should be reviewed and evaluated for maintenance and improvement.

2. Personnel problems arise on a regular basis and require fair, unbiased resolution. The decision to bring a new employee in or to rotate established personnel often follows some concrete guidelines, which are meant to maintain a level of impartiality. In all fairness, the choice is always hard, but the welfare of the patients and the quality and efficiency of the laboratory take precedence over personal circumstances or childish threats.

   A simple compromise may encompass all of the above. By splitting the day and evening shift positions between the two qualified and deserving employees, the initial conflict may be resolved but could create a new problem when the night shift position is left open. Hiring from outside may resolve the problem but could cause feelings of resentment toward the new employee as well as the person who hired them. Other approaches may be to consider the candidates and to make an informed choice, or to give each candidate the opportunity to work for a trial period or to have an outside evaluator conduct the interviews and make a recommendation. These alternatives may sound very matter of fact, but decisions affecting the lives of others are very difficult.

   Carefully consider the needs of the institution, the patients, the laboratory, the departments, and finally the individuals involved. Qualifications, productivity, and attitude should also be scrutinized. The cost of training, retraining, or replacing personnel round out factors that could ultimately affect the final resolution.

   Personnel policies, particularly those associated with hiring, should be evaluated on a regular basis to ensure that the employees as well as the institutions maintain the highest level of quality. Probationary periods afford employers and employees an opportunity to rectify adverse situations.

3. Health-care professionals agree that patient care is their primary focus, but opinions vary about the best way to attain the quality care desired. Physicians and nurses have more direct contact with patients, which may explain their concerns about the length of time it takes a laboratory to perform sample analysis. Each patient sample is treated with the same care and skill by the laboratory personnel, but the circumstances of a person's well-being dictate the priority and necessity of requested tests.

   This case focuses on that point because emergency patients are sometimes in dire need of care that hinges on laboratory results. Satellite laboratories, such as the one suggested, to resolve the problem in this case have a unique set of problems associated with compliance and competency, not to mention the outrageous cost of establishing a laboratory.

   On the surface the idea is quite reasonable, but upon further investigation the cost of equipment, personnel, and training in conjunction with the expenditure of time reveal a more complex and less attractive resolution. It would seem more reasonable to utilize the resources for an upgrade of the present laboratory to include more personnel and newer technology.

   Both solutions supplied will require time to implement, and the patients should not have to wait to receive quality care. A short-term addition to these scenarios may be to offer overtime or incentives to the current laboratory staff, have overlapping shifts during peak periods, or even rehire some retired techs to work during the peak times to reduce the turnaround time. Also, evaluate where delays are occurring before, during, and after analysis.

   If it is concluded that expansion or improvement is needed. Time should be spent at designated intervals during the long process to validate, modify, or discard the resolution model.

Chapter 31, Preanalytical, Analytical, and Postanalytical Phases

ANSWERS FOR QUESTIONS

1. D. Preanalytical—formulation of clinical question and choices made regarding clinical testing

2. E. Analytical—specimen preparation, analysis of specimen, and quality control

3. A. Postanalytical—analysis of effect of testing data on patient outcomes

4. The preanalytical component is critical because the clinical question is formulated here. The medical technologist/clinical laboratory scientist can provide information regarding the types of tests available to address the question, the efficiency and cost of the different types of tests, and the specimen required. This information must be considered in the present health-care environment to avoid unnecessary costs and unnecessary delay in answering the clinical question because the wrong test was selected. Specimen preparation, analysis of the specimen, and quality control are analytical components of the job. Consultation with the physician regarding the action taken and the effect on the patient as a result of the testing data provided are examples of the postanalytical component.

CASE COMMENTARY

1. Anytime anyone questions the laboratory results, the questioning should be taken seriously. These findings should be investigated. Colonies counts could be correlated to actual clinical findings. The literature could be reviewed, and one would find that studies have already shown that in healthy young women a colony count of less than 100,000 cfu/ml may be significant. This is primarily a postanalytical situation. You are correlating laboratory information with patient outcomes.

2. The situation is primarily a preanalytical situation. You as the laboratorian realize that the Clinitest tablet examination should indicate if a reducing substance is present, although it will not identify the substance. Therefore, Clinitest tablet negative specimens would not need to have paper chromatography analysis, because it would be negative for reducing substances. Communications with the physicians prior to receiving orders would prevent unnecessary testing.

3. Because the reference test for Tryoponin I is the "gold standard," and the turnaround time is eight hours, this would be the preferred test. This is primarily a preanalytical situation, and communications with the physicians would prevent unnecessary testing. Perhaps you might discuss with the chief technologist the deletion of in-house CK isoenzyme testing due to the volume and tech time. You might want to investigate the possibility of bringing the Tryponin I testing in-house.

4. This can be considered a preanalytical situation because there seems to be an ordering error on the patient. However, it could also be an analytical situation because a procedure for handling this type of situation needs to be implemented. And it could also be considered a postanalytical situation because the ordered tests revealed that additional testing is needed in order to produce good patient outcomes.

5. When a trend develops, something in the test procedure is gradually failing. One should check the instrument and supplies, such as reagents. This is an analytical situation that could impact patient outcomes.

Chapter 32, Instrument Selection

ANSWERS FOR QUESTIONS

1. a. Characteristics of the laboratory including such factors as the lab test menu needed in the future, the current and future lab workload, the test mix of the lab, the work-flow situation (e.g., what STAT capabilities are needed) and labor considerations such as minimal sample loading times, walk-away features, instrument quality control features and data generation features, ease of troubleshooting, and maintenance downtime.
   b. An additional consideration is the instrument's impact upon the lab environment: its size, special electrical or plumbing needs, and the amount of heat generated during operation.
   c. Also, as part of the assessment, quality of performance issues should be addressed and should include setting minimum standards for instrument performance factors including linearity, sensitivity, specificity, accuracy, precision, and stability of electronics and of reagents used.

2. The manager, supervisors, individuals who will be using the instrument, representatives of the administration, planners, LIS officer, safety officer, pathologists, and physicians

3. Costs to be considered include: purchase or leasing, labor per test, reagents, reagent stability factors, installation costs, impact on heating/cooling/plumbing services, labor for maintenance and troubleshooting, quality control calibrators, storage of reagents, service contracts, depreciation, disposables, and consumables.

4. Networking with others who have used the instrument will supply information to the manager regarding advantages and disadvantages of the instrument as viewed by those who have hands-on experience with the instrument. Discussions can verify manufacturer's claims.

CASE COMMENTARY

1-5. These cases have been selected to allow you to develop a needs assessment for the laboratory described. Utilizing instrumentation textbooks and manufacturer's literature, you can conduct research on the cases to help determine which instrument you think best meets the needs of a specific lab. You do not have to do all cases, instead you may wish to focus on cases for the types of lab settings in which you are interested. The teacher may need to supply some materials, especially related to the specific instruments you should consider, if time is limited. Textbooks may not discuss the instruments newly available in the marketplace. Most important is the justification for the choice; less important is the actual instrument chosen because several instruments may be acceptable for the criteria developed. Therefore, there are no absolutely correct answers to the cases.

These cases may be done individually or in groups to simulate teamwork. The first stage of solving the cases involves doing a needs assessment with the limited information supplied in the case. Look for key needs such as menu size, throughput needed, STAT capabilities, and so on. Determine the most critical needs. Second, do your research using vendor literature, vendor Web sites, and perhaps speaking with the sales representative in your area. During the research stage, you may wish to discuss your choices with area technologists to try a networking approach to gathering information.

The next stage is to match the needs to the characteristics and features of the instrument discovered in your research. You should narrow your possible choices to two to three instruments. Next, examine factors such as costs for the instruments you are considering.

Finally, you (or your team) should make a decision and discuss what made you select that one specific instrument. Could you explain to your employees what factors lead to the final selection?

Chapter 33, Establishing Preventative and Corrective Maintenance Programs

ANSWERS FOR QUESTIONS

1. Preventative maintenance (PM) is a planned program of specific tasks to be performed at specific intervals to prevent the failure of laboratory instruments. Corrective maintenance is simply the repair/replacement of parts when a failure occurs in an instrument. Failure is not planned nor scheduled, and the activities needed for correction will vary depending on the problem.

2. PM is beneficial for the laboratory because it reduces instrument failure rates, which in turn reduces lost production time and employee idle time. PM helps to prolong the life of the instrument. It also reduces personnel exposure to safety hazards. Instrument maintenance contributes to the stability and reliability of laboratory results. Less instrument failures result in fewer delays in providing health care to patients.

3. Service contracts are essential for major instruments that are now too complex electronically and mechanically for the average technologist to repair. The contract provides for knowledgeable service personnel to do timely repairs that are beyond the scope of in-house repairs.

4. To establish a PM program, the supervisor should first inventory all equipment. Second, a form should be developed to record the results of all PM activities performed at specified intervals. The supervisor should assign personnel to assume responsibility for each instrument and then train the personnel in both performing the tasks and documenting the tasks performed. The supervisor should ascertain that the tasks have been completed and documented according to the schedule. Finally, the supervisor and the manager should evaluate the PM and repairs to determine if any correlations exist between poor PM and the quality of lab data generated.

5. C. Corrective maintenance is simply the repair/replacement of parts when a failure occurs in an instrument.

6. The process of locating the malfunction is known as troubleshooting. There are numerous sources that outline steps in beginning the troubleshooting process. The process should follow logical steps and assumptions rather than random repair attempts. Before the problem can be located, it must be defined clearly. In addition, the most obvious and common solutions should be attempted before more exotic faults are considered.

CASE COMMENTARY

1. The supervisor has only a limited amount of information to determine what is happening in this situation. She knows that the problem occurs once a month early on Sundays. The instrument checks indicated that the problem was an electrical one. First, the supervisor and instrument operators should examine all the electrical connections to the instrument—is the cord damaged or frayed, are the breaker boxes normal, and so on. Next, the supervisor should contact the physical facilities director to determine if the hospital experienced a power surge or an electrical failure of any kind during the time period.

   Suppose the supervisor did these checks and was unable to locate any indication of a problem. She decided to discuss the problem with the individuals on the weekend night shift. Both technologists were also baffled by a problem that occurred on three occasions without warning. The supervisor asked them to try to remember anything unusual that occurred on those Sunday mornings. One of the technologists commented that the night had been extremely quiet—in fact so quiet that housekeeping had been able to complete waxing of the entire floor in the chemistry section instead of only doing a small portion as was usual. The supervisor asked the techs how often the floors were waxed, and they commented that the waxing was done once a month. From this offhand comment the supervisor was able to determine from the housekeeping department that a new floor buffing machine had been purchased three months ago and that the lab floors were waxed early on Sunday mornings. She was able to discuss the issue with the housekeeper and found that he was using the floor buffer on the same electrical circuit as the instrument, causing power fluctuations when the buffing machine was turned on. He commented that in the intensive care unit the new machine had actually caused blown fuses. The vendor of the instrument verified that the instrument was very sensitive to power fluctuations and should always be installed on a separate circuit or with a heavy-duty surge protector. If power became erratic, the instrument might experience failure in certain circuits. After the failure, if the electrical self-check procedure was utilized, the instrument could reset itself rapidly if the voltage and current were steady again.

   Finally, the Sunday morning mystery was solved.

2. Immediately the speed of the cytocentrifuge should be checked with a tachometer. Also, the timing should be checked with a stopwatch. Because the cellular elements are fragmented and distorted, the speed may be too high or the timing too long. It appears that the cytocentrifuge has not been added to the PM records and no maintenance has been done on the instrument since it was purchased. The cytocentrifuge should definitely be added to the PM list and the speed and timing checked monthly and recorded. The maintenance performed should be recorded in the maintenance records.

Chapter 34, Organization and Time Management

ANSWERS FOR QUESTIONS

1. The first step in organization is to set goals and define tasks.
2. The main list is a list of all tasks to be done in no particular order, and the secondary list is derived from the main list but list tasks in order of importance. One might use the main list to list all tasks that need to be accomplished in a week. The secondary list is then arranged according to importance, with top priority items performed at the beginning of the week.

3. Computer and mind.

4. Time savers are
   1) Set goals—Make goals specific and measurable.
   2) Set priorities—Do the most important (highest priority) tasks *first*.
   3) Organize—Arrange workload to accomplish what is expected.
   4) Delegate—Free up time for handling more important tasks.
   5) Get started—Do it now. The sooner it is started, the sooner it will be finished.

5. Time wasters are
   1) Procrastination—Putting off until later, what should be done *now*.
   2) Interruptions—Results may be delayed due to frequent interruption by telephone and by people.
   3) Clutter—Mental or work-space clutter may hinder processing.
   4) Disorganization—Not knowing where to begin.
   5) Lack of goals—Not knowing what is important to do, or not knowing when or how to do it.

   Decide what is important, do what needs to be done now, minimize interruptions, and keep an uncluttered work space.

CASE COMMENTARY

1. There is a lack of organization on the part of the administrative technologist that causes the clutter and the constant activity. Your evaluations are good, so the administrative technologist does not believe that time must be spent with you. Instead the administrative technologist spends time with the problem employee. The problem with this approach is that the administrative technologist is not taking time to reward your good performance. This may not motivate some good employees. Organizational approaches that the administrative technologist might take would be to have the secretary hold all calls while in conference and plan adequate time for the evaluation through advanced scheduling. All the time wasters, including procrastination, interruptions, clutter, disorganization, and lack of goals, seem to be present. It also appears that the administrative technologist could benefit from goal setting, prioritizing, organizing, and delegating.

2. This administrative technologist is using techniques such as goal setting, prioritizing, organizing, and delegating.

Chapter 35, The Laboratory Information System: Choosing the Right One

ANSWERS FOR QUESTIONS

1. Five benefits of an LIS are: reduce time-consuming paper work, store patient data, store quality control data, provide immediate access to results, reduce chance of an assay being run on the wrong patient when barcode is used.

2. B. Selecting the LIS team to evaluate the system is the first step.

3. An RFP provides the vendor with detailed information about what the laboratory will require from the system, what kind of service will be expected during and after installation, and what financial limitations exist.

4. LIS managers and other staff at other hospitals that are using the prospective systems should be contacted to ascertain input regarding their experiences with the proposed systems. Other members of the hospital medical staff should be consulted regarding their specific needs from the laboratory.

5. Visits to other laboratories are critical because valuable information regarding the specific operation, advantages, and disadvantages of each system can be evaluated in a particular setting. Matching the LIS to the hospital situation is critical, and hospitals of similar size and operation can provide information regarding the suitability of the system that the vendor cannot provide.

CASE COMMENTARY

1. The new LIS apparently does not fully service the entire emergency department. Each section should have easy access to a printer where all reports will print upon release by the laboratory. A proper LIS team including members from the laboratory staff and even the medical staff would have recognized this need and would have provided more printers.

2. If the urinalysis reports are confusing, they may need to be reconfigured to make them easier to read. Again, a proper LIS team should have included representatives from the medical staff who could have provided input about how reports should be configured.

3. There seems to be a problem with the interface between the chemistry instrument and the new LIS, meaning that a possibly expensive reconfiguration of the interface may have to be done, or the chemistry department may have to learn to live with the delays. Problems with this system and this particular instrument may have been discovered if the LIS team had been able to do some research—in particular through discussions with other users of the instrument and/or system.

4. One of the most important features of an LIS company is the service it provides once the system is in place. It is critical for the team choosing the LIS to check with several customers of the company for their opinions about the company's service record.

5. The LIS should be set up to print lists of pending/overdue tests for each department. These lists should be checked, at a minimum, at the end of each shift to make sure that no orders are missed. Better input from the laboratory before the system was put into place would have ensured that this was done from the beginning.

   Obviously, there should have been more input from the laboratory and the medical staff about which system would have best served everyone. Although cost is an important factor in the choice, a bad system can do more harm than good. Also, it is very important to get the opinions of other laboratorians who have used a particular system before the final decision is made to purchase that system.

Chapter 36, Epidemiology in the Clinical Laboratory

ANSWERS FOR QUESTIONS

1. Epidemiology is the medical science that investigates variability in disease occurrence. It may be defined as the study of the determinants and distribution of disease in populations. Epidemiology, in essence then, investigates the who, what, where, and when of disease outcomes.

2. E. The overall purpose of epidemiology is to provide the basis for public health disease prevention and control measures for groups at risk of disease.

3. F. Epidemiology is used: 1) in public health planning, 2) for disease surveillance, 3) to evaluate health programs and medical technologies, and 4) to perform etiological research.

4. Clinical laboratories provide essential screening and diagnostic test services used to assess the health status of the public. Further, epidemiology methods are routinely applied in the clinical laboratory to assess the quality and accuracy of these tests as well as to monitor mandatory disease reporting to state agencies.

5. a. validity: measures how closely the test value is to the true measure.
   b. "gold standard": the most accurate measure currently available.
   c. sensitivity of a test: ability of the screening test to detect positives among the truly diseased, is calculated $a/(a + c)$, and is measured as a proportion (0.0–1.0).
   d. specificity of a test: the ability of a screening test to detect negatives among the truly nondiseased, is calculated $d/(b + d)$, and is measured as a proportion (0.0–1.0).
   e. reliability: repeatability of results.
   f. interrater reliability: measures the degree to which two or more assessors agree on test results.
   g. kappa statistic: measures the agreement level between two raters once chance agreement has been taken into account.
   h. surveillance: the ongoing systematic collection, analysis, and interpretation of data for the purpose of health improvement.

6. These predictive value measures are more appropriately used to decide whether or not a screening test is useful for the population at hand.

7. The Notifiable Infectious Disease Surveillance Program was established through the Centers for Disease Control and Prevention (CDC) to monitor the incidence of specific infectious conditions throughout the United States.

8. The clinical laboratory plays a basic and crucial role in this important CDC surveillance program, serving as the link between the physician's test request and result reporting to the local and state health department, where, at the latter, counts for each condition are tabulated and forwarded to the CDC for national reporting. In addition, the laboratory must also ensure that the information accompanying each report is complete, accurate, and sent within the imposed time limit.

CASE COMMENTARY

1. Yes, you need to take immediate action regarding this situation. The microorganism appears to be Group B beta hemolytic streptococcus, which has been implicated in nosocomial infections in the hospital. The microorganism is usually resident in the mother and transferred to the baby at birth. Because these are isolates from blood cultures and there are four babies with the microorganism, you would immediately contact the infection control officer of the hospital. Actions must be initiated immediately to treat the infected babies, to isolate the source of the microorganism, to prevent further spread of the microorganism, and to determine whether all the babies have the same microorganism. This is not considered a reportable microorganism.

2. Your presentation should include the fact that the present screening test offered by the laboratory is highly sensitive, but not very specific. The Western Blot is used as a confirmation test for the screening test because it is highly specific, but not as sensitive. The screening test is used because it is desirable to detect any possible positive in the screened patients; however, there are a good number of false positives found because of the high sensitivity level. Also the screening test is used because the cost to the patient is low, whereas the cost of the Western Blot is high. The present procedure is to perform the screening test, which if negative ends the testing at a low cost to the patient. But if the screening test is positive, the Western Blot is performed, and the cost is significantly higher. The materials and personnel required to perform the Western Blot in-house plus the low volume of testing would make the Western Blot more expensive in-house than sending out to the reference laboratory.

Chapter 37, Accreditation

ANSWERS FOR QUESTIONS

1. A. It is the approval of an institution, portion of an institution, or program regarding minimum acceptable criteria.

2. D. All of the above

3. JCAHO: The JCAHO was formed in 1951 by the American College of Physicians, The American Medical Association and the American College of Surgeons. Its primary purpose was to provide voluntary accreditation for the hospital. In 1953 the first "Standards for Hospital Accreditation" was published.

    CAP: The CAP was established in December 1946 by a committee of the American Society of Clinical Pathologists to accredit clinical laboratories.

    AABB: AABB was established to promote the highest standard of care for patients and donors in all aspects of blood banking, and their accreditation program was developed for this purpose.

    NAACLS: The purpose of NAACLS is the accreditation of the educational programs of clinical laboratory science.

4. CLIA '88 covers all laboratories performing laboratory testing regardless of where these labs are based. This includes private labs, hospital-based labs, and physician office labs. CLIA '88 also established minimum requirements that must be met in order to perform laboratory

testing. The requirements cover quality assurance, quality control, proficiency testing, record retention, complexity of tests (high, moderate, and waived), job categories, and personnel requirements to perform testing, supervise, and direct laboratory services.

CASE COMMENTARY

1. This is a simple problem to fix. You simply enroll the lab in an acceptable proficiency testing program for this particular analyte. There are several acceptable programs for this: CAP and COLA (for physician office laboratories). CAP is the one used in most hospitals. You must provide a purchase order documenting purchase of the program and the response from the agency indicating enrollment in the program. JCAHO requires you to respond to all type I recommendations within six months of the survey date. Because you have six months, you may even be able to send a completed proficiency test report back with your response.

2. This problem may be easy to fix. After your CAP inspection you will have thirty days to respond to all phase II and phase I deficiencies. For phase I deficiencies you simply have to make a statement that this is being taken care of and that you should be in compliance with the next inspection. Phase I does not require any documentation to be sent to CAP as follow up. On phase II deficiencies you must send documentation that you are in compliance. To take care of this deficiency, you must have your engineering or biomed department do a thorough inspection of all equipment and all electrical plugs used for that equipment. This is documented on the maintenance sheets, and the copy of the form showing that this is complete is sent as documentation that satisfies that particular regulation. On the documentation, you must put the number of the deficiency at the top of the document so that the inspector will know what standard or regulation the documentation addresses.

3. This is not as easy to fix as it may seem. A phase II deficiency in space cannot be easily addressed or fixed. The inspector will usually not issue such a phase deficiency unless there is a serious compromise in patient care or employee safety due to the space issue. This also involves either complete renovation or building of a new lab if this occurs in subsequent years. This may be easy to answer if your department is already included in an expansion program that is ongoing at your institution. You can simply have the CEO write a letter stating this fact and when the projected completion date is expected. A copy of the completed plans for the project may also be required. The inspector would then give you time to complete the project. If your department is not already included in the expansion plan, then other avenues must be explored. These include a letter from the CEO stating that the hospital will be exploring the possibility of expansion of the laboratory and the expected completion date. There may be a possibility the lab could be located to another area in the interim to gain space (note: this is not easy to do because of the technology needed to run the department). The CAP may require you to build or relocate the laboratory to more space within the next two years or lose accreditation. This is not, however, usually done. If the hospital can show that they are truly working on solving the problem, the accrediting agency will usually allow time to complete the project.

4. The regulation requires that you have remote alarms on the refrigerators in case someone is not in the blood bank and the alarm sounds. Most blood banks have audible alarms both in the department and at a remote area. This remote area can be either in security or at the public broadcasting exchange (PBX) area. This allows the lab to be called when the alarm sounds at the remote area, thus guaranteeing that blood bank personnel are aware of the problem. To fix this issue you would need to have the blood bank alarms attached to an alarm in either the security area of PBX operator area. This would then be documented by a purchase order for the work, documentation of completion of the work, and a copy of the record or temperature checks to show the alarms are operating properly.

Chapter 38, Legal Considerations

ANSWERS FOR QUESTIONS

1. human resource department (personnel department)
2. the job announcement and the job description
3. E. arrest record, marital status, number of children, religious affiliation
4. If a laboratorian was hired to do drug testing that would be used in legal cases, it might be permissible to determine if the laboratorian had previous drug related convictions. The job should be carefully analyzed to be sure that the information is essential.
5. collective bargaining unit
6. E. confidentiality, reimbursement procedures, specimen chain of command

CASE COMMENTARY

1. Yes, the technologist would be personally liable; however, the institution would not be liable because the technologist did not follow the procedure established by the institution.
2. Because the candidate voluntarily gave the information and was not asked for the information, the interviewer has not done anything illegal. However, this information should not be repeated or used in making the hiring decision.
3. No, the results should not be given to the nurse, because the nurse in this case is the patient. The results should be reported directly to the physician.
4. The employer cannot legally deny employment based on the lack of a specific certification unless the employer can demonstrate the need for a specific certification.
5. If the technologist followed the procedure, then an accident occurred. The technologist can be liable, thus the reason for personal professional liability insurance. If the technologist did not follow proper procedures, then this would not be considered an accident, but something more serious. The questions for the institution might be whether this was a predicable accident, whether the institution took precautions to prevent it, and whether the accident was handled properly.

Chapter 39, Consulting

ANSWERS FOR QUESTIONS

1. professional or technical
2. technical, knowledge of literature, synthesize a large volume of material, communications, basic marketing, self-management, and business skills.
3. General issues are

   scope: addresses the purpose of the consulting business. One should decide exactly what services will be offered.

liability: addresses assessing personal, professional, and product liability.

capital: addresses how much money will be needed to establish the consulting business and where it will be obtained.

publications: addresses the types on publications used in the consulting business.

marketing: addresses the advertisement of the consulting business, including target audience.

Specific issues are:

proposal: addresses the activities of the project including time table and cost.

contract: a legal document defining the duties of the consultant and the client.

fees: addresses the fees for each activity and how the fees will be paid.

CASE COMMENTARY

1. First, the consultant should be technically prepared. In order to gather the technical information needed for this consulting job, the medical technologist/clinical laboratory scientist should consult current publications such as biological safety recommendations for the Centers for Disease Control, state regulations, journal articles, hospital association recommendations, and so on. Also the consultant might decide to contact several other hospitals in order to examine materials that have already been developed. Second, because this would provide a large volume of material, the consultant must synthesize the material so that it is concise, organized, and understandable. Third, as the material is synthesized, the consultant should predict how future activities will impact the waste disposal recommendations. After all the material is gathered, the consultant is ready for the meeting. As the committee develops the recommendations, the consultant should always think creativity.

2. One should always be sure that the business card contains all the information anyone would need for making contact. This business card looks pretty, but there is no information as to how to contact the consultant.

3. Before beginning a consulting business, one should assess the market to determine if there is a need for the service. In this case, the local private laboratory is only a phone call away if the physician has any questions regarding the specimen needed for testing, and the information is free to the physician.

4. Often consulting businesses start after one has performed a service for one individual and realizes that others need the same expertise. First, you decide the scope of your consulting practice—are you going to just develop procedure manuals or do more? Second, consider whether you need to incorporate. Consult a small business lawyer to determine whether this is the direction you should take. Third, decide what expenses you initially will incur and determine where the funds will be derived. Fourth, develop a brochure describing you consulting business, business cards, stationary, and so on and distribute to possible clients in the area.

    For the physician that has just requested your services, develop a proposal establishing what is to be done, the time frame for development, the costs, and so on. Meet with the physician regarding the proposal to be sure that you both agree on the job to be done. Modify the proposal as necessary. Use the proposal information to develop a contract that delineates the agreement including the job, your duties, time table, client's responsibilities, cost, payment method, and so on. Provide the contract to the physician. After the contract is signed, complete the consulting job. Materials that you develop for this consulting job may often be modified for the next consulting job and used; therefore, care should be taken with the first experience, as materials may be used in the future, and you are developing a reputation for your work.

Chapter 40, Establishment of a Continuing Education Program

ANSWERS FOR QUESTIONS

1. Schwabbauer states that continuing education includes educational activities not normally associated with an academic degree.

2. NCA requires twelve contact hours per year to maintain certification.

3. Six variables that must be considered when implementing a CEP are:
   a. Establishing a need
   b. Establishing a task force to implement
   c. Working with an established budget
   d. Researching types of CEPs
   e. Issuing credits
   f. Monitoring effectiveness

4. External clients are individuals or groups external to the laboratory such as physicians, nurses, patients, or anyone living in the community. Examples of external client educational programs are providing continuing education activities and coordinating science fairs.

5. P.A.C.E.® means Professional Acknowledgment of Continuing Education.

6. 14 contact hours = 1.4 CEUs.

   1 contact hour = 0.1 CEU; therefore 14 contact hours × 0.1 CEU = 1.4 CEUs

7. Participants should be surveyed to assess clearness of presentation, adequacy of time, and relationship to needs.

8. 1.0 CEU = 10 contact hours

   0.1 CEU = 1 contact hour; therefore 1.0 CEU = 10 contact hours

CASE COMMENTARY

The following is a "proposed solution" to the case history. It is not the only correct solution, but it should be used as a guideline for selecting appropriate and cost-efficient methods. The three continuing education items that should be considered followed by a brief narrative are listed below:

- External speakers—The speaker of the session may be videotaped and rebroadcast to employees who were unable to attend the initial airing of the teleconference. Written consent from both the speaker and facility is required for rebroadcast. The only cost is videotaping and rebroadcasting.
- Audiocassettes—Ima is correct on her suggestion. As the explanation summarizes in the case, posttests accompanying the audiocassettes may be copied and graded for in-house continuing education credit using the provided answer sheet. But only the original six posttests may be submitted to the primary continuing education provider at no cost for P.A.C.E.® or CLME credit. As an idea, because the laboratory is a thirty-member technical staff, employees may be placed on a rotational basis to receive P.A.C.E.® or CLME credit from the primary continuing education provider (two audiocassettes and six posttests/month for one year—one technical member of the staff will receive P.A.C.E.® or CLME credit once every five months).

At this point, the amount of money spent on continuing education totals $470 from the allocated $775 budget.

- Magazine subscription—This is an excellent idea for continuing education. As the explanation summarizes in the case, each employee could be furnished a copy of the free publication. The posttest accompanying the continuing education article may be completed by the employee and returned with the $18 fee to the primary education provider for official continuing education credit. The education officer could develop her own evaluation system for any articles read and give the employees continuing education credit in-house.

The total amount of money spent is $535 from the allocated budget of $775. This is well under the budget. The remaining $240 may be set aside in the budget for other avenues of continuing education throughout the next year.

A chart below summarizes the spending of the allocated $750.

Continuing Education Project	Cost
External speaker	$ 95.00
Audiocassettes	$375.00
Magazine subscription	$ 65.00
Total	$535.00

Chapter 41, Construction and Delivery of an Instructional Unit

ANSWERS FOR QUESTIONS

1. Educational level, prior knowledge, previous experience, and biases

2. *Lecture.* Advantage: Timely information, summarize material, supplement other information, large number of learners. Disadvantage: Vast amounts of material, not needed when information is in printed form.

   Discussion. Advantage: Learner-centered, builds increased levels of thinking, develops affective domain. Disadvantage: Not useful for imparting new information.

   Demonstration. Advantage: Teaches skills, procedures, techniques; usually needs another form of instruction to support it. Disadvantage: Small number of learners, must be followed by controlled practice.

3. *Flip Chart.* Advantage: Effective for discussion, holds attention, building of ideas. Disadvantage: Information on chart must match verbal communication or learners are confused.

   Printed Material (e.g., charts, diagrams, and tables not found in the textbook).

   Advantage: Should accompany outline and objectives, needed for learner. Disadvantage: Too much material in handouts.

   Overhead Projector. Advantage: Easy to use, saves class time, aids visual learners. Disadvantage: Excessive use does not allow for eye contact with learners, too much information may be included preventing good listening.

LCD Projector. Advantage: Allows color and movement. Disadvantage: Visuals may be too distracting, possible electronic failure.

4. a. What is the learner to do?
   b. Under which conditions should the learner accomplish the objective?
   c. What are the criteria to show achievement of the objective?

5. a. cognitive domain: intellectual outcomes, knowledge-based
   b. psychomotor domain: motor skills
   c. affective domain: interests, attitudes, appreciation, and the development of a value system

6. a. cognitive
   b. psychomotor
   c. affective

7. A **goal** is an achieveable statement of broad direction. It allows the instructor to target the purpose of the educational unit and provides the base upon which measurable objectives are constructed. An **objective** is a specific statement of what the learner is expected to know or to be able to do after a period of instruction; it is totally learner-based.

    Goal: The student (or employee) will develop phlebotomy skills.

    Objective: Following a demonstration and discussion regarding the materials necessary for performing a phlebotomy procedure, the student will assemble all the required materials accurately.

8. E. Laboratory, lecture, demonstration, and role-play might all be used to teach one how to perform a Gram stain.

9. F. Lecture, demonstration, and role-play would be appropriate teaching strategies for the student or employee to learn how to interact professionally with patients.

10. B. Use of the word *understanding* is not measurable

11. A. Good objective

CASE COMMENTARY

1. The first step would be to directly communicate with the student and identify why she looks puzzled. Exploring the way she learns best will allow the instructor to either adjust the teaching strategy for the entire class or to suggest various other ways that she can receive the information. If the rest of the class appears to be learning, the format should not be changed. If there is an academic development office at the institution, the learner may benefit from various studying/note-taking techniques. The instructor should always aim to offer the opportunity for optimal learning for each individual.

2. It is usually difficult for a more experienced individual to take instruction from a younger, less experienced person. The instructor must take into account the target population even if it is only one person. An additional problem might be that the instructor is a clinical laboratory scientist and the learner is a technician.

    The learner may be apprehensive, and the instructor should have some introductory communication before beginning the demonstration. Having printed materials is also helpful. If the learner doesn't appear to understand during the presentation, another verbal communication, perhaps accompanied by flow charts or diagrams, should take place.

    Although the instruction time may be limited, sometimes it is beneficial to break instruction into smaller time frames. This allows for smaller amounts of material to be processed. Additional time should always allow for a period of review at the beginning and a short summary at the end. Always construct a lesson plan/unit that includes using goals, objectives, teaching strategies, printed material, and media prior to beginning.

3. Anytime an instructional unit is given, a lesson plan should be made. A forty-five-minute session is fairly short; however, learners should be presented with objectives and other relevant printed material. It would also be helpful to know if the students have already had chemistry and biology or if they are interested in a health science career. If it is a special interest group, the objectives could be written at a higher taxonomic level.

    Working with high school students presents a challenge because the instructor has to keep their interest. A short lecture or explanation of the urinalysis procedure followed by a demonstration and student practice might be an effective way to provide instruction.

Chapter 42, Measurement and Evaluation Strategies for an Instructional Unit

ANSWERS FOR QUESTIONS

1. Measurement is concerned with the application of an instrument or instruments (i.e., a tool produced to measure the intended outcome) to collect data for some specific purpose. Evaluation is using the measurement data for appraisal with specific purposes or aims in mind.

2. Reliability is a demonstration of consistent measurement from test to test and over multiple times. Validity measures relevant tasks.

3. Norm-based education describes performance in terms of position in a group of peers. Competency-based education evaluates performance in terms of a specific behavior.

4. Formative—evaluation during instruction

    Diagnostic—evaluation of learning difficulties during instruction

    Summative—evaluation of learner achievement at the end of instruction

5. *Essay.* Advantage: Observe information and organization. Indication of ability to analyze and synthesize. Disadvantage: Small amount of material. Difficulty in objectivity. Increased time to score.

    True/False. Advantage: Easy to construct. Easy to grade. Acceptable for formative period. Disadvantage: Can be ambiguous and irrelevant. Can guess; 50/50 chance. No assurance of learner's knowledge.

    Matching. Advantage: Easy to construct. Disadvantage: Only for taxonomic Level 1 questions.

    Multiple Choice. Advantage: Versatile. Easy to score. Administered to large groups. Format of certification examinations. Disadvantage: Time consuming to construct.

6. Item analysis is an effective tool that examines the agreement of the learner's answers with the acceptable responses for specific items on measurement instrument/examination.

7. *Anecdotal Record.* Advantage: Supplements and validates other observations. Good for formative period. Disadvantage: Bias may result. Time consuming.

    Checklist. Advantage: Simple to use. Works well in clinical situation. Disadvantage: Time consuming if feedback is to be immediate. May be subjective if its use is not explained.

8. Objectivity is extremely important in evaluation methods that use one of the observational techniques. Several errors can occur.
   - Bias—evaluators tend to evaluate all students the same. Generosity error occurs at the high end of the scale; the evaluator is usually trying to avoid confrontation from the learners. Severity error places all learners at the bottom of the scale. Central tendency error avoids both ends of the scale and makes every learner average.
   - Halo—the evaluator rates on the general impression of a learner, which affects all evaluation characteristics. If the evaluator likes the learner, all areas will be marked very high; if the learner is not liked, all areas will be low even if that learner has earned a better evaluation. This error differs from the bias because each learner is evaluated differently.
   - Logical—similar ratings are given for areas perceived to be related. An example would be giving a learner an excellent evaluation for the psychomotor domain because he always earns the highest mark on the cognitive examinations.

   Proper design and use of measurement instruments followed by communication with those individuals who will be using them can eliminate most of these errors.

9. Guidelines to be followed when performing affective domain evaluation include
   - publish the objectives.
   - monitor the students before evaluation.
   - confront any problems.
   - offer assistance to the student.
   - determine the severity of a problem before evaluation.

10. C. All distractors (answer choices) are not grammatically correct.

11. B. The question does not match the objective.

12. This is a halo error because the evaluator has rated using her general impression of the learner (i.e., the learner is an excellent baby-sitter; therefore, she must be an excellent student).

13. This is a bias error showing central tendency because the evaluator is avoiding both ends of the rating scale, thus making all students average.

CASE COMMENTARY

1. The entire curriculum for chemistry must be reviewed. Start with the objectives to make certain that they cover all the competencies that have set up for the learner. Make a blueprint that addresses a match of the measurement instrument's questions to the objectives. Check to see that various taxonomic levels are covered.

   Identify the faculty. Are individuals teaching different topics? If this is the first time that the class hasn't met the national mean, consider that the examination may have changed. Review the descriptors that come with the program report.

2. This is an example of evaluation bias. The faculty member might want to be liked by every learner or is afraid of repercussions if a lower grade is given. She may be a wonderful teacher, but if every student receives an "A," there might be a problem.

   Review the curriculum and ascertain if there is a variety of taxonomic levels for the questions. Investigate the type of measurement instrument(s) used. Are they appropriate for the subject?

   Most importantly, communicate with the instructor. Review the grading policy and the criteria she utilizes to determine the grade.

3. This also might be an example of evaluation bias. Review the competencies with the instructor. Determine if the evaluator is expecting too much of the learner. Stress that a learner is supposed to reach entry level competency, and describe in detail what that means for the evaluation process. Encourage the use of an anecdotal record to demonstrate the reason for the lower evaluations.

   Talk to the students. Have them evaluate the instructor. Is she at fault? Are effective teaching strategies that provide the required knowledge base being used? Remember, the measurement instrument is based on the objectives.

   Compare the class' performance in the various areas of hematology. If they are meeting expectations in these areas, the problem is probably the instructor. Try to avoid using her as an instructor.

4. The content of an evaluation should never be a surprise. The summative evaluation should never be the only one in a unit. Poor performance on formative instruments may necessitate diagnostic evaluation, but the learner would know that his performance was not up to minimal standards. Anecdotal records and critical incident reporting would be very helpful in this case. It would also be mandatory if the student chose to appeal the evaluation.

Index

A

AABB. *See* American Association of Blood Banks
AACC. *See* American Association for Clinical Chemistry
Abbott Laboratories, Web site, 196
ABN. *See* Advanced beneficiary notice
About, Inc., Web site, 126, 210
Abstract, 64
Abstract random, 70
Abstract sequential, 70
Abuse. *See* Fraud
Accreditation, 227–231
Accuracy test, 158–159
Adjusted patient days, 135, 137
Advanced beneficiary notice (ABN), 130
Advanced Instruments, Inc., Web site, 196
Advance for Administrators of the Laboratory, Web site, 143
Advance for Medical Laboratory Professionals, Web site, 143
Advertisement, job, 18–25
    key elements of, 18, 22
    sample, 23
Advertising. *See* Marketing
Advocate standards of excellence, 1
Affective domain evaluation, 259–260
African American population, 45
Age Discrimination in Employment Act, 46, 233
Ageism, 44–45
Air War College and Ira C. Eaker College, Web site, 70
Alaska Department of Labor and Workforce Development, 22
Alliance Training, Cultural Awareness Can Improve Your Business, Web site, 47
American Association for Clinical Chemistry, Clinical Laboratory News, Web site, 131, 191
American Association for Clinical Chemistry (AACC), 2, 156
American Association of Blood Banks Buyer's Guide, Web site, 195
American Association of Blood Banks (AABB), 2, 63, 106, 227, 229
American Institute of Stress, The, 57
American Marketing Association, Boston Chapter of, 113
American Medical Association, Web site, 234
American Medical Technologists (AMT), 2
American Society for Clinical Laboratory Science (ASCLS), 1, 63, 131, 191, 234
    Code of Ethics, 4–6
American Society for Clinical Pathology (ASCP), 2, 63, 243
American Society for Clinical Pathology Board of Registry (ASCP Board of Registry), 233
American Society for Microbiology (ASM), 2
American Society of Hematology, 2
American Society of Microbiology (ASM), 63
Americans with Disabilities Act, 233
AMS. *See* American Society for Microbiology
AMT. *See* American Medical Technologists
Analytical, phase of patient care, 189–191
Andrews Telecommunications, Web site, 96
Anecdotal examination, 258
Anti-kickback statute, 113
Appeal procedure. *See* Correction, employee
Applicability, 141
Arnold Sanow, MBS, CSB, Web site, 88
Articles. *See* Journal, professional
ASCLS. *See* American Society for Clinical Laboratory Science
ASCP BOR. *See* American Society for Clinical Pathology Board of Registry
ASCP. *See* American Society of Clinical Pathologists
Asian population, 45
Association for Conflict Resolution, Web site, 92
Authority, 80
Authority-compliance management, 79
Autonomy, 5

B

Baby Boomer, 45
Balanced Budget Act, 45, 121
Ball Street University Teaching Strategies, Web site, 186
Barrier protection, 106–107
Beckman Coulter, Web site, 196
Beckman Synchron CX3, 134
Behavior, 92
Beneficence, 5
Berkeley Lab, Biohazardous Waste Management, Web site, 108
Billable procedures, 135
Biohazardous waste, 107–108
Biological hazards, 105
Biomedical Clinical Pathology, Web site, 191
Blood-borne pathogens plan, 104
Body of Knowledge, 1
Braley Consulting Services, Inc., Web site, 214
Budget, 121–128
    adhering to, 125–126
    assumptions, 121–122
    for Continuing education program (CEP), 242
    cost per test/cost per unit of service, 125
    forecast of expenses, 122–123
    goals, 121
    laboratory objectives, 121
    monitor, 124
    sample, 123–124
    variance, 124
Building a House for Diversity: A Fable About a Giraffe and Elephant–A Diversity Fable, 46
Business Owner's Toolkit, 22

C

California Department of Health Services, Web site, 230
CAP. *See* College of American Pathologists
Capital expenses, 122
CAP method. *See* College of American Pathologists
CAP Workload Recording
    calculations, 136
    unit, 134–135
Cardiopulmonary Resuscitation (CPR), 107
Care-delivery process, 178
Career Development Center, University of Wisconsin, Milwaukee, 14, 30
Cash purchase, 122
Catherwood Library, School of Industrial & Labor Relations, Cornell University, 47
CDC. *See* Center for Disease Control and Prevention
Center for Disease Control and Prevention (CDC), 221, 242
    Division of Laboratory Science, Web site, 181
    Morbidity and Mortality Weekly Report, Web site, 223
    National Center for Infectious Disease, Web site, 223
    surveillance program. *See* Notifiable Infectious Disease Surveillance program
    Wonder, Web site, 223
Centers for Medicare and Medicaid Services (CMS), 113, 131, 229–230
CEP. *See* Continuing education program
Certificate of Accreditation, 229
Certificate of Registration, 229
Certificate of Waiver, 229
Certification, 233
CEU. *See* Continuing education units
Change, 51–54
    dimensions of, 51
    embracing, in organization, 85
    facts about, 51
    how to manage, 51–52
    process that drives, 51
    understand resistance to, 52
Change Management Resource Library, The, 52
Chart of accounts, 122
Checklist
    employee orientation, 33–34
    validation of competency checklist, 33–40
Chemical
    hazards, 105
    hygiene officer (CHO), 108
    hygiene plan (CHP), 104
Chronological resume format, 11
Civil Rights Act, 45, 233
Cleveland State University, Web site, 75
CLIA '88. *See* Clinical Laboratory Improvement Amendments
Clinical laboratory
    employees and students, 105
    supervisor, 105
    technician (CLT), 241
Clinical Laboratory Improvement Amendments (CLIA '88), 180, 227, 229
Clinical Laboratory Management Association, 63, 126
Clinical laboratory safety, 103–111
    barrier protection, 106–107
    employees and students, 105
    first aid, 107
    general safety, 104–105
    hazard warning labels, 107
    material safety data sheets (MSDS), 105
    Occupational Safety and Health Administration (OSHA) requirements, 103–104
    record keeping, 108
    safety director, 104–105
    supervisor, 105
    types of hazards, 105–106
    waste disposal, 107–108
Clinical Laboratory Science, 63
Clinical laboratory science (CLS), 241

Clinical Laboratory Science Internet Resources, Web site, 181
Clinical Leadership and Management Review, 63
Clinical safety officer, 105
CLS. *See* Clinical laboratory science
CLT. *See* Clinical Laboratory technician
CMS. *See* Centers for Medicare and Medicaid Services
Coalition of Healthcare eStandards, Inc., Web site, 143
Code of Ethics, 1, 4–5
Code of Federal Regulations, 180
Code of Federal Regulations publications, 103
Coefficient of variation, 169
Coefficient of variation (%CV), 157–158
Cognitive domain measurement, 257–258
Collaboration, 70
Collective bargaining, 233
College Grad.com, Web site, 14
Collegegrad.com, Web site, 27
College of American Pathologists (CAP), 106, 116–117, 134–135, 227–230
College of William and Mary, Training and Technical Assistance Center, Web site, 88
Color Code, The, 46
Communication
    affective, 69
    business, 61
    defined, 68
    and interpersonal relationships, 68–72
    intrapersonal, 70
    mediums of, 69
    model of, process, 68
    purposes of, 69
    skills, 238
    style of, 70
    written, 61–67
Communication, management issues regarding, 61–102
    conflict management, 91–94
    customer satisfaction, 99–102
    and interpersonal relationships, 68–72
    leadership, 78–84
    motivation, 73–77
    professional writing, 61–67
    teambuilding, 85–90
    telephone etiquette, 95–98
Comparison study, 155–164
Competency-based education, 256, 258
Competency-based evaluation, 33, 37–38
Competition, 112–113
Concrete random, 70
Concrete sequential, 70
Confidence interval, 169
Confidentiality, 233–234
Conflict
    management, 91–94
    sources of, 70
Conflict Management Group, Web site, 92

Consulting, 237–240
    aspects of, business, 238
Consulting Academy, Web site, 239
Continuing education program (CEP), 241–246
    budget for, 242
    issuing credit for, 243
    need for, 241–242
    task force to implement, 242
    types of, 242–243
Continuing education units (CEU), 241
Contractual agreement, 142–143
Corporate culture, 78–80
Correction, employee, 41–43
Corrective maintenance, 204. *See also* Preventative maintenance, 204
Cost per test, 125
Cost per unit of service, 125
Country club management, 79
CPR. *See* Cardiopulmonary Resuscitation
CPT. *See* Current procedural technology
Criteria-based evaluation, 33, 35–36
Critical incident, 258
Culture, 45–46. *See also* Corporate culture
Current procedural technology (CPT), 130
Customer satisfaction, three R's, 99
Customer service, 99–100

D

David G. Rhodes Associates, Inc., Web site, 161
DB Program Diversity Training, Web site, 47
Decentralization, 80
Deepthunder, Web site, 186
Delegating role, manager's, 34
Delegating situation, 80
Delegation of authority, 80
Delivery system options, 113
Deontological ethics, 5
Departmentalization, 80
Department of Agricultural Environment and Development Economics, Ohio State University, 35
Department of Epidemiology and Biostatistics, University of California, San Francisco, Web site, 223
Department of Human Resources, Southern Illinois, University at Carbondale, The, 42
Department of Veteran Affairs, Mediator Skills, Web site, 70
Depreciation, 141
Diagnostic evaluation, 256
Diagnostic Related Group (DRG), 121
Diagnostic validity, 160
Dilemma, ethical, 6
Discipline. *See* Correction, employee
Discrimination, 46. *See also* Diversity

Distress, 56
Distress, ethical, 6
Diversity, 44–50
    African American population, 45
    ageism, 44–45
    Asian population, 45
    Baby Boomers, 45
    Building a House for Diversity: A Fable About a Giraffe and Elephant–A Diversity Fable, 4
    Color Code, The, 46
    culture, 45–46
    gender equality, 45
    Generation X, 44–45
    Generation Y, 44–45
    Hispanic population, 45
    Latin American population, 45
    Mexican American population, 46
    nationalities and origins, 45–46
    Native American population, 46
    outside workplace environment, 44
    Pacific Islanders, 45
    physically or mentally challenged, 46
    religious, 46
    sexual harassment, 46
    sexual orientation, 46
    teamwork and, 44–45
    in workplace environment, 44
Diversity Central, Web site, 47
DRG. *See* Diagnostic Related Group

E

Eagle's flight, Web site, 81
Education programs, 1. *See also* Accreditation; Instructional unit; Measurement
EEOC. *See* Equal Employment Opportunity Commission
Electrical hazards, 106
E-mail, 62
Emergency Medical Treatment and Active Labor Act (EMTALA), 233
Employee
    competency validation form, 34, 37–38
    correction and discipline, 41–43
    evaluation, 33–40
    interview and selection process, 26–32
    orientation checklist, 33–34, 37
    orientation form, 34, 37
    recruitment of new, 149
    rewards, 34
    teams, 56
Empowerment. *See* Authority
EMTALA. *See* Emergency Medical Treatment and Active Labor Act
Engineering controls, 106
Environmental Protection Agency (EPA), 107
EPA. *See* Environmental Protection Agency; Equal Pay Act

Epidemiology, 217–226
Equal Employment Opportunity Commission (EEOC), 45, 47
Equal Pay Act (EPA), 45, 233
Equipment lease agreement, 122
Error. *See* Random error; Systematic error
Essay questions, 257
Ethics, professional, 4–8
Etiquette. *See* Telephone etiquette
Eustress, 56
Evaluation
    affective domain, 259–260
    anecdotal, 258
    critical incident, 258
    of instructional unit, 255–263
    item analysis, 258
    multiple choice, 257–258
    observational techniques, 259
    practical, 258
    psychomotor domain, 258–259
    role playing, 259
    self-, 258–259
    simulation, 258–259
    true/false, 257
Evaluation, employee
    competency-based, 33, 37–38
    criteria-based, 33, 35–36
    evaluator, 33–34
Exception principle, 80–81
Expenses, 122
Experience Based Learning, Inc., Web site, 92

F

Facilitator, team, 87
Fair Labor Standards Act (FLSA), 233
Family and Medical Leave Act (FMLA), The, 233
FDA. *See* Food and Drug Administration
Federal Register, 229
Federal Register, 180
Fidelity, 5
Finance. *See* Budget
Fire safety, 105
First aid, 107
FLSA. *See* Fair Labor Standards Act
FMLA. *See* Family and Medical Leave Act, The
Food and Drug Administration (FDA), 156
Formal group, 80
Formative evaluation, 256
Forming phase, of team development, 85
Fraud, 129–133
    alerts, 130–131
    model compliance plan (MCP), 129–130
    training, 131
F test, 158

G

Generalist organization, 2
Generation X, 44–45
Generation Y, 44–45
Genethics.ca, Web site, 6
Gideon Information, Inc., Web site, 223
Glass Ceiling Commission, 45
Goal, defined, 247
Gold standard, defined, 218
Government of Ontario, Canada, Ministry of Education, Web site, 30
Group purchasing organization (G.P.O.), 143
Growth needs, 73
Guaranteed sale, 141
Guide to Accreditation, A, 229

H

Hazard Communications, 104
Hazards, laboratory, 105–106
Hazard warning labels, 107
HCFA. *See* Health Care Financing Administration
Health and Human Services Office of the Inspector General (OIG), 129–130, 131
Health Care Financing Administration (HCFA), 229
Healthcare Product Comparison System, Web site, 195
Healthcare Publishing News, Nelson Publishing, Inc., Web site, 143
Health Department of Western Australia, Web site, 126
Health Insurance Portability and Accountability Act (HIPAA), 213, 233–234
Hersey-Blanchard model, 34
Hersey-Blanchard Situational Management Theory, 80
Herzberg's Two Factory Theory, 74
HIPAA. *See* Health Insurance Portability and Accountability Act
HIS. *See* Hospital information system
Hispanic population, 45
Hospital information system (HIS), 212–213
Human Resources (HR), 26
Humboldt State University, Web site, 251
Hygiene factors, 74

I

Imaginative communication, 69
Impoverished management, 79
Improvement model, 179
Inappropriate communication, 69
Informative communication, 69
Institute for Healthcare Improvement, Web site, 181
Institutional issues, 233–234
Instructional unit
    construction and delivery of, 247–254
    educational objectives, 247–249
    lesson plan for, 247
    measurement and evaluation strategies of, 255–263
    media support for, 250–251
    teaching strategies, 250
    See also Education
Instrument, 194–200
    research, 195–196
    selection of, 256–257
    sources for refurbished/used instruments, 196
    See also Laboratory instruments
Interaction between institution and individual, 78–79
Interactive Learning Paradigms, Inc., Web site, 108
International Classification of Diseases, 130
International Committee of Medical Journal Editing, Web site, 64
International Management Technologies, Inc., Web site, 101
International Organization for Standardization, Web site, 181
International Society for Clinical Laboratory Technologists (ISCLT), 2
International Stress Management Association, 57
Interpersonal communication, 70
Interrater reliability-kappa, evaluation of, 219–220
Interrator reliability, 219
Interview, employment, 26–32
    dress code, 27
    interviewee preparation for, 26–27
    interviewee questions during, 28
    interviewer preparation for, 27–28
    interviewer questions during, 27–28
    legal considerations, 232–233
    psychological profiling, 28
    purpose of, 26
    thank-you letter, 28
Intrapersonal communication, 70
ISCLT. *See* International Society for Clinical Laboratory Technologists
Issues
    job, 232
    management, 1–59
Issues in Health Care, Web site, 6
Item analysis, 258

J

JCAHO. *See* Joint Commission on Accreditation of Health Care Organizations
Job description, 18–25
    legal consideration, 232–233
    sample, 18–21
    sections of, 18
Job Link USA, Web site, 30
Joint Commission on Accreditation of Health Care Organizations (JCAHO), 106, 227–230

Journal, professional, 63
    article format of, 63–64
    process of article acceptance for, 64
    publications editor, 64
    volunteer-peer reviewers, 64
Journal of Clinical Microbiology, 63
Journal of the International Federation of Clinical Chemistry and Laboratory Medicine, The, 191
Journal of The Society for Healthcare Epidemiology of American, Slack, Incorporated, Web site, 223
Justice, 5

K

Kappa statistics, 219–220

L

Laboratory
    characteristics of, 194
    environment, 194–195
Laboratory information system (LIS), 195, 212–216
Laboratory instruments, 194–200
    evaluation of performance quality, 195
    features of, 195
    maintenance of, 201
    needs assessment, 194
    selection of, 194–200
    See also Corrective maintenance; Instrument selection; Preventative maintenance (PM)
Laboratory Management Index Program (LMIP), 135, 138
Laboratory processes, quality, 180
Laboratory testing services
    fraudulent coding and billing, 129–130
Latin American population, 45
Leadership, 78–84
Leadership situation
    types of, 79–80
Legal considerations, 232–236
    institutional issues, 233–234
    personnel issues, 232–233
Letter
    as business communication, 61–62
    resume cover, 13
    sample, 62
    thank-you, 28–29
Levey-Jennings chart, 169–172
Linearity measurement, 157
LIS. *See* Laboratory information system
Listening, 69
LMIP. *See* Laboratory Management Index Program
Locus of authority, 6

M

Mailing, resume, 14
Maintenance programs, 201–207
    equipment management, 201
    preventative maintenance (PM), 201–207
Managed Care On-Line, Web site, 126
Management
    continuum of, styles, 79–80
    Hersey-Blanchard model of, roles, 34
    style, 79
    types of, 79
    See also Conflict management
Management, quality, 177–183, 178
Management by Objectives (MBO), 34
Marketing, 112–115
Martin's Rugby Coaching Archive, Web site, 88
Maslow's hierarchy of needs, 73–74
Matching examination, 257
Matching institution with individual model, 78–79
Material safety data sheets (MSDS), 105
MBO. *See* Management by Objectives
MCP. *See* Model compliance plan
Mean value, calculation of, 167
Measurement
    of instructional unit, 255–263
    See also Test method evaluation
Median value, calculation of, 167
Medical technology/clinical laboratory science, 1–2
Medical University of South Carolina, Web site, 223
Memo, 61–62
Memo, sample, 62–63
Mentally challenged, 46
Metamyelocyte Corporation, 156
Method evaluation statistics, aspects of, 156–161
Method validation, 155
Mexican American population, 46
Middle-of-the-road management, 79
MindData, Web site, 35
Model compliance plan (MCP), 129–13
Mode value, determination of, 168
Motivation Maslow's hierarchy of needs, 73–74
Motivators, 74
MSDS. *See* Material safety data sheets
Multiple-choice examination, 257–258

N

National Accrediting Agency for Clinical Laboratory Sciences (NAACLS), 1, 227, 229–230
National Bureau of Standards (NBS), 156
National Committee for Clinical Laboratory Standards (NCCLS), 108, 116–117, 156
National Council on Measurement and Education, Web site, 260

National Credentialing Agency for Laboratory Personnel, Inc. (NCA), 1–2, 45, 233
National Fire Protection Association (NFPA), 107
Nationalities and origins, 45–46
National Laboratory Training Network (NLRN), 242
National Labor Relations Act (NLRA) of 1935, 233
National Labor Relations Board (NLRB), 233
Nationally notifiable infectious diseases, 222
Native American population, 46
NBS. *See* National Bureau of Standards
NCA. *See* National Credentialing Agency for Laboratory Personnel, Inc.
NCCLS. *See* National Committee for Clinical Laboratory Standards
Net Preference, 74
Netster, Web site, 30
NFPA. *See* National Fire Protection Association
NLRA. *See* National Labor Relations Act of 1935
NLRB. *See* National Labor Relations Board
NLRN. *See* National Laboratory Training Network
Nonmaleficence, 5
Nonverbal communication, 69
Norm-based education, 256, 258
Norming phase, of team development, 85
Notifiable Infectious Disease Surveillance program, 221

O

Objective
  defined, 247–248
Observational techniques, 259
Occupational Exposure to Blood-borne Pathogens, 104
Occupational Exposure to Hazardous Chemicals in Laboratories, 104
Occupational Safety and Health Act of 1970, 55
Occupational Safety and Health Administration (OSHA), 103–104, 108
Office of Clinical & Biological Safety, Michigan State University, NSPA Chemical Hazard Labels, Web site, 108
Olympus, Web site, 196
One Minute Manager, The, 41
On-Line Consultant Software, Laboratory Information Systems (LIS) Directory, Web site, 214
Online Writing Lab, Purdue University, Web site, 64
Operational expenses, 122
Oral presentation, 64
Organization, professional, 1–2
Organization, time management and, 208–211
Organizational skills, 209
Orientation
  employee, 33–34, 37
  relationship, 79
  task, 79
OSHA. *See* Occupational Safety and Health Administration

Outreach program, development of, 112–115
Overcommunicating, 69
Overtime, 150

P

Paauwerfully Organized, Web site, 210
P.A.C.E. *See* Professional Acknowledgment of Continuing Education
Pacific Islanders, 45
Paired t-test, 158–159
Paraverbal communication, 69
Pareto principle, 179
Participating role, manager's, 34
Participating situation, 80
Pearson Education, Web site, 186
People Solution Strategies, Web site, 101
Peppers and Rogers Group, Web site, 113
Perception, 74
Performing, phase of team development, 85
Personal protective equipment (PPE), 104–107
Personnel issue, 232–233
Persuasive communication, 69
Phelps Dunbar, Counselors at Law, Web site, 234
PHI. *See* Protected health information
Physical hazards, 106
Physically challenged, 46
Physiological and safety needs, 73
Plan/Do/Check (Study)/Act, 178–179
Planning, 180
Policy Manual, University of North Texas, 42
Postanalytical phase, of patient care, 189–191
Postcard, reply, 13–14
Poster presentation, 64
PPE. *See* Personal protective equipment
Practical examination, 258
Preanalytical phase, of patient care, 189–191
Precision test, 157–158
Predictive value, 219
Presentation
  oral, 64
  poster, 64
  resume, 14
Preventative maintenance (PM), 201–207
  accreditation organizations, 202, 204
  defined, 202
  instrument manuals, 202
  log sheet, 203
  regulatory requirements, 202
  repair costs, 202
  training, 202, 204
Pricing, competitive, 113
Principles, of ethics, 5
Privacy. *See* Confidentiality
Problem solving, 184–188

Procedure, 106–107
    analytic, 116–117
    billable, 135
    manual, 116
    for patient confidentiality, 234
    postanalytic, 116–117
    preanalytic, 116
    quality control (QC), 208–209
    sample, 120
    writing in NCCLS format, 116–120
    See also Current procedural technology
Productivity measurement, 149
Profession, entry into to, 1
Professional Acknowledgment of Continuing Education (P.A.C.E.), 243
Professionalism, 1–3
Professional Management and Marketing, Web site, 113
Professional organization, 1–2
Professional stress management program, 56–57
Proposal, 61–62
Protected health information (PHI), 233
Psychological profiling, 28
Psychomotor domain evaluation, 258–259
Publications editor, 64
Public health surveillance, 220–221
Public relations, 99–102
Purchase order, 145
Purchase order requisition, 143, 144
Purchasing, 140–147
    buying power, 143
    capital, 141–142
    group purchasing organization (G.P.O.), 143
    operational supplies, 140–141
    purchase order, 145
    purchase order requisition, 143, 144
    services, 142–143

Q

Quality, 141–142
    defined, 177
    improvement, 180
Quality circle, 87–88
Quality control (QC), 165–172, 212
    and assessment, 180
    procedures, 208–209
Quality Talk, Web site, 101

R

Radioactive hazards, 106
Random error, 160
Range, determination of, 168
Reagent rental agreement, 122, 124
Recognition and dignity, 1

Record keeping, of laboratory safety, 108
Reference intervals, normal (healthy), 160–161
Reference method, 156
References, resume, 14
Refurbished/Used Laboratory Instruments, sources for, 196
Rehabilitation Act of 1973, 233
Relationship orientation, 79
Reliability, defined, 219
Religion, 46
Request for proposal (RFP), 213
Research topics, for professional journal articles, 63
Respiratory Protection, 104
Resumé
    abbreviations used in, 9, 11
    chronological, format, 11
    cover letter, 13
    functional, format, 11
    function of, 9
    parts of, 9
    preparation of, 9
    presentation and mailing, 14
    references, 14
    reply postcard, 13–14
    sample, 10–13
    style or form of, 9, 11
Retraining, 34
Reviewers, volunteer peer, 64
Rewards, employee, 34
RFP. *See* Request for proposal
Rice University Human Resources, 22
Ritualistic communication, 69
Role playing, 259
80/20 rule. *See* Pareto Principle

S

Safety. *See* Clinical laboratory safety
Safety director, 104–105
San Francisco State University, Response Sets in Learning and Problem Solving, Web site, 186
Scalar principle, 80–81
Scandinavian Society for Clinical Chemistry and Clinical Physiology (SCCCP), 156
Scheduling, employee
    employee self-scheduling, 150
    non-traditional, 150
    overtime consideration, 150
    productivity measurement, 149
    recruitment of new employees, 149
    sample schedule, 150–151
    standard unit of measure, 148
    work flow analysis, 149–150
Scientific articles. *See* Journal, professional
Screening test validity, 218–219
Selection process, employee, 26–32

Self-actualization, 73
Self-directed team. *See* Quality circle
Self-evaluation, 258–259
Self-scheduling, employee, 150
Selling role, manager's, 34
Selling situation, 80
Sensitivity, 218. *See also* Test method evaluation
Sensitivity measurement, 218
Sexual harassment, 46, 233
Sexual orientation, 46
Shaw Resources, Customer-Inspired Management Systems, Web site, 101
Simulations, 258–259
Situation. *See* Leadership situation
Skewed distribution, 167
Skylight Professional Development, Web site, 186
Slope/linear regression, 159
SNA Consulting, Web site, 131
Social needs, 73
Social Security Amendments of 1965, 228
Social system, 78
Solucient, Web site, 126
Southern Illinois University, Dr. Gordin C. Brunner II, Web site, 75
Southern Texas State University, Web site, 96
Span of control, 80
Specialist organizations, 2
Specialization. *See* Departmentalization
Specificity, 218. *See also* Test method evaluation
Staffing performance report, weekly, 135–136
Standard deviation, calculation of, 168–169
"Standards for Hospital Accreditation," 228
Standard unit of measure, 148
Stark Law, 113
State of Wisconsin, Department of Employment Relations Reference Library, 52
Statistical parameters, 160
Steering committee, 87
Storming phase, of team development, 85
Straight-line depreciation, 141
Stress
    management, 55–59
    options in dealing with, 55–56
    symptoms of, 55
    techniques to relieve, 55
    types of, 56
Stress Management for Students, National University of Singapore, 57
Summative evaluation, 256
Surveillance compliance, 220–221
Systematic error, 160

T

Task list, 208–209
Task orientation, 79

Teaching strategies, 250
Teal Trust, The, 88
Team
    benefits from implementation of, building, 86
    early stages of, development, 86
    facilitator, 87
    leader, 87
    phases of, development, 85
Teamwork
    diversity and, 44–45
Teleological ethics, 5
Telephone etiquette, 95–98
Telling mode, manager's, 34
Telling situation, 80
Termination, employee, 34, 233
Test method evaluation, 155–164
    accuracy, 158–159
    analytical sensitivity, 159
    analytical specificity, 159–160
    diagnostic validity, 160
    linearity, 157
    normal (healthy) reference intervals, 160–161
    precision, 157–158
Test method(s)
    reference method and, 156
    switching, 155–156
TGCI, the Grantsmanship Center, Web site, 35
Thank-you letter, 28–29
Through the Patient's Eyes, 177
Time, savers and wasters, 209
Time and materials, 142–143
Time management, organization and, 208–211
Title VII of the Civil Rights Act, 46
Training
    on fraud and abuse issues, 131
    preventative maintenance (PM), 202, 204
Transfusion, 63
True/false measurement, 257

U

Undercommunicating, 69
Unity of command, 80
University of Human Resource Services, Indiana University, 42
University of Illinois, Sexual Orientation in the Workplace, Web site, 47
University of Kansas, Department of Communication Studies, Web site, 70
University of Louisville College of Business and Public Administration, Web site, 96
University of Pittsburgh
    Guide to Budgets and Budgeting, Web site, 126
    Medical Center Blood Bank, 55
    School of Medicine, Department of Pathology, Web site, 161

University of Southern Mississippi, The, 47
University of Texas Health Science Center at Houston, The, 22
University of Washington, Web site, 251
U.S. Department of Labor, Occupational Safety and Health Administration, Web site, 108
U.S. Employee Laws, Web site, 234
U.S. News, Web site, 30

V

Validation of competency checklist, 33–40
Value, 141–142
Variance, calculation of, 168
Veracity, 5
Verbal communication, 69
VHA, Web site, 126
Virginia Polytechnic Institute and State University, Web site, 210
Virtual Hospital
    University of Iowa, Web site, 143
    Web site, 191, 243
Vocational Rehabilitation Act of 1973, 46
Vroom's Expectancy Theory, 33, 74

W

Waste disposal, 107–108
Wesley E. Sime, Department of Health and Human Performance, University of Nebraska, Lincoln, 57
Westgard
    examples of, rules, 171
    QC, Web site, 161, 181
    quality control, Web site, 191
Who Moved My Cheese, 51
Word processing program, 61–62
Work, management issues regarding, 103–263
    accreditation, 227–231
    analytical components of patient care, 189–193
    budgeting and finance, 121–128
    clinical laboratory safety, 103–111
    consulting, 237–240
    continuing education program (CEP), 241–246
    employee scheduling, 148–154
    epidemiology, 217–226
    evaluation of test methods, 155–164
    fraud and abuse, 129–133
    instructional unit construction and delivery, 247–254
    instructional unit measurement and evaluation strategies, 255–263
    instrument selection, 194–200
    laboratory information system (LIS), 212–216
    legal considerations, 232–236
    maintenance programs, 201–207
    organization and time management, 208–211
    problem solving, 184–188
    procedures in National Committee for Clinical Laboratory Standards (NCCLS) format, 116–120
    purchasing, 140–147
    quality control, 165–172
    quality management, 177–183
    work recording, 134–139
Work flow analysis, 149–150
Workplace
    diversity in, 44–50
    types of, structure and function, 80
Workplace, management issues regarding, 1–59
    change, 51–54
    diversity, 44–50
    employee correction and discipline, 41–43
    employee evaluation, 33–40
    ethics, 4–8
    job description and advertisement, 18–25
    job interview, 26–32
    resume, 9–17
    stress management, 55–59
Work practices. *See* Procedure
Work recording, 134–139
    adjusted patient days, 135, 137
    billable procedures, 135
    College of American Pathologists (CAP) method, 134–135
    Laboratory Management Index Program, 135, 138
    staffing performance report, 135–136
Work team. *See* Team
Writing. *See* Communication; Procedures
Writing Solution, Inc., Web site, 64